Atlas of

Clinical Andrology

Dedication

This Atlas is dedicated to all scientists conducting physiological and clinical research leading to assisted conception and improved quality of life.

Atlas of
Clinical Andrology

by
ESE Hafez and SD Hafez
Co-Directors, *Reproductive Health Center*
Kiawah Island, South Carolina, USA

Taylor & Francis
Taylor & Francis Group
LONDON AND NEW YORK

First published in the United Kingdom in 2005
by Taylor & Francis,
an imprint of the Taylor & Francis Group,
2 Park Square, Milton Park
Abingdon, Oxon OX14 4RN, UK

Tel.: +44 (0) 20 7017 6000
Fax.: +44 (0) 20 7017 6699
Website: www.tandf.co.uk

British Library Cataloguing in Publication Data

Data available on application

Library of Congress Cataloging-in-Publication Data

Data available on application

ISBN 1-84214-266-6

Distributed in North and South America by

Taylor & Francis
2000 NW Corporate Blvd
Boca Raton, FL 33431, USA

Within Continental USA
Tel.: 800 272 7737; Fax.: 800 374 3401
Outside Continental USA
Tel.: 561 994 0555; Fax.: 561 361 6018
E-mail: orders@crcpress.com

Distributed in the rest of the world by
Thomson Publishing Services
Cheriton House
North Way
Andover, Hampshire SP10 5BE, UK
Tel.: +44 (0) 1264 332424
E-mail: salesorder.tandf@thomsonpublishingservices.co.uk

Composition by Siva Math Setters, Chennai, India
Printed and bound by Antony Rowe Ltd., Chippenham, Wiltshire, UK

Contents

Acknowledgements

The authors are extremely grateful to Betty Hafez, executive editor of the international journal *Archives of Andrology*, for her editorial skill and the very hard work needed to coordinate all the activities related to review and proofread the manuscripts before publication. She was also responsible for summarizing the tables in an easily readable form and for giving full descriptions to the captions of the figures. Without her efforts there would be no Atlas. In particular we thank Ms Cindy Lloyd of Yorktown Street, James Island, SC for her elegant secretarial and clerical help. We are indebted to several academics who have allowed us to include their valuable illustrations and research results in the Atlas, particularly Professor Carl Pinkert (University of Alabama, Birmingham, Alabama, USA). We thank the staff of the publishers Taylor & Francis Medical Books for giving generously of their intellect and expertise. We acknowledge especially Mr Nicholas J. Dunton and Ms Dinah Alam for their sound advice and hard work. We are greatly indebted to friends and colleagues who made the writing of this Atlas such a satisfying experience.

Sincere thanks are due to the American Society of Andrology, the Society for the Study of Reproduction and the American Society of Andrology for giving permission to use illustrations from their journals. Dr Jane M. Morrell, R&D Manager of Nidacon AB International, of Göteborg, Sweden was kind enough to provide us with original illustrations of the various procedures used in the purification of semen samples, and, for freezing and thawing of human sperm, CryoProtec®. Finally, we would also like to thank those who answered our questions on the phone, via e-mail or in personal conversation.

ESE Hafez and SD Hafez
January 2005

Preface

Andrology, the science of the physiology, pathology and microbiology of male reproduction, is a field not well established in medicine, in science or in the public consciousness. Unlike gynecology, the science of andrology is a young discipline and is currently generating some amazing new insights, as well as many new puzzling questions. Only in the past 20–25 years have researchers begun to specialize in andrology.

Remarkable advances have been accomplished in assisted reproductive technology: *in vitro* fertilization micromanipulation of reproductive products, intracytoplasmic insemination, intrauterine insemination and *in vitro* manipulation of semen.

A few groups of enthusiastic researchers have devoted special attention to human andrology, and rapid development is anticipated owing to the application of modern technology, which has advanced so spectacularly in recent years.

This Atlas includes the most recent research findings in male endocrinology, neuroendocrinology, growth factors, sperm quality/fertility, male immunology and molecular andrology. Recent advances in molecular genetics have a significant impact on the precision of assessing the psychopathological processes of spermatogenesis, Sertoli cells, seminal plasma, sperm capacitation and fertilization. The chapters of this Atlas are multidisciplinary in nature, and in their range and depth they reflect our intention to bridge the gap between basic and clinical science. There are chapters devoted to laboratory techniques, and morphological, anatomical, biochemical, immunological, hereditary and microbiological parameters and their clinical application. Emphasis is placed on specific aspects as related to health and disease in men, e.g. hereditary aspects of prostate diseases, erectile dysfunction and unexplained infertility.

The Atlas covers three main areas in biomedical sciences: reproductive physiology, reproductive dysfunction and modern assisted reproductive technology. Emphasis is placed on endocrine mechanisms of the testes, spermatogenesis, sperm maturation, motility and transport in the male/female reproductive tract, capacitation and fertilization. The functional ultrastructure of spermatozoa is presented, as shown by transmission electron microscopy, scanning electron microscopy and atomic force microscopy.

ESE Hafez and SD Hafez
Reproductive Health Center
Kiawah Island,
South Carolina, USA

Introduction

Extensive investigations have been conducted on the physiopathology and ultrastructure of the testes, accessory sex organs, epididymis, molecular andrology, prostate in health and disease, spermatozoa, testicular dysfunction, anomalies of sperm and debris in seminal plasma, genetic andrology, genetic bioengineering, micromanipulation of gametes and blastocysts and assisted conception (Barboza *et al.*, 2004; Bastacky *et al.*, 1995; Beernink, 1984, 1986; Beernink and Ericsson, 1982; Berry *et al.*, 2000; Bourgeon *et al.*, 2004; Brinster, 1992; Brinster and Avarbock, 1994; Chen *et al.*, 2000, 2003; Cote *et al.*, 2002; Escalier, 2003; Foote, 1982; Foote and Oltenacu, 1980; Forsling, 1984; Gronberg *et al.*, 1997, 2000; Hansen, 2000; Holstein *et al.*, 1981; Korenman *et al.*, 1990; Matsui *et al.*, 1992; Neuhausen *et al.*, 1999; Palmiter *et al.*, 1980; Pinkert *et al.*, 1997, 1998; Pursel and Rexroad, 1993; Rexroad and Hawk, 1994; Rivilin *et al.*, 2004; Valeri and Azzouzi, 2000; Wilmut *et al.*, 1997; Wood *et al.*, 1993; Xu, 2000).

Little is known, however, regarding erectile dysfunction, ejaculatory dysfunction, pathophysiology of capacitation, acrosome reaction and fertilization, immunological andrology, cardiovascular anomalies and infectious diseases.

Section I Reproductive Physiology

1

Endocrinology of reproduction in men

Gametogenesis in men extends from fetal life to active reproductive life, and involves reserve stem cells and stem cell spermatogonia (Figure 1.1). Several endocrine glands are involved in the reproductive physiology of men (Figures 1.2 and 1.3; Table 1.1). The hypothalamus produces gonadotropin-releasing hormone (GnRH), which stimulates the release of follicle stimulating hormone/luteinizing hormone (FSH/LH). These pituitary peptides stimulate steroidogenesis in the testes (Figure 1.4; Table 1.2), which is under neurological control (Figures 1.5 and 1.6). There is a functional organization of the hypothalamic–pituitary–gonadal axis, which involves feed-forward and feedback loops. In particular, prostaglandin biosynthesis has a major role in various aspects of reproductive physiology and pathology of reproduction in men. Extensive studies have been conducted on the molecular parameters of reproductive mechanisms (Figure 1.7). The clinical/physiological interactions between these hormones and various growth factors are summarized in Tables 1.3 and 1.4.

Hormones or reproduction may be classified according to either their biochemical structure or mode of action. The biochemical structure of hormones includes lipoproteins, polypeptides, steroids, fatty acids and amines. Polypeptide hormones (FSH, LH, oxytocin) have a molecular weight of 300–70 000 Da. Steroids (estrogens, testosterone) are derived from cholesterol and have a molecular weight of 300–400 Da. Fatty acids are derived from arachidonic acid and have a molecular weight of about 400 Da, while amines are derived from tyrosine.

HYPOTHALAMUS

The hypothalamus consists of the region of the third ventricle, extending from the optic chiasma to the mammillary bodies. There are neural connections between the hypothalamus and the posterior lobe through the hypothalamic hyperphysical tract, and vascular connections between the hypothalamus and the anterior lobe. Arterial blood enters the pituitary by way of the superior hyperphysical artery and inferior hyperphysical artery. The superior hyperphysical artery forms capillary loops at the median eminence and pars nervosa. From these capillaries, blood flows into the hypothalamohypophyseal portal system. Part of the venous outflow from the anterior pituitary occurs by retrograde back flow, which exposes the hypothalamus to high concentrations of anterior pituitary hormones. This blood flow provides the pituitary gland with the negative-feedback (short-loop) mechanism of regulating the functions of the hypothalamus.

PITUITARY GLAND

The pituitary gland, located in the sella turcica, is divided into anterior, intermediate and posterior lobes. The anterior pituitary has five different cell types secreting six hormones. By cell type, the somatotropes secrete growth hormone, corticotropes secrete adenocorticotropic hormone, mammotropes secrete prolactin, thyrotropes secrete thyroid-stimulating hormone and gonadotropes secrete FSH/LH.

Neural communication involves neurotransmitters released at synaptic junctions from nerve cells that act across narrow synaptic clefts.

Testosterone, produced by the testes, has effects on most tissues throughout the body, including the brain. Within the brain, testosterone has a prominent role in the organization, programming and activation of neural circuits. In particular, testosterone exerts a

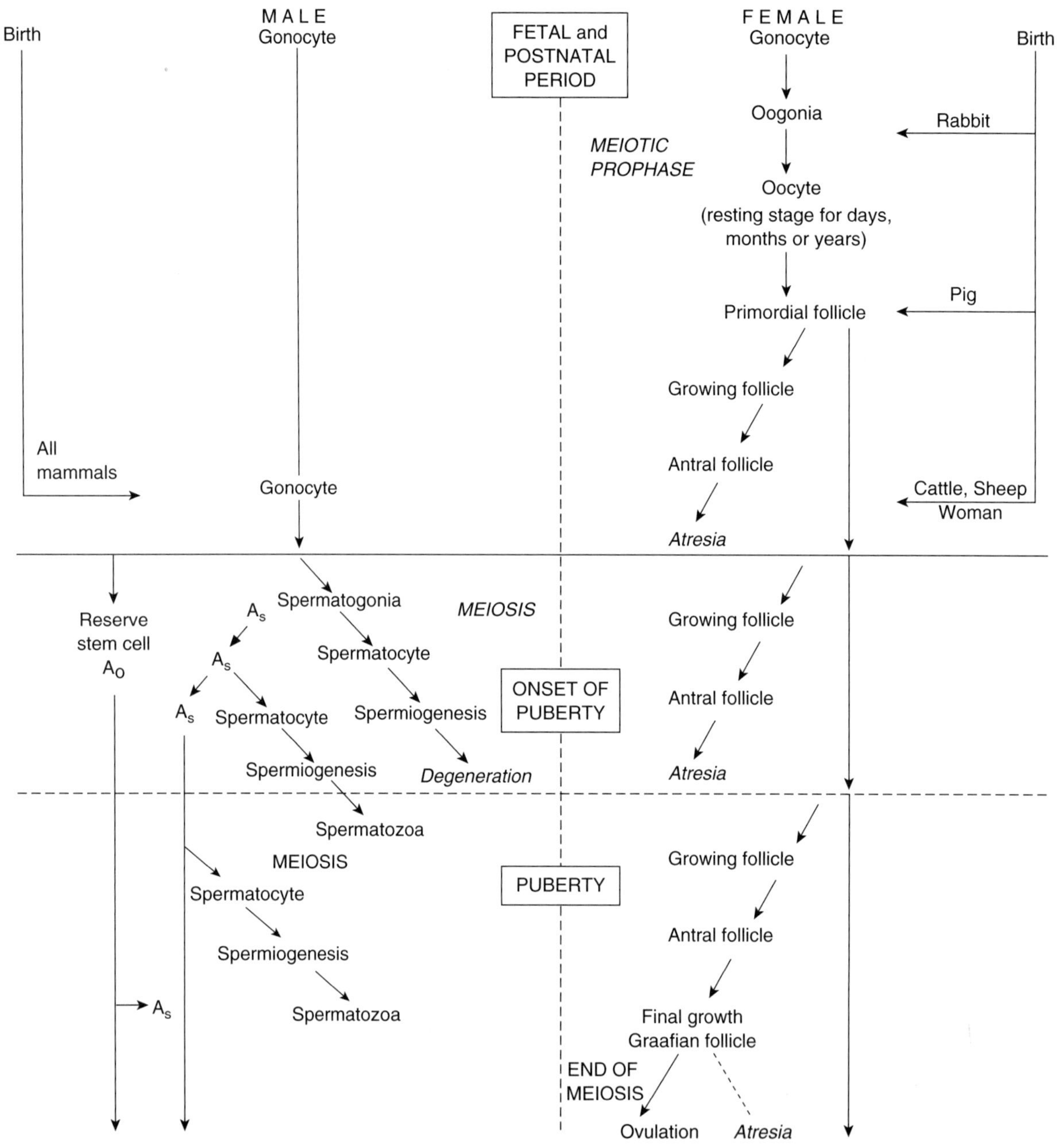

Figure 1.1 Comparison of gametogenesis in male and female mammals from fetal life to active sexual life. A_o, reserve stem cells; A_s, stem cell spermatogonia (adapted from Hafez and Hafez, 2000; Hafez *et al.*, 2003)

negative-feedback effect on GnRH secretion by the brain, which in turn affects the secretion of LH from the pituitary gland. The action of testosterone on the brain also affects behavior, including reproductive behavior.

ANTI-MÜLLERIAN HORMONE (AMH)

Anti-Müllerian hormone/Müllerian inhibiting substance (AMH/MIS) has a key role in the formation of the urogenital system. Embryos of both sexes possess two pairs of genital ducts. In males, the Wolffian or mesonephric ducts give rise to the epididymides, vas deferentia and seminal vesicles, whereas in females the Müllerian or paramesonephric ducts give rise to the oviducts, uterus and upper portion of the vagina. For normal male development, the Müllerian ducts must regress. In contrast, females must retain their Müllerian ducts; Wolffian ducts degenerate in the absence of testicular androgens. The regression of the Müllerian ducts is induced by AMH/MIS, a member of the transforming growth factor (TGF)-β super family of growth and differentiation factors.

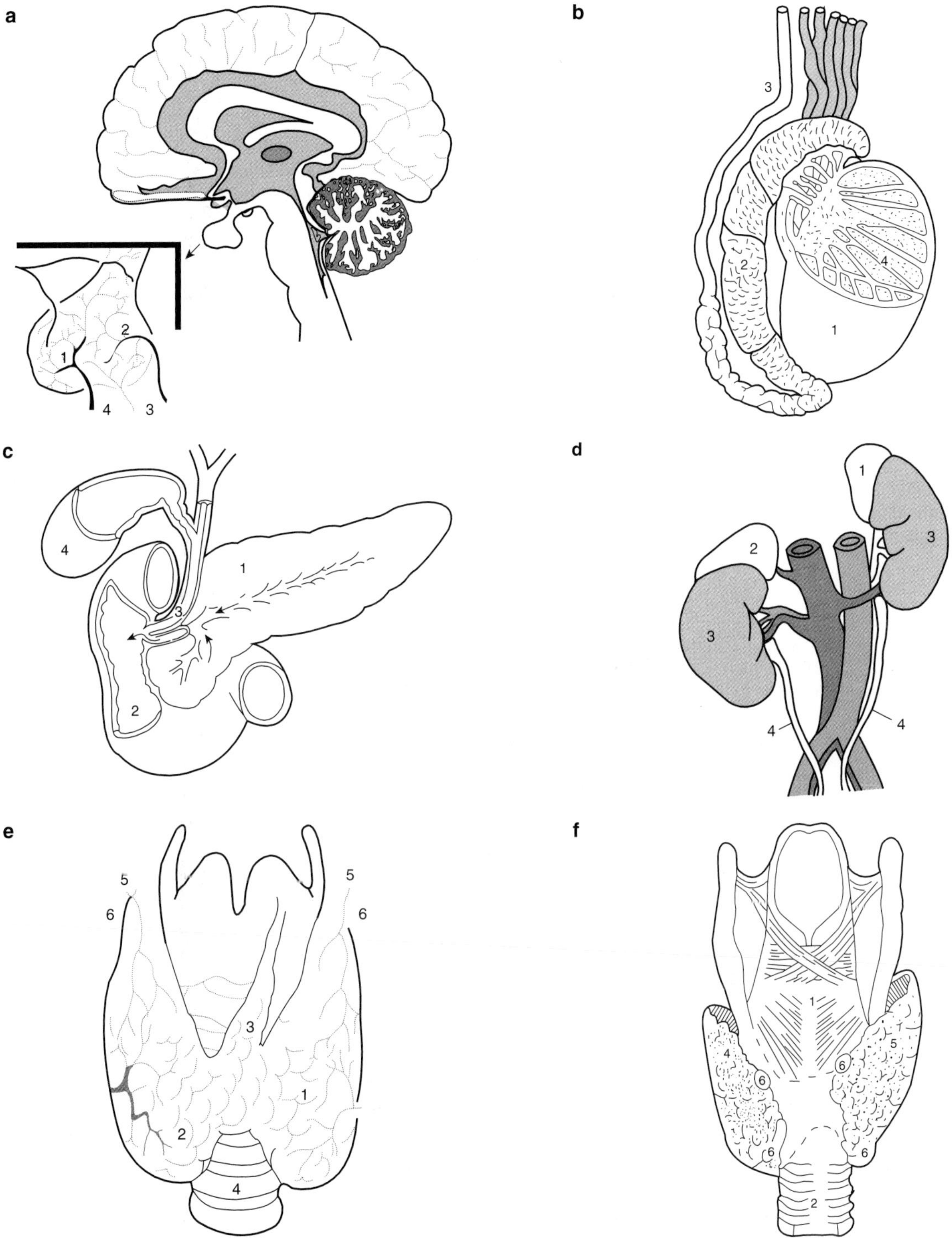

Figure 1.2 Some endocrine glands involved in the reproductive physiology of men. (**a**) The pituitary gland and the brain. The pituitary has an anterior portion (1), which produces several hormones that affect other endocrine glands, and a posterior portion (2) that is attached to the hypothalamus by a stalk. Blood vessels (3) carry hormones to the pituitary and away from it (4). Hormones of the posterior pituitary are involved in blood vessel tone and water metabolism. (**b**) The testis (1) is the site of sperm and hormone production. Male germ cells originating in tubules of the testis pass into the epididymis (2) and the seminal duct or vas deferens (3). Hormone-producing tissue (4) produces the principal masculinizing hormone, testosterone, which enters the bloodstream. Sperm and seminal fluids are transported into the posterior urethra. (**c**) The pancreas (1) produces digestive enzymes, which drain from collecting channels into the duodenum (2), in proximity to the bile duct outlets (3) from the gallbladder (4). The pancreas also produces a hormone, insulin, in islet cells that are independent of the enzyme-producing structures. Insulin enters directly into the bloodstream. (**d**) The adrenal glands (1, 2), kidneys (3) and ureters (4). (**e**) The thyroid gland, showing lobes (1–3), trachea (4) and (5, 6). (**f**) The thyroid (4, 5), parathyroid (6), trachea (2) and musculature (1)

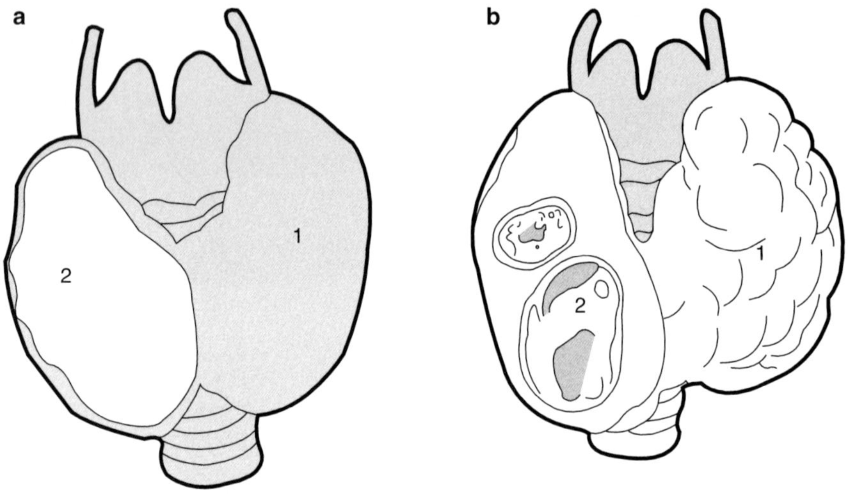

Figure 1.3 Thyroid gland. (**a**) Colloid goiter, frequently called 'simple goiter', is a soft, diffuse, symmetrical enlargement of the thyroid gland due to large deposits of thyroid hormone of poor quality, as may be caused by deficiency of iodine in the diet. The diagram shows an external view of the left lobe (1) and a cross-section of the right lobe (2) of a thyroid with colloid goiter. (**b**) Nodular, or adenomatous, goiter is so-called because of masses that may distort the surface (1) and interior (2) of the thyroid gland. Often there are no constitutional symptoms and only mild disfigurement, but it is possible for some adenomas to become toxic and produce symptoms of hyperthyroidism

Table 1.1 Hormones secreted by reproductive organs

Hormone	*Structure and source*	*Principal functions*
Estrogen	18-carbon steroid, secreted by the theca interna of the ovarian follicle	Promotes sexual behavior; stimulates development of secondary sex characteristics, anabolic effects
Progesterone	21-carbon steroid, secreted by the corpus luteum	Acts synergistically with estrogen in promoting estrous behavior
Testosterone	19-carbon steroid, secreted by Leydig cells in the testis	Develops and maintains accessory sex glands; stimulates secondary sexual characteristics, sexual behavior, spermatogenesis; possesses anabolic effects
Relaxin	Polypeptide hormone with α and β subunits secreted by the corpus luteum	Dilates cervix; causes uterine contractions
Prostaglandin $F_{2\alpha}$	20-carbon unsaturated fatty acid, secreted by almost all body tissues	Causes uterine contractions assisting sperm transport in the female tract and parturition
Activins	Proteins, found in follicular fluid in female and rete testis fluid in male	Cause regression of the corpus luteum (luteolytic); stimulate FSH secretion
Inhibins	Proteins, found in Sertoli cells in male and the granulosa cells in female	Inhibit release of FSH to a level which maintains species specific number of ovulations
Follistatin	Protein, found in ovarian follicular fluid in the female	Modulates the secretion of FSH

During male development, Sertoli cells of the testes secrete AMH, which signals (through its type II receptor expressed in mesenchymal cells adjacent to the Müllerian duct) the epithelium to induce regression. In male fetuses, AMH expression reaches peak levels during the period of Müllerian duct regression. However, expression continues after Müllerian duct regression is complete, but at reduced levels, declining to very low levels after puberty. In contrast, the ovaries do not synthesize AMH during fetal stages, creating a permissive environment for female reproductive tract differentiation. It is localized to the granulosa cells of preantral and small and large antral follicles, but is not detected in primordial follicles, atretic follicles and corpora lutea. AMH has inhibitory effects on granulosa cell proliferation, aromatase

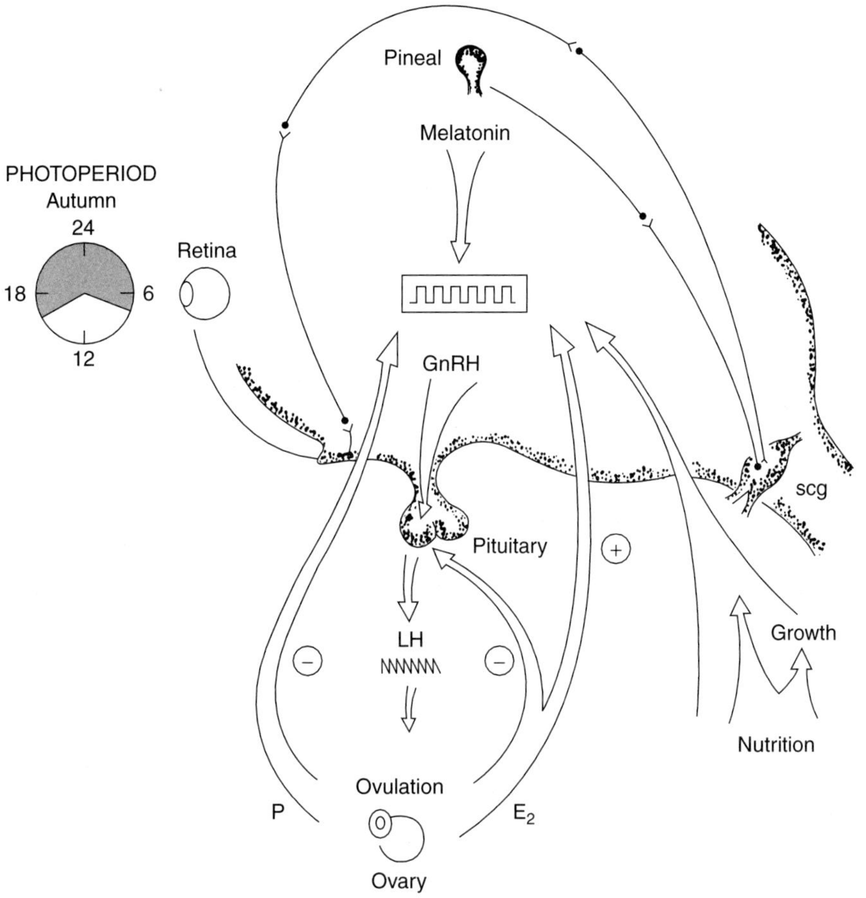

Figure 1.4 FSH steroid/gonadal peptide regulation of testicular function. The hypothalamus produces GnRH, which stimulates the release of LH/FSH. These pituitary peptides stimulate steroidogenesis. Estradiol/progesterone regulate pituitary/hypothalamic signals. Pituitary peptides (activin, inhibin and follistatin) regulate pituitary release of FSH alone. scg, soluble guanylyl cyclase

Table 1.2 Altogether, the pituitary gland produces a number of hormones of diverse effects. Disorders of the pituitary gland are those of too much or too little hormone production

Syndrome	*Hormone involved*	
Acromegaly	Growth stimulating hormone (somatotropin)	too much
Gigantism	Growth stimulating hormone (somatotropin)	too much too early
Dwarfism	Growth stimulating hormone (somatotropin)	too little
Thyrotoxicosis	Thyroid stimulating hormone	too much
Masked myxedema	Thyroid stimulating hormone	too little
Cushing's disease (of pituitary origin)	Adrenal cortex stimulating hormone (ACTH)	too much
Adrenal insufficiency (of pituitary origin)		too little
Sexual precocity Sexual infantilism	Ovary and testis stimulating hormones (gonadotropins)	too much too early
Panhypopituitarism	All pituitary hormones	too little
Syndrome of persistent lactation	Prolactin	too much
Diabetes insipidus	Antidiuretic hormone	too little

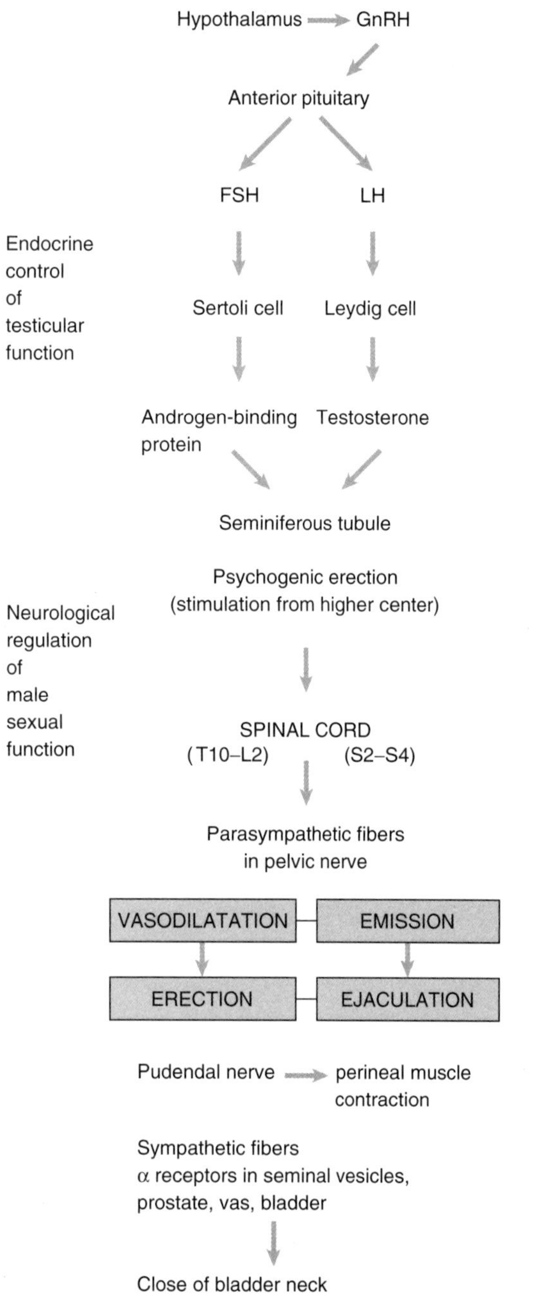

Figure 1.5 Endocrine control of testicular and neurological regulation of male sexual function (courtesy Professor A. A. Acosta)

activity and expression of the LH receptor. AMH is an indirect regulator of primordial follicle recruitment, via a decrease in FSH and an increase in inhibin (Pask *et al.*, 2004).

FSH/LH/ACTIVIN

LH and FSH are produced in pituitary gonadotrophs, and are composed of two non-covalently linked subunits, α and β. The α-subunit, called lipoprotein hormone α-subunit, is common to LH and FSH, and the β-subunit is specific to each hormone. The synthesis of each β-subunit is the rate-limiting step in LH and FSH production, and is regulated by the complex interaction of multiple factors, including activin and GnRH.

Activin, a member of the TGF-β family of growth factors, was originally identified as a factor in ovarian fluid that stimulated the secretion of FSH from pituitary gonadotrophs. Activin increases FSH-β subunit synthesis at the transcriptional level. The expression of activin is not limited to the ovary; it is also secreted within the pituitary gland, where it exerts an autocrine/paracrine effect. Activin physiologically regulates the production of LH as well as FSH. GnRH activates the LH-β promoter via the mitogen-activated protein (MAP) kinase pathway; activin A-induced activation of the LH-β promoter is independent of the MAP kinase pathway (Yamada *et al.*, 2004).

RECOMBINANT FSH

The introduction of recombinant human FSH (rFSH) is a milestone for fertility treatment. Compared with its older relatives, urinary human menopausal gonadotropin and urinary FSH (uFSH), rFSH has the clear advantages of a high level of purity, batch-to-batch consistency and better availability; however, rFSH remains much more expensive than the older products. The conclusion from a meta-analysis of 12 randomized trials was that rFSH is superior to uFSH in terms of clinical pregnancy rate per cycles started. Recombinant FSH was also more effective than uFSH in inducing multifollicular development. The higher effectiveness of rFSH has been demonstrated in studies that compared treatment with the same IU dose, and in studies that compared treatment with 150 IU of rFSH versus 225 IU of uFSH. The higher effectiveness of rFSH is probably due to a more basic hormone profile, compared with uFSH; the basic isohormones exhibit higher *in vitro* bioactivity than the acidic isohormones. A prospective randomized controlled trial was performed in humans to compare the three common IVF protocols: a short protocol and two long protocols in which GnRH agonist is started at either the early follicular phase or the mid-luteal phase. The two long protocols had the same implantation and pregnancy rates, which were better than with the short protocol (Ravhon, 2002).

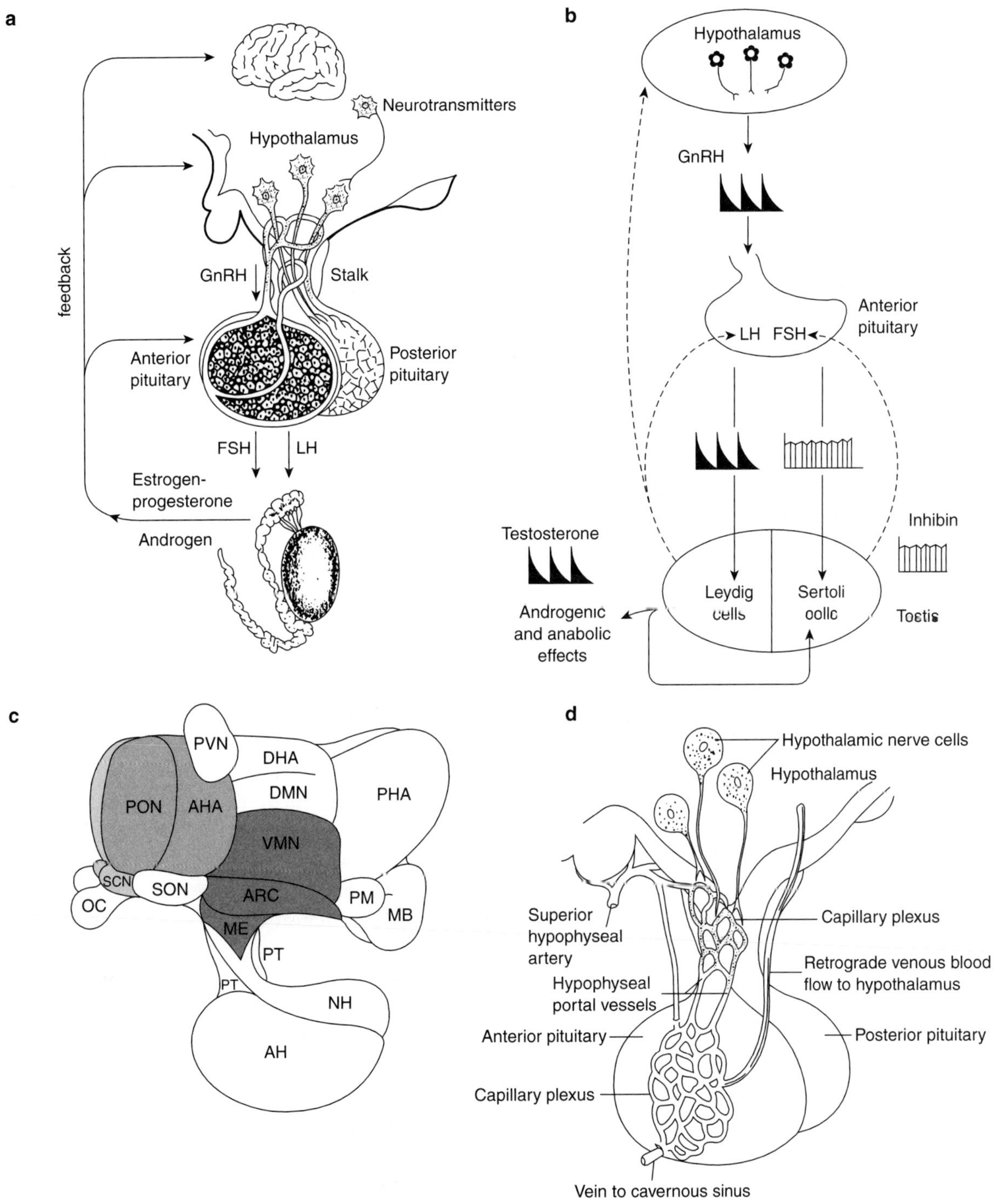

Figure 1.6 (**a**) Endocrine–neuroendocrine relationship between the hypothalamus, pituitary gland and gonad (ovary–testis). Hypothalamic neurosecretory materials (GnRH) are transported by the portal blood capillaries to the cells of the anterior pituitary. FSH and LH stimulate the testis. (**b**) Hypothalamus, anterior pituitary and testis inter-relationships. Solid arrows indicate stimulatory effects, dashed arrows indicate inhibitory effects. (**c**) Schematic drawing of hypothalamic nuclei and the pituitary. AH, adenohypophysis; AHA, anterior hypothalamic area; ARC, arcuate nucleus; DHA, dorsal hypothalamic area; DMN, dorsal medial nucleus; ME, median eminence; MB, mammillary body; NH, neurohypophysis; OC, optic chiasma; PHA, posterior hypothalamic area; PM, premammillary nucleus; PON, preoptic nucleus; PT, pars tuberalis; PVN, paraventricular nucleus; SCN, suprachiasmatic nucleus; SON, supraoptic nucleus; VMN, ventromedial nucleus. (**d**) Hypothalamic–pituitary–gonadal complex. Hypothalamic nerve cells release neurohormones into the portal vessels for transport to the anterior pituitary via the hypothalamohypophyseal vessels. Solid particles in nerve cells represent neurohormones. Blood is transported by the retrograde venous system back to the hypothalamus

a

b

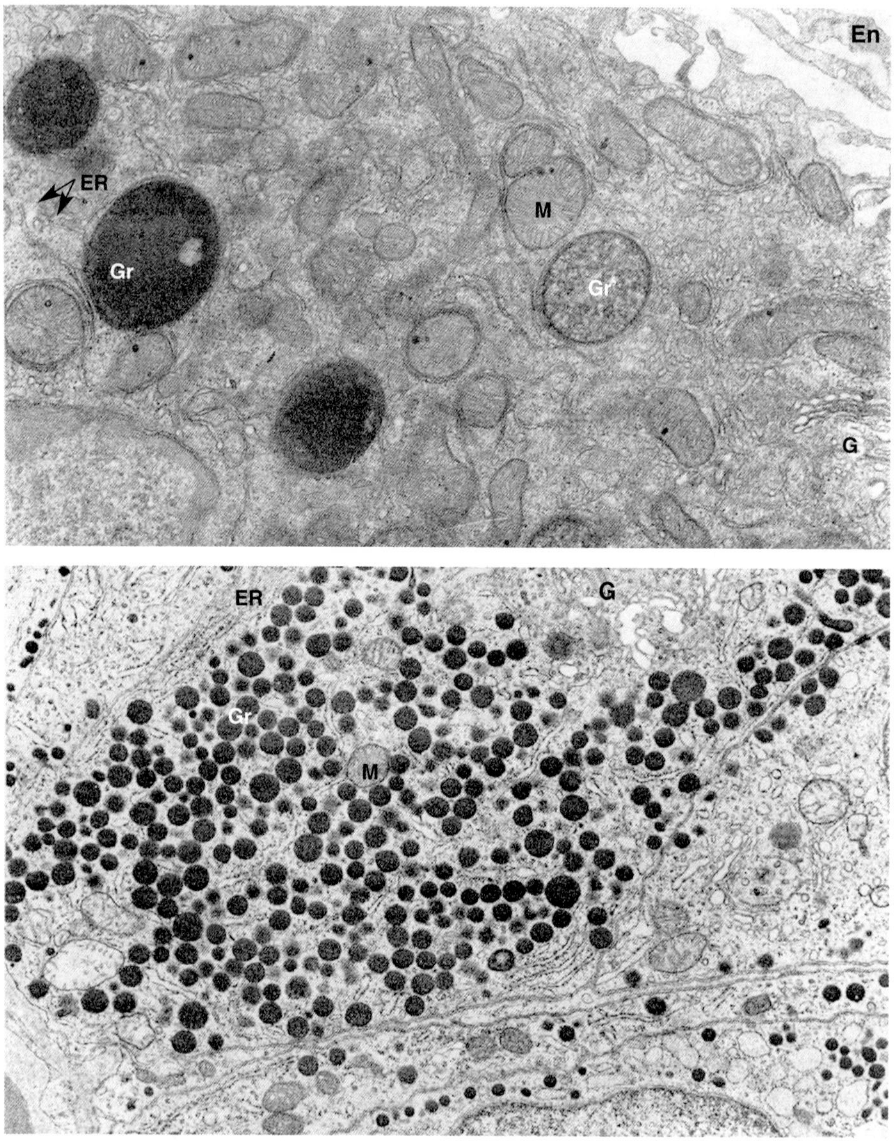

Figure 1.7 (**a**) Interstitial cell (TEM). ER, endoplasmic reticulum; G, Golgi complex; Gr, spherical granule; M, mitochondria; En, endothelium. (**b**) Anterior lobe of the pituitary (TEM): somatotrophs and gonadotrophs. ER, endoplasmic reticulum; G, Golgi complex; Gr, cytoplasm granules; M, mitochondria

LEPTIN

The peptide leptin is produced primarily by adipocytes, and achieves hormonal status by virtue of its secretion into the bloodstream. Its role in reproduction includes important effects on the hypothalamus to induce release of LH-releasing hormone, thereby triggering gonadotropin release and leading to development of the reproductive tract and induction of puberty.

Steroidogenesis depends on the supply of its precursor, cholesterol, derived from intracellular and extracellular sources. Intracellular levels are tightly controlled by regulation of the uptake, storage and synthesis by a unique family of transcription factors known as the sterol regulatory element-binding proteins (SREBPs). These transcription factors are localized to the endoplasmic reticulum. Upon depletion of cholesterol, the membrane-bound proteins are cleaved by proteases, releasing a 68-kDa transcription regulator. The mature SREBPs enter the nucleus, where they bind to sterol regulatory sites located in the promoter regions of genes involved in cholesterol homeostasis and transport. Circulating leptin has an effect on the gene expression profile and phenotype of white adipose tissue.

Table 1.3 Differential diagnosis of azoospermia/endocrine profile

	Algorithm endocrine evaluation			
Category	*LH/nl*	*FSH*	*Testosterone*	*Diagnosis*
Hypergonadotropic azoospermia	↑	↑	↓	Testicular dysfunction
Hypogonadotropic azoospermia	↓	↓	↓	Abnormal hormonal stimulation/endocrine evaluation
	nil	nil	nil	Normal testicular unexplained obstruction
Eugonadotropic azoospermia	Normal LH Normal FSH Normal testosterone			Obstruction Maturation arrest Sertoli cell only syndrome Ejaculatory dysfunction Sexual dysfunction
Differential diagnosis of azoospermia based on ejaculate volume/fructose presence	Normal semen volume, fructose positive			Endocrine evaluation (+) sperm
	Low semen volume and/or fructose negative			Post-ejaculatory urine (–) sperm

MELATONIN (*N*-ACETYL-5-METHOXYTRYPTAMINE)

Melatonin, the principal hormone of the pineal gland, is also found in plants, but at much lower concentrations than in animals. This hormone is involved in setting the timing (entertainment) of circadian rhythms, as well as regulating seasonal responses to changes in day length in seasonally breeding mammals (sheep, goats, horses, camels) – so called photoperiodic responses. Photoperiodic responses include changes in reproductive status, behavior and body weight. Melatonin is synthesized endogenously by the pinealocytes of the pineal gland. The essential amino acid L-tryptophan is a precursor in the synthesis of melatonin.

Melatonin synthesis displays a circadian rhythm that is reflected in serum melatonin levels. The rhythm is generated by a circadian clock located in the suprachiasmatic nucleus (SCN) of the hypothalamus. The SCN clock is set to the 24-hour day by the natural light–dark cycle. Light signals through a direct retinal pathway to the SCN. The SCN clock sends circadian signals over a neural pathway to the pineal gland, which drives rhythmic melatonin synthesis. The neural input to the gland is norepinephrine, and the output is melatonin. Melatonin may be indicated for some forms of insomnia and other sleep disturbances, and can abolish some of the symptoms.

The effects of hormones are typically mediated through receptors. Two forms of high-affinity melatonin receptors and one form of a low-affinity receptor have been identified. The high-affinity ML1 receptors are designated Mella and Mellb. The low-affinity receptor is designated ML2. Melatonin has anti-apoptotic activity in the thymus, as well as in cultured dexamethasone-treated thymocytes (a standard model for the study of apoptosis). Its anti-apoptotic activity is thought to occur via down-regulation of the glucocorticoid receptor.

HORMONE RECEPTORS/ REPRODUCTION

GnRH is a hypothalamic decapitate, which has a central role in the regulation of reproduction by stimulating the synthesis/secretion of pituitary LH/FSH. This effect is mediated through high-affinity receptors belonging to the G-protein-coupled seven transmembrane receptor family. GnRH receptors are also found in the testes, ovary, brain, adrenal gland and placenta, as well as hormone-dependent cancers, in addition to the pituitary. Analysis of the primary structure of the GnRH receptor has been performed to permit comparative analysis of such receptors and to evaluate the second messenger transduction mechanisms of the GnRH receptor, through which the effects of GnRH are mediated.

GnRH receptors of various species have been cloned and sequenced. The mammalian GnRH receptor encodes a single polypeptide of 327/328 amino acids, and the non-mammalian receptor

Table 1.4 Growth factors in andrology (data from Tanji *et al.*, 2001)

Growth factor	*Physiological role in andrology*	*Reference*
HGF	Multifunctional growth factor induces mitogenesis, dissociation and motility of epithelial and endothelial cells *in vitro*, and acts as a morphogenetic factor for tubular epithelium. Expressed in the mesenchyme, whereas the HGF receptor, c-MET, is expressed in epithelium. Expression of c-MET is unregulated by androgen deprivation.	Humphrey *et al.*, 1995 Pisters *et al.*, 1995
KGF	Secreted by fibroblasts and specifically promotes keratinocyte proliferation. In prostate, it is expressed and secreted by normal stromal cells. Only epithelial cells express the BEK/FGFR-2 receptor that binds KGF, suggesting that this growth factor controls epithelial cell proliferation in a paracrine manner. It is a potent mitogen for normal prostatic epithelial cells *in vitro* and promotes the growth of these cells under serum-free conditions. Prostatic stromal cell-derived KGF exhibits the properties of an andromedin, which may indirectly mediate control of epithelial cell growth and function by androgen.	Cunha *et al.*, 1995 Finch *et al.*, 1989 Story *et al.*, 1992 Sugimura *et al.*, 1996 Yan *et al.*, 1992
IGFs	Polypeptide with amino acid sequence and functional homology to insulin; proteins are produced by a variety of tissues, and the regulation of their production and function is extremely complex. There are 2 IGF peptides (IGF-1 and IGF-2), 2 cell surface receptors and at least 6 specific high-affinity binding proteins that modulate IGF actions. The mitogenic effect of IGFs is due to their ability to facilitate the transfer of cells from the G_1 phase to the S phase in the cell cycle. Produced only by the stromal cells, and normal epithelial cells, particularly basal cells, express IGF-1 receptors, suggesting a paracrine pathway. Have important mitogenic effects in the prostate and are essential for the development of the prostate. Expression of IGF regulated with other growth factor pathways, EGF, FGF and TGF-β.	Alarid *et al.*, 1994 Cohen *et al.*, 1994 Fiorelli *et al.*, 1991 Stile *et al.*, 1979
TGF-β	Multifunctional polypeptides regulate cellular differentiation and functions. At least 5 isoforms of TGF-β have been identified, but only types 1, 2 and 3 are present in mammalian cells. The polypeptides contain 112 amino acids and share about 80% sequence homology. TGF-β predominates in all tissues, whereas the expression of TGF-β2 and -β3 is more tissue restricted. TGF-β1 is expressed in smooth muscle cells, which are located adjacent to epithelial cells. Play dual roles of both stimulator and inhibitor in male reproductive organs. TGF-βs induce proliferation of mesenchymal cells and inhibit the growth of epithelial cells and inhibit DHT-dependent epithelial branching morphogenesis of seminal vesicles. TGF-β1, -β2 and -β3 are important for fetal development and are expressed at high levels in 17-day murine urogenital sinus mesenchyme, but not to play a role in regulating cell growth through the antiproliferative effects of EGF/TGF-β. On epithelial cells can counterbalance the mitogenic effects of various growth factors, thus having a role in growth regulation; associated with castration-induced prostate cell apoptosis. Normal prostate tissues have TGF-β receptors and generally respond to TGF-β through reduction in proliferation. TGF-β receptors are predominantly expressed in epithelium. Three types of receptors identified according to molecular weight. Only type I and II receptors have a direct role in TGF-β signal transduction. Type II receptors bind to TGF-β and then recruit type I receptor.	Cunha *et al.*, 1995 Graycar *et al.*, 1989 Kondaiah *et al.*, 1990 Massague *et al.*, 1990 Schurrmans *et al.*, 1988 Story *et al.*, 1996 Tanji *et al.*, 1994 Timme *et al.*, 1986 Wrana *et al.*, 1994
EGF TGF-α	Related polypeptides, which consist of 53 and 50 amino acids, respectively, share about 35% sequence homology and bind to same cell surface receptor. They have roles in embryogenesis, cell differentiation and angiogenesis. EGF is secreted by both normal and malignant cells, while TGF-α is produced by tumor cells. Human prostate epithelial cells require EGF in serum-free medium for growth in primary culture, and normal human fetal prostatic fibroblasts can replicate in response to this growth factor. Regulated by androgens and may be an important factor in an autocrine or paracrine mode of regulation. Exert their effects through their receptor (EGF-R), present in epithelial cells of male sex accessory organs. Their ability to interact with the same receptor is accounted for by their sequence homology. The differences in action of the 2 ligands may be due to different conformational changes induced within the receptor by the binding of each ligand. Androgens down-regulate EGF-Rs in prostate. TGF-α plays a role in prostatic differentiation and maintenance of epithelial integrity rather than proliferation. TGF-α expression occurs predominantly in stroma, whereas its receptor is expressed by epithelial cells, suggesting a paracrine mode of regulation.	Cohen *et al.*, 1994 Lee *et al.*, 1985 Nishi *et al.*, 1996 Rappolee *et al.*, 1988 St Arnaud *et al.*, 1988 Traish and Wotiz, 1987 Ullrich *et al.*, 1984

encodes a protein of 379 amino acids. The predicted mammalian/non-mammalian receptor proteins contain seven transmembrane domains and belong to the G-protein-coupled receptor family. The mammalian GnRH receptor is 38% homologous to the non-mammalian GnRH receptor at the amino acid level. When expressed in COS-7 cells or HEK293 cells, the isolated GnRH receptor cDNA invokes GnRH-activated second messenger systems. The gene encoding the GnRH receptor is composed of three exons and two introns, and contains multiple transcriptional start sites and regulatory sequences in the 5' flanking region. Studies suggest that idiopathic hypogonadotropic hypogonadism may be the result of single or multiple mutations in the GnRH receptor gene. Future studies should lead to a better understanding of the mechanisms involved in the transcriptional regulation of the GnRH receptor gene in the pituitary, extra-pituitary tissues and cancers.

Sperm capacitation/acrosome reaction/fertilization involve sperm receptors on plasma lemma, oocyte receptors located on the zona pellucida (ZP_3; ultrastructural interactions involve ZP_2) and inner acrosomal membrane receptors. Immunochemical parameters, using monoclonal antibodies to acrosin, exhibit an abnormal pattern of weak fluorescence in the post-nuclear region.

FUTURE RESEARCH IN ENDOCRINOLOGY

The Center for Scientific Review of the National Institutes of Health reviews individual studies in the following research areas of endocrinology, metabolism, nutrition and reproductive sciences:

(1) Pituitary, thyroid and adrenal physiology and pathophysiology

(2) Cancers of the endocrine system

(3) Growth, development and disorders of endocrine organs and their products

(4) Neuroendocrinology

(5) Reproductive neuroendocrinology, including development of the hypothalamic–pituitary–gonadal axis and mechanisms underlying the biorhythms of reproductive hormones

(6) Hormone interactions with other organ systems and tissues

(7) Hormones and immunobiology

(8) Pediatric and developmental endocrinology

(9) Endocrinology of aging

(10) Endocrine pharmacology and toxicology, including the effects of endocrine disrupters and xenobiotics

(11) Endocrine-related disorders of the male and female reproductive systems

(12) Hormones, stress and the autonomic systems

(13) Hormone based therapies

(14) Comparative endocrinology

(15) Animal models of endocrine disorders

2

Functional ultrastructure of testis and epididymis

The genetic control of testis determination involves several genes: Tdy (testis determining factor), Sry (Y chromosome-specific gene), Sox6 (Sry-related gene), Sox9 (Sertoli cell-determining factor), TAZ83 (coding at early to mid-pachytene germ-cell stage), TAZ4 (testis-specific gene located on chromosome 11) and TNZ1 (expressed in neonatal Leydig cell) (Table 2.1).

SPERMATOGENESIS

The seminiferous epithelium, which lines the seminiferous tubules, is composed of two basic cell types: Sertoli cells and developing germ cells. The germ cells undergo a continuous series of cellular divisions and developmental changes, beginning at the periphery of the tubule and progressing towards the lumen. The stem cells, called spermatogonia, divide several times before becoming spermatocytes. The primary spermatocytes duplicate their DNA and undergo progressive nuclear changes during meiotic prophase known as preleptotene, leptotene, zygotene, pachytene and diplotene before dividing to form secondary spermatocytes, known as spermatocytogenesis. Without further DNA synthesis, the resultant secondary spermatocytes divide again to form the haploid cells known as spermatids (Figure 2.1). The spermatids then undergo a progressive series of structural and developmental changes to form spermatozoa.

Spermiogenesis

The round spermatids are transformed into spermatozoa by a series of progressive changes collectively known as spermiogenesis. The changes include condensation of nuclear chromatin, formation of the sperm tail or flagellum apparatus, and development of the acrosomal cap. The various developmental stages of spermatic transformation are divided into

Table 2.1 Genetic control of testis determination

Gene	*Role during testis development*
Tdy (testis determining factor in mice)	Act on supporting cell lineage and induce differentiation of supporting cells to Sertoli cells
Sry (a Y chromosome-specific gene)	Different homologs of Sry have a common open reading frame which has 41% homology to a DNA-binding motif HMG box; Sry encoded protein might have DNA-binding activity
Sox6 (Sry-related gene), Sox5	Overlapping functions in the adult mouse
Sox9	A critical Sertoli cell differentiation factor
TAZ83	Coding at early to mid-pachytene germ-cell stage
TAZ4	Testis-specific gene located on chromosome 11
TNZ1	Expressed in neonatal Leydig cells

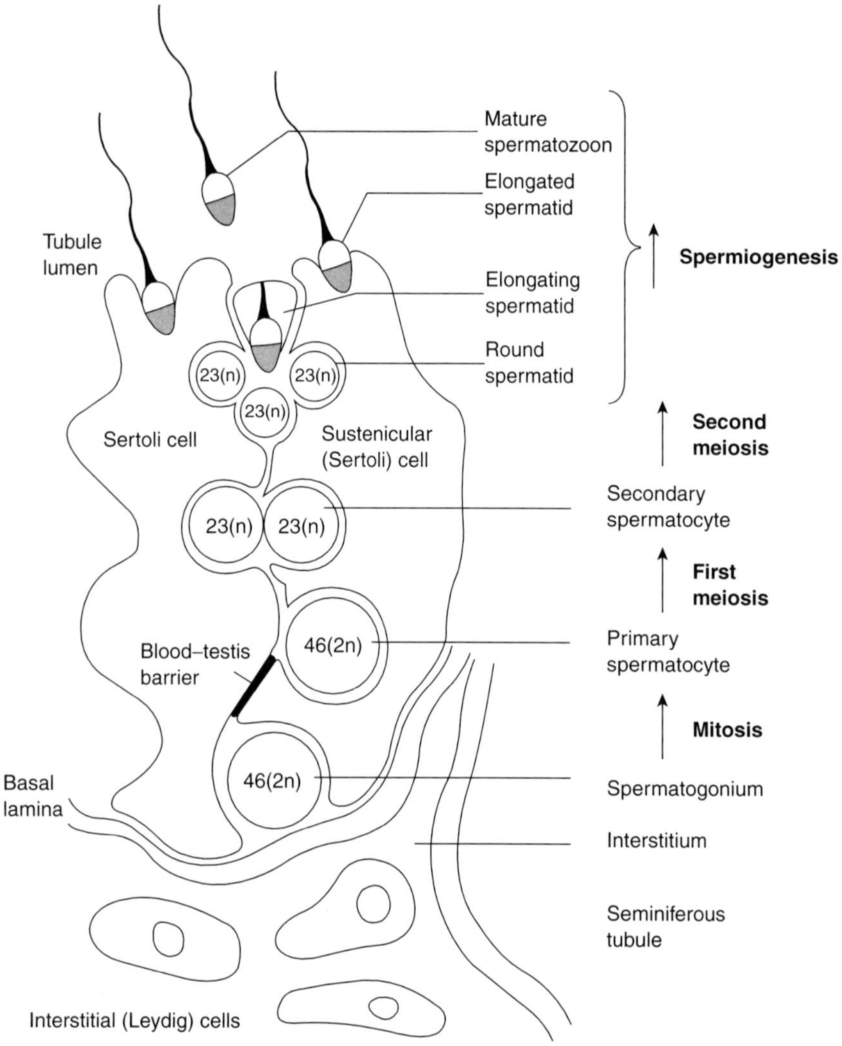

Figure 2.1 Spermatogenesis occurs within the seminiferous tubules of the testis, where all stages of sperm cell are nurtured by Sertoli cells. As spermatogenesis proceeds, the sperm cells migrate from the basal lamina to the lumen of the seminiferous tubule. Diploid spermatogonia proliferate mitotically to give rise to primary spermatocytes, and these divide meiotically to yield haploid secondary spermatocytes. The secondary spermatocytes undergo a further meiotic division and, hence, each primary spermatocyte gives rise to four round spermatids, each of which is destined to differentiate into a functional mature spermatozoon

four phases: Golgi body formation, cap formation, acrosomal and maturation phases. The reshaping of the nucleus and acrosome of each spermatid, initiated during the previous phase, produces the spermatozoon. Within the nucleus, the chromatin granules undergo progressive condensation as the transitional proteins are replaced by protamines which form a fine homogeneous material that uniformly fills the entire sperm nucleus.

During the later stages of spermiogenesis, the Sertoli cell shapes the cytoplasm remaining after elongation of the spermatid into a spheroidal lobule called the residual body. This lobule of cytoplasm, which remains connected to the elongated spermatid by a slender thread of cytoplasm, is also interconnected with other residual bodies by intercellular bridges that result from the incomplete division of the germ cells during spermatogenesis. Formation of the residual body completes the final maturation, and the elongated spermatids are ready for release as spermatozoa into the lumen of the seminiferous tubule (Figure 2.2).

Spermiation

Spermiation is the process by which the elongated spermatids, that are oriented perpendicularly to the tubular wall, are gradually extruded from the Sertoli cells into the lumen of the tubule. The lobules of residual cytoplasm, through which groups of spermatids are connected by intercellular bridges, remain embedded in the epithelium. Extrusion of the spermatozoa components continues until only a slender stalk of cytoplasm connects the neck of the

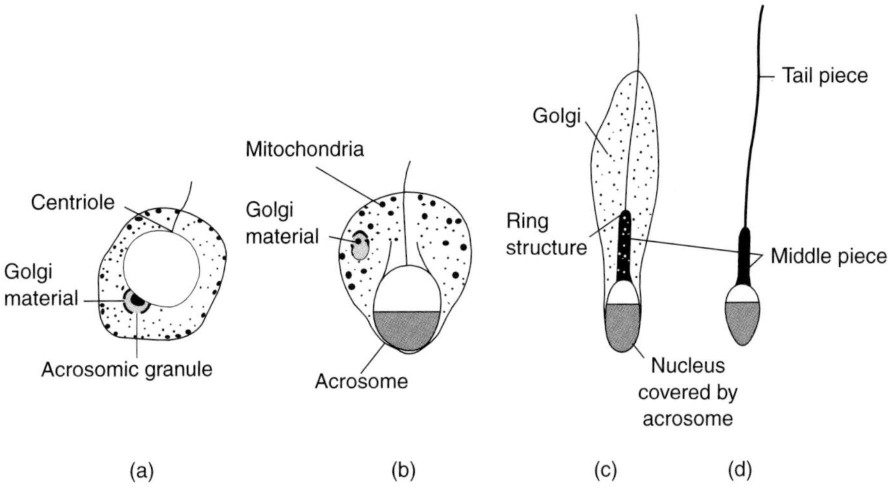

Figure 2.2 Spermiogenesis. Maturation of round spermatid into spermatozoa: (a) round spermatid, (b) elongating spermatid, (c) elongated spermatid and (d) spermatozoon. From Fleming and King (2003), with permission

spermatid to the residual body. Breakage of the stalk results in formation of the cytoplasm droplet in the neck region of the released spermatozoon (proximal droplet) and retention of the interconnected residual bodies. Following release of the spermatozoa the residual bodies are phagocytosed by the Sertoli cells to recycle the protoplasmic components. Not only do the Sertoli cells phagocytose the residual bodies remaining from the spermatogenic process, but they also remove considerable numbers of degenerated germ cells. Because the spermatogenic process is relatively inefficient, large numbers of potential sperm degenerate before maturation.

Regulation of spermatogenesis

Spermatogenesis is a complex multistage process that involves formation of spermatogonia from germ stem cells, spermatogonial renewal and differentiation into primary spermatocytes, meiosis by which diploid spermatocytes develop into haploid spermatids, and spermiogenesis in which round spermatids mature into sperm. Spermatogenesis is a well-coordinated developmental program in which the different steps are defined by a cell type- and stage-specific induction or repression of the expression of specific genes. Many of these genes are expressed predominantly or exclusively in cells during spermatogenesis and their regulation can involve control at the transcriptional or post-transcriptional level. Various hormones, signaling pathways, transcription factors and interactions with the local environment play a critical role in regulating the different stages in this differentiation program. The identification of cell type- and stage-specific genes provides excellent tools to dissect the differentiation program and to study the mechanisms by which spermatogenesis is controlled. The germ cell-specific transcription factor cyclic adenosine monophosphate (cAMP) responsive element modulator (CREM) appears to be a key factor in the regulation of the expression of a number of postmeiotic genes. Several members of the nuclear receptor family (estrogen, retinoid and peroxisome proliferation activated receptors) are implicated in the regulation of specific stages of spermatogenesis.

The two compartments of the testes, the seminiferous tubules and interstitium, are under the hormonal control of gonadotropins, acting on either Sertoli cells or Leydig cells. During spermatogenesis, the different cell types and, in particular, germ cells express four specific sets of genes, which are regulated at either the transcriptional or transductional level. Some of these genes are detected exclusively in haploid cells, whereas others are initially expressed before or during meiosis and continue to be expressed in spermatids:

(1) Male germ cell-specific gene homologs (e.g. glyceraldehyde-3-phosphate dehydrogenase);

(2) Unique genes expressed exclusively during spermatogenesis;

(3) Germ cell-specific alternate transcripts leading to specific isoforms;

(4) Genes regulated developmentally during germ-cell differentiation (e.g. cAbl proto-oncogene).

Leydig cells also secrete non-pathogenic products, including growth factors, cytokines and vasoactive peptides, which contribute to the intercellular communication between Leydig, Sertoli and tubular cells. Testosterone initiates and maintains spermatogenesis.

Spermatogenic wave

The stages of the cycle within the seminiferous epithelium change not only with time, but also along the length of the tubular loop. At any one stage, a portion of tubule is adjacent to other portions of tubule in stages just preceding or following it in time. This sequential changing in cycle stage along the length of the tubule is known as the wave of the seminiferous epithelium. Examination of a loop of seminiferous tubule along its length also reveals that the wave involves a sequence of stages beginning with the less-advanced stages in the middle of the loop to progressively more-advanced stages nearer the rete testis (Figures 2.3–2.6; Table 2.2).

Transferrin receptor

Intracytoplasmic sperm injection (ICSI) using testicular sperm is a valid option for the treatment of infertile couples in whom the male partner has azoospermia; however, testicular epididymal sperm extraction (TESE) may not be successful in all patients. Transferrin is the major secretory product of Sertoli cells, and is present in high concentrations in the seminal plasma of fertile men. Transferrin receptor is a transmembrane lipoprotein composed of two identical disulfide-linked 90-kDa subunits, providing iron for cell proliferation and differentiation. A soluble form of the transferring receptor (sTfr) can be detected in seminal plasma, probably originating from spermatocytes/spermatids (El-Garem *et al.*, 2003). Measurement of sTfr in the seminal plasma of patients with azoospermia may contribute to the etiological diagnosis of this condition. In combination with serum follicle stimulating hormone (FSH), this measurement may help to predict the outcome of TESE.

Seminal plasma

Primordial germ cells (PGCs) proliferate and migrate towards the genital ridges to become enclosed by Sertoli cells. These germ cells are then called gonocytes. The proliferative activity of gonocytes is different from that of PGCs in that, after division, the daughter cells remain connected by an intercellular bridge. Moreover, gonocytes differ structurally from PGCs.

Gonocytes and A spermatogonia are not identified by their morphology. Hence, at the start of spermatogenesis germ cells called gonocytes, but as they develop further they are said to be a mixed population of A_s, A_{pr} and A_{al} spermatogonia, and the more-differentiated A_1 spermatogonia. Several researchers developed a monoclonal antibody to recognize a marker that is specifically expressed by the quiescent gonocytes until birth. It would appear that gonocytes are specific to fetal testes, whereas A_s, A_{pr} and A_{al} spermatogonia of adult testes arise after birth. The development of gonocytes towards A_s, A_{pr} and A_{al} spermatogonia, therefore, occurs during the quiescent period of germ cells, around the time of birth.

Most seminal plasma is produced by the prostate and seminal vesicles, while the testis and epididymis contribute less than 5% of the total semen volume. A low ejaculate volume reflects abnormality of the prostate or seminal vesicles. Fructose is produced by the seminal vesicles; thus the absence of fructose indicates either ejaculatory duct obstruction or seminal vesicle aplasia/hypoplasia. The latter can occur with cogenital bilateral absence of the vas deferens, which can be differentiated from ejaculatory duct obstruction by physical examination.

Blood–testis barrier

The seminiferous tubules are not penetrated by blood or lymph vessels. In addition, the developing germ cells within the tubules are protected from chemical changes in the blood by a specialized permeability barrier. This blood–testis barrier has two principal components: the incomplete or partial barrier of the myoid cells that surround the tubule; and the unique junctions between adjacent Sertoli cells.

In the testis, the blood–testis barrier (BTB) is located near the basal lamina, which effectively divides the epithelium into basal and adluminal compartments. During late stage VII through to early stage IX of the epithelial cycle, preleptotene and leptotene spermatocytes residing in the basal compartment adjacent to the basement membrane must traverse the BTB to gain entry to the adluminal compartment in order to develop into haploid spermatids. Without this timely movement of developing preleptotene and leptotene spermatocytes across the BTB, spermatogenesis is halted, leading to infertility.

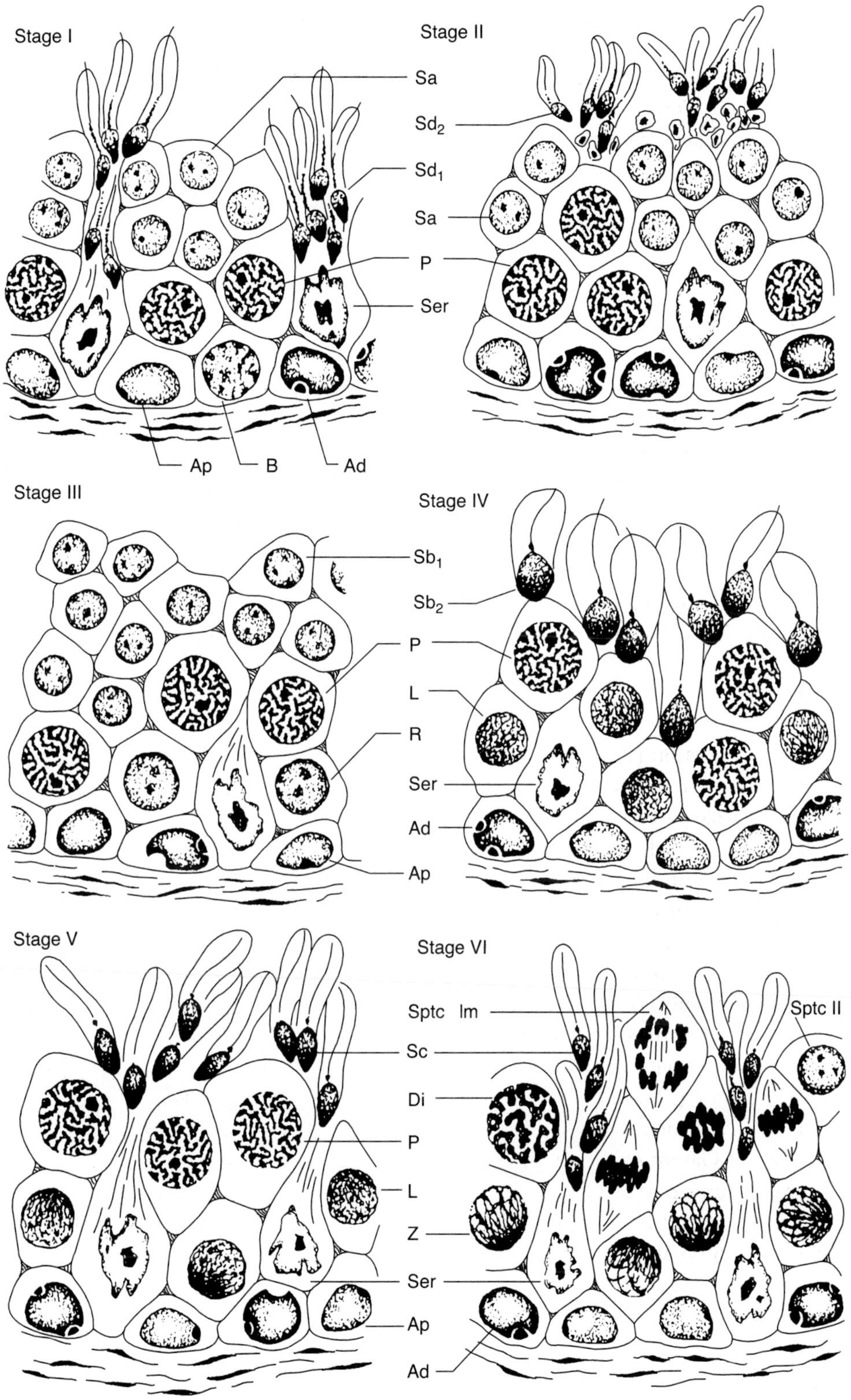

Figure 2.3 Diagrammatic illustration of the cellular composition of the six stages of the cycle of the seminiferous epithelium in man. The stages are labeled (I)–(VI) and correspond to cell associations which succeed one another in time in any given area of the seminiferous tubule according to the sequence from left to right. After stage VI, stage I reappears and the sequence starts over again. The spaces allotted to the stages of the cycle are proportional to their relative durations. Ad, type A dark spermatogonium; Ap, type A pale spermatogonium; B, type B spermatogonium; R, preleptotene; L, leptotene; Z, zygotene; P, pachytene; Di, diplotene primary spermatocytes; Sptc Im, primary spermatocyte meiosis; Sptc II, secondary spermatocyte; Sa, Sb, Sc, Sd, spermatids; Ser, Sertoli cell (adapted from Hafez and Hafez, 2000)

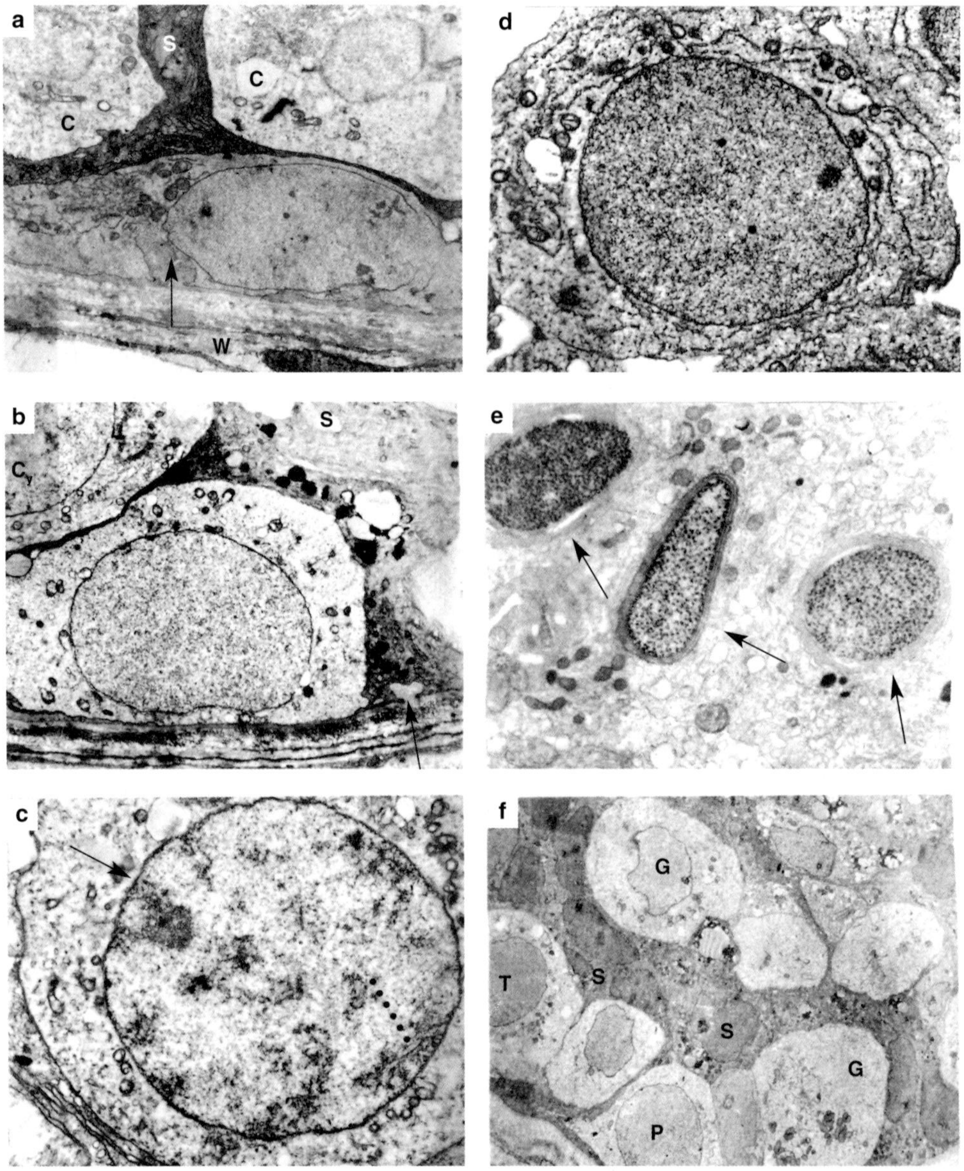

Figure 2.4 Transmission electron microscopy of normal human testis. (**a**) Type A spermatogonium attached to tubular wall (W, arrow). Sertoli cell cytoplasm (S) expands between two primary spermatocytes (C) and spermatogonium (10 200×). (**b**) Type B spermatogonium attached to basal lamina (arrow). Sertoli cell cytoplasm (S) interposed between this cell and primary spermatocyte (C_y) (6375×). (**c**) Primary spermatocyte: arrow points to short complex formed by sex chromosome cores (7800×). (**d**) Secondary spermatocyte endoplasmatic reticulum appears as flat saccules with localized dilatations, arranged concentrically around the nucleus (12 000×). (**e**) Three maturing spermatids; condensing chromatin has 'tigroid' appearance (6000×). (**f**) Immature testis in a 4-year-old boy: gonocyte-like cell (G), transitional spermatogonium (T) and primitive (P) spermatogonium (1350×)

The BTB creates a unique microenvironment for germ cell development; it segregates immunologically most of the germ-cell antigens, except those residing on spermatogonia and preleptotene/leptotene spermatocytes, from the systemic circulation, and maintains cell polarity. BTB dynamics *in vitro* and/or *in vivo* are regulated by cytokines, such as transforming growth factor (TGF)-β_3 and tumor necrosis factor (TNF)-α, via two defined signaling pathways:

(1) TGFβ/MEKKs (MAP (mitrogen-activated protein)/ERK kinase kinase)/p38 MAP kinase;

(2) TNFα/integrin-linked kinase (ILK)/glycogen synthase kinase (GSK).

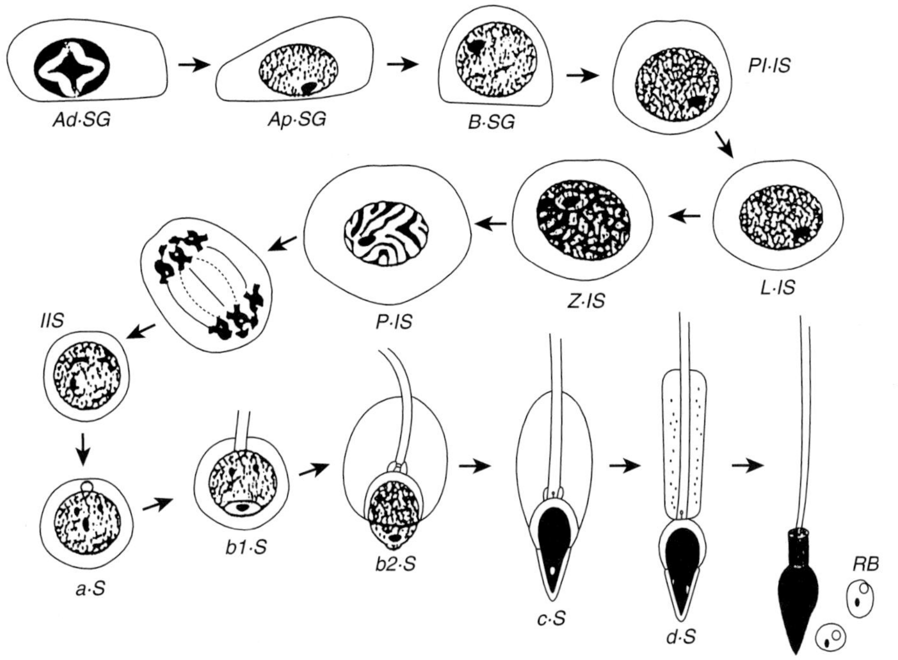

Figure 2.5 Stages of human spermatogenesis. Mature spermatozoa are obtained following mitotic, meiotic and post-meiotic phases. The cell types shown are spermatogonium type A dark (Ad-SG) and type A pale (Ap-SG), spermatogonium type B (B-SG), preleptotene (P1), leptotene (L), zygotene (Z) and pachytene (P) primary spermatocytes (IS), secondary spermatocytes (IIS), spermatids (S) at different stages of mutation (a, bl, b2, c, d) and mature spermatozoa with residual bodies (RB)

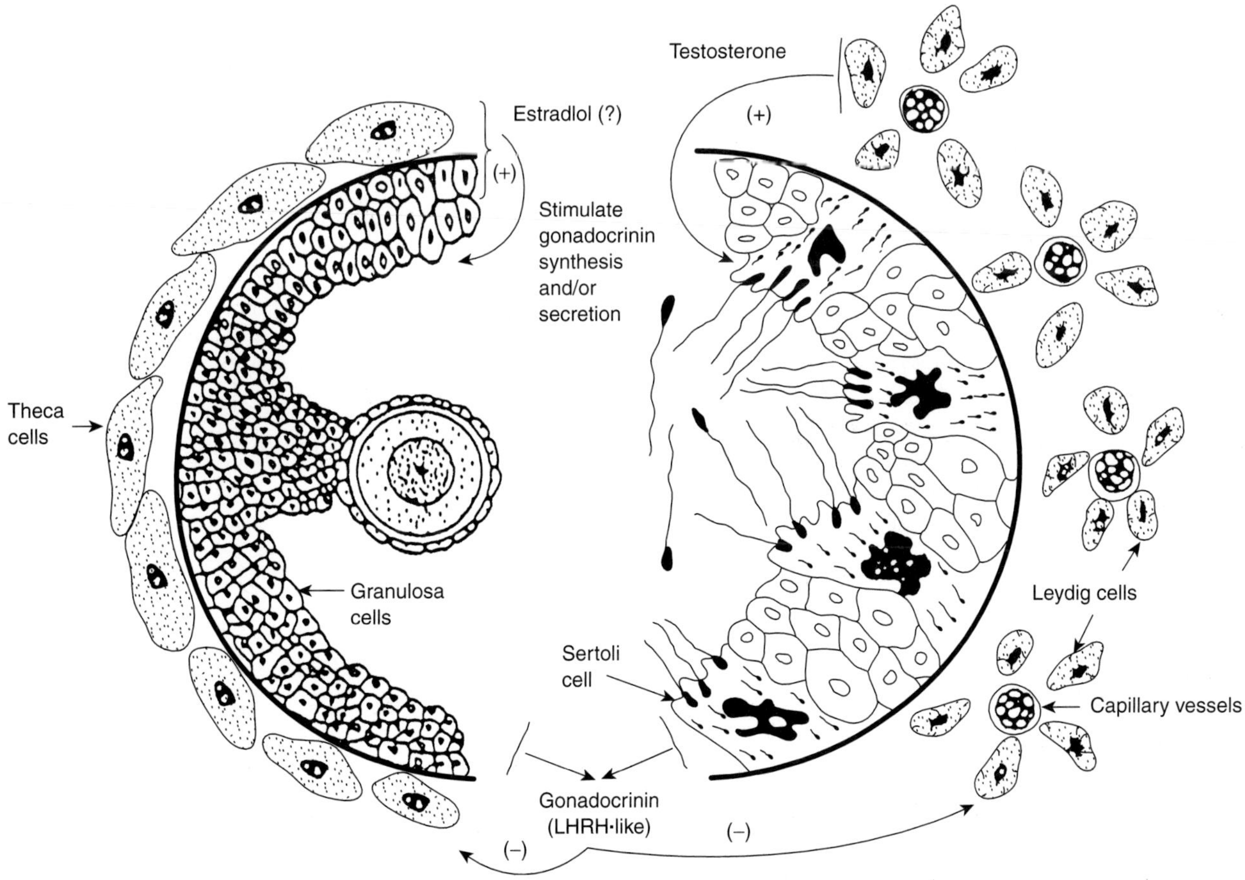

Figure 2.6 Seminiferous tubule showing Leydig and Sertoli cells

Table 2.2 Cytological characteristics of germinal epithelium

Adulthood	
A spermatogonia	Attachment to basal lamina; oval nucleus with one or more corpuscles, finely granular chromatin that can be more deeply stained when nuclear 'vacuole' is present
B spermatogonia	Attachment to basal lamina can be complete, partial or almost absent round nucleus with fine chromatin; heterochromatic granules and one or two less conspicuous nucleoli
Primary spermatocytes	No attachment to basal lamina; nucleus with filamentous (leptotene or thick pachytene chromosomes; the sexual pair can appear to be heterochromatic ('sex vesicle'); pachytene spermatocytes with large nucleoli are large germ cells
Secondary spermatocytes	Smaller nucleus, fine chromatin; similar to those of young spermatids although larger; infrequently recognized
Spermatids	Round nucleus with fine chromatin or small, elongated, deeply chromatic nucleus; presence of acrosome granule or head cap, both PAS positive; flagellum soon becomes evident, as well as 'manchette'; when mature forms are free in lumen (spermatozoa), discarded cytoplasms appear as residual bodies
Sertoli cell	Large cell with numerous extensions between germ cells; nucleus large and polymorphous, showing infoldings of nuclear membrane; large nucleolus with eosinophilic core
Prepuberty	
Gonocyte	Very large cell with basophilic cytoplasm situated in core of germinal cord without attachment to basal lamina; degeneration frequently seen; disappearing progressively after birth
Intermediate type	Large cells, similar to gonocytes but showing attachment to basal lamina; gradually disappearing during infancy
Primitive type spermatogonia	Smaller oval cell with light basophilic cytoplasm; round nucleus with fine chromatin showing 1 or 2 nucleoli; practically the only genial type when puberty starts
Immature supporting cell	Scarce cytoplasm with poorly defined limits; elongated nucleus with palisade-like arrangement; 1 or 2 small nucleoli; frequently dividing during infancy

PAS, periodic acid-Schiff

Myoid layer

The basement membrane or tunica propria that surrounds the seminiferous tubules contains a layer of contractile myoid cells. In some species the majority of the cell junctions of this layer are sealed by tight apposition of the adjacent cell membranes. This barrier, however, is not well developed in the bull, ram or boar and may be relatively unimportant in the testis of farm animals.

Sertoli cell junctions

The principal permeability barrier between the blood and testis is thought to be the complexes at junctions between adjacent Sertoli cells (Figures 2.7 and 2.8). These Sertoli–Sertoli junctions, which are situated near the cellular base, contain multiple zones of adhesion (tight junctions) where the opposing membranes are fused. They consist of a basal compartment containing spermatogonia and preleptotene spermatocytes, and an adluminal compartment containing the more advanced stages of spermatocytes and spermatids, which freely communicates with the lumen of the tubule.

Nitric oxide and nitric oxide synthase

Nitric oxide (NO) and nitric oxide synthase (NOS) play a pivotal role in epithelial barrier function in many organs, including the testis, and in spermatogenesis. BTB function is maintained by intricate regulatory mechanisms. In addition to hormones and cytokines, nitric oxide (NO) is a putative tight junction regulator in the testis; tight junction dynamics are regulated by three tight junction integral membrane proteins via three possible signaling pathways.

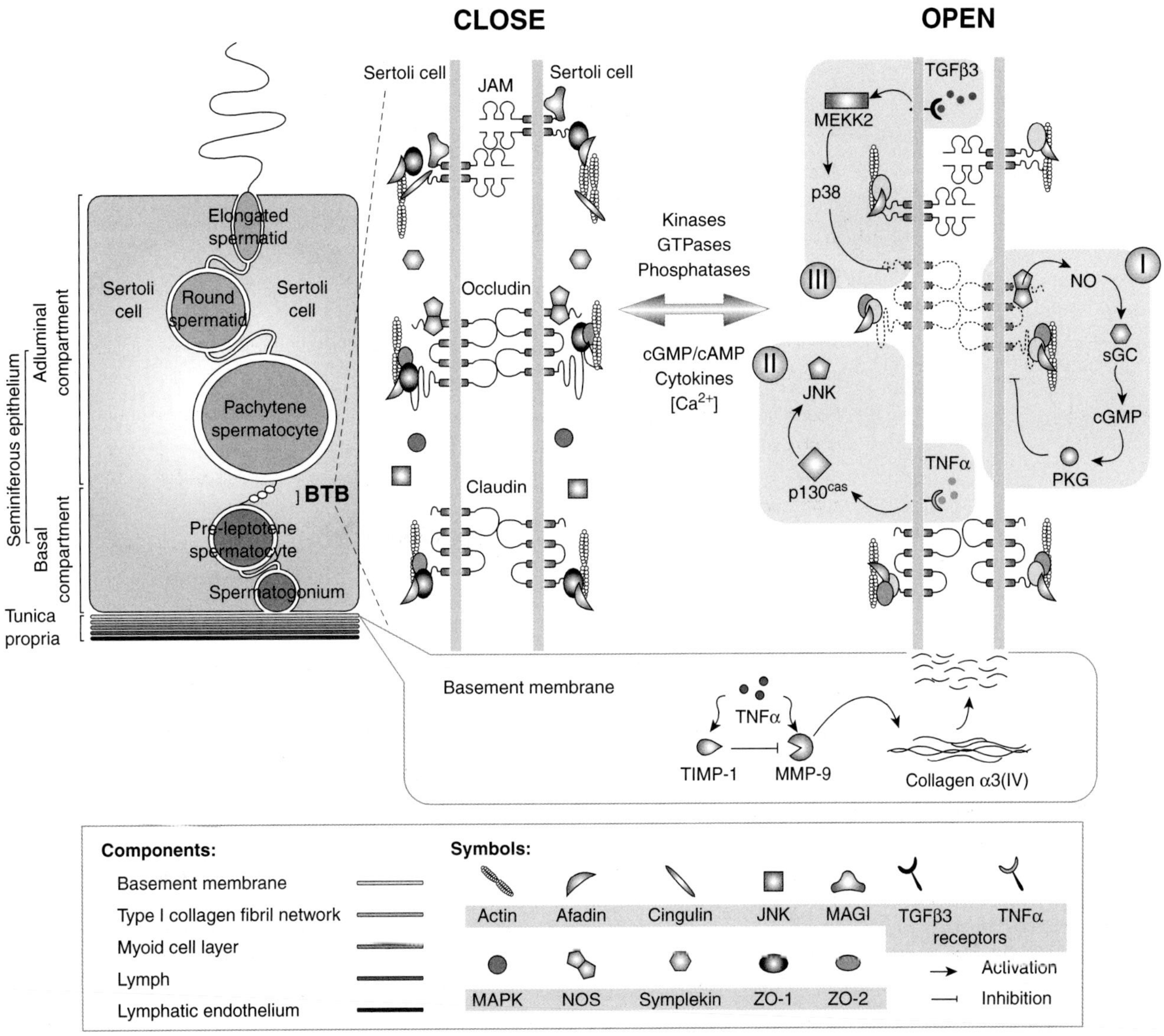

Figure 2.7 Nitric oxide (NO)/nitric oxide synthase (NOS) and tight junctions in the testis. The three tight junction-integral membrane proteins (JAM, occludin and claudin) are shown at the site of the blood–testis barrier, as well as the three possible signaling pathways (I–III) that regulate the opening and closing of the Sertoli cell tight junctions. (I) NO stimulates soluble guanylate cyclase (sGC) to synthesize cyclic guanosine monophosphate (cGMP), leading to tight junction disruption. The cGMP can also activate protein kinase G (PKG), which, in turn, can affect tight junction dynamics via its effects on occludin, reducing the level of occludin at the site of Sertoli cell tight junctions, thereby opening up the tight junction barrier. (II) Tumor necrosis factor-α (TNFα) activates the integrin-linked kinase (ILK)/glycogen synthase kinase (GSK)/p130^{cas}/c-Jun *N*-terminal kinase (JNK) signaling pathway which, in turn, affects the level of occludin. Transforming growth factor-β_3 (TGFβ_3) activates mitogen-activated protein (MAP)/ERK kinase kinase 2 (MEKK2) and p38 MAP kinase to perturb Sertoli cell tight junctions via its effects on the level of occludin and zonula occudens (ZO)-1 at the site of the blood–testis barrier. BTB, blood–testis barrier; TIMP-1, tissue inhibitor of metalloproteinase-1; MMP-9, matrix metalloproteinase-9; MAGI, membrane-associated guanylate kinase with inverted orientation. From Lee and Cheng (2004), with permission

Two other tight junction-integral membrane proteins, namely CAR and CRBI, are found in other epithelia. Sertoli cell tight junctions that constitute the BTB physically divide the seminiferous epithelium into adluminal and basal compartments. Underneath the basal compartment is the tunica propria, which is composed of a non-cellular and a cellular zone. The cellular zone includes the basement membrane. In the testis, the basement membrane is a modified form of extracellular matrix composed largely of type

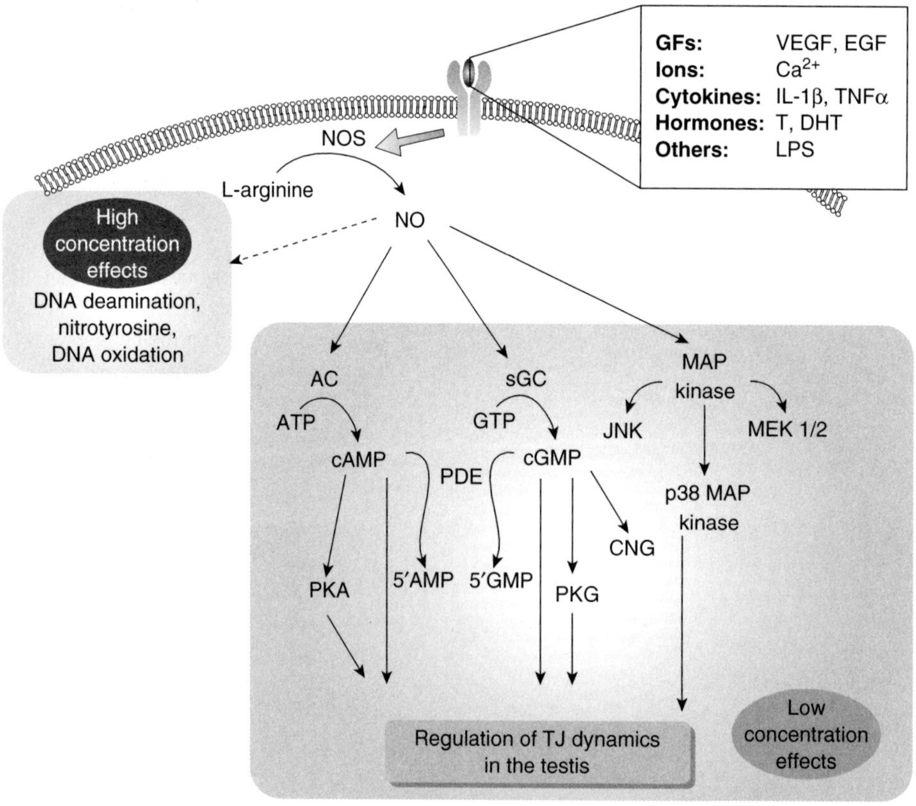

Figure 2.8 Nitric oxide (NO) and nitric oxide synthase (NOS) effects on tight junctions in the testis. A low concentration of NO (<1 μmol/l) can stimulate other cellular downstream signaling pathways. In addition, NO can activate soluble guanylate cyclase (sGC) and adenylate cyclase (AC) to synthesize cyclic guanosine monophosphate (cGMP) and cyclic adenosine monophosphate (cAMP), respectively. The cAMP activates protein kinase (PKA). Likewise, the cGMP has more diverse effects by activating phosphodiesterase (PDE), cyclic nucleotide-gated channel (CNG) and PKG. Both cAMP and cGMP are known regulators of Sertoli cell tight junction (TJ) dynamics. PDE can negatively control the levels of cAMP and cGMP. In addition, NO can stimulate mitogen-activated protein (MAP) kinases, such as p38, c-Jun *N*-terminal kinase (JNK) and MAP/ERK kinases 1 and 2 (MEK 1/2). In the testis, cAMP/PKA and cGMP/PKG are putative regulators of tight junction dynamics. DHT, 5α-dihydrotestosterone; EGF, epidermal growth factor; LPS, lipopolysaccharides; VEGF, vascular epithelial growth factor; T, testosterone; GFs, growth factors; IL, interleukin. From Lee and Cheng (2004), with permission

Table 2.3 Epididymal sperm maturation, capacitation and acrosome reaction

Maturational stage	*Quality*
Sperm gain fertilization potential	Ability of testicular sperm to move is due to immaturity of plasma membrane
Development of sperm motility	Transfer of substances: glycerol-3-phosphorylcholine a forward motility protein from the epididymal fluid
Maturation of sperm plasma	Sperm unable to move progressively or interact with and fertilize eggs
Membrane	Sperm attain motility in caput epididymis or corpus epididymis according to species
Maturational sperm structures	Sperm do not gain fertilization potential simultaneously in same region
	Most sperm attain full fertilization potential in cauda, major sperm storage site
Deposit, storage, ascent in female tract	Sperm fertilization potential is evaluated by: (1) sperm's ability to fertilize zona-free hamster eggs; (2) motility patterns; (3) surface characteristics; and (4) structural stability of head/tail Epididymis/vas deferens secrete specific components necessary for functional maturation

IV collagen, laminin, heparin sulfate proteoglycan and entactin, which is adjacent to the seminiferous epithelium; behind this is a layer of type I collagen fibrils. The cellular zone is made up of a layer of myoid cells; behind this lies the lymphatic endothelium. The three classes of tight junction-integral membrane proteins, namely occludins, claudins and JAMs, interact with adaptors, such as zonula occludens (ZO)-1, ZO-2, afadin, cingulin and membrane-associated guanylate kinase with inverted orientation (MAGI), tethering actin filaments to the tight junction-integral membrane proteins and recruiting proteins to the BTB site (Figure 2.7).

REACTIVE OXYGEN SPECIES IN SEMEN

Extensive investigations have been conducted on phagocytosis, which is an oxygen-dependent process. During non-specific immunological defense, the activity of pentose phosphate is dramatically increased leading to the formation of reduced nicotinamide adenosine dinucleotide phosphate (NADPH). NADPH is also generated in leukocytes by oxidation of glucose-6-phosphate. As NADPH is needed to reduced the oxygen bound to membrane-based cytochromes, the oxygen demand is strongly increased (respiratory burst). During this process oxygen is converted into superoxide anions, hydrogen peroxide, monomolecular oxygen and hydroxyl radicals, which are effective microbicidals, by several types of phagocytic cells (neutrophils, eosinophils, basophils and macrophages).

SPERM MATURATION IN EPIDIDYMIS

During epididymal maturation, membrane lipids in the sperm undergo distinct physical and chemical alterations, including changes in the distribution pattern of intramembranous protein (lipoprotein) particles in the sperm plasma membrane of epididymal sperm (Table 2.3). The plasma membrane contains both membrane-integrated and surface-adsorbed proteins. Some of these intrinsic proteins change their location in or on the plasma membrane during sperm maturation. These dynamic changes occur throughout the male reproductive tract, but most actively in the caput and corpus epididymis leading to the sperm becoming fertilizable. During the maturation of epididymal sperm, some surface lipoprotein, either membrane-integrated or membrane-adsorbed,

Table 2.4 Chemical and biological parameters that are regulated during epididymal development

S-adenyl-L-methionine decarboxylase
Alcohol dehydrogenase C2
Alkaline phosphates
3α-Hydroxysteroid dehydrogenase
5α,5β-Reductase
α-Mannosidase
Angiotensin-converting enzyme
Angiotensin II receptors
Anionic sites in basement membrane
Androgen-binding protein
Androgen receptor
Apolipoprotein E
Aquaporin-1
Bcl-2
β-Hexosaminidase
17β-ol-dehydrogenase
Beta-trace
Bone morphogenetic protein 7
Brush-border membrane antigens
CFTR
Clusterin/SGP-2/TRPM-2
Cytokeratins and vimentin
Dehydrogenase and hydrolase activities
Δ4,5α-Reductase
Desmin
E-cadherin
4-ene steroid 5α-reductase
Estradiol-binding protein
Estrogen receptor
Estrogen receptor α
γ-Glutamyl transpeptidase
General protein secretion
Glutathione peroxides
Glutathioine S-transferase
Yo subunit
Glycoconjugates
Glycoproteins 83 and 49
Guanidinoacetate methyltransferase
H^+ ATPase
HE 1 and HE 4
Immobilin
Insulin-like growth factor-1
Keratins
Lactic dehydrogenase
Lectin binding
Low-density lipoprotein-2/megalin
Matrilysin
Metallothionein-3
MUC 6 mucin gene
Neutral β-glycosidase
Neural cell adhesion molecule
Neurotrophins and receptors
Occludin
Ornithine decarboxylase
Proopiomelanocortin

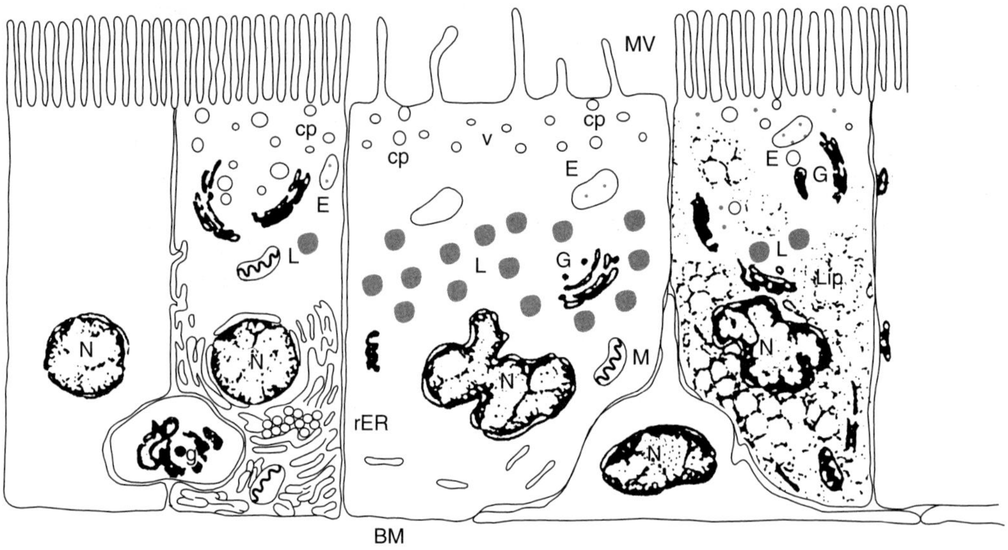

Figure 2.9 Principal cell of the caput epididymis on the left and of the corpus epididymis on the right, with a clear cell in between, as visualized by electron microscopy. A halo cell and a basal cell are also shown. Principal cells of both regions contain coated pits (cp), endosomes (E), lyosomes (L) and elaborate Golgi apparatus (G). Rough endoplasmic reticulum (rER) occupies the basal region of the principal cell of the caput, while numerous lipid droplets (Lip) occupy the cytoplasm of the principal cells of the corpus region. The clear cell shows few microvilli (MV), but numerous coated pits, small apical vesicles (v), endosomes and lysomes, all of which are involved in endocytosis. The halo cell is inserted between adjacent principal cells, located basally, and contains small dense core granules (g), while the basal cell stretches inself along the basement membrane (BM). M, mitochondria; N, nucleus. From Robaire (2002), with permission

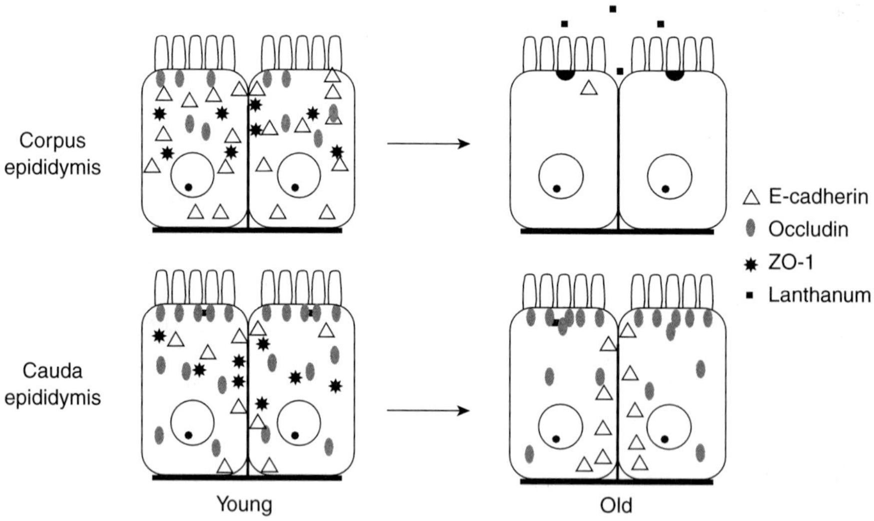

Figure 2.10 Age-related changes in the expression of E-cadherin, occludin and zonula occludens (ZO)-1, as well as in the permeability of lanthanum in the Brown Norway rat corpus and cauda epididymis. From Robaire (2002), with permission

are located over the entire sperm head. Other proteins are restricted to the acrosomal or postacrosomal region of the head (Table 2.4). These lipoproteins/polypeptides stabilize the plasma membrane and prevent premature acrosome reactions. Maturational interactions of epididymal sperm are not limited to those involving the sperm head; adsorption and/or integration of several specific glycoproteins and peptides occurs on or in the plasma membrane of the tail (Figures 2.9–2.11).

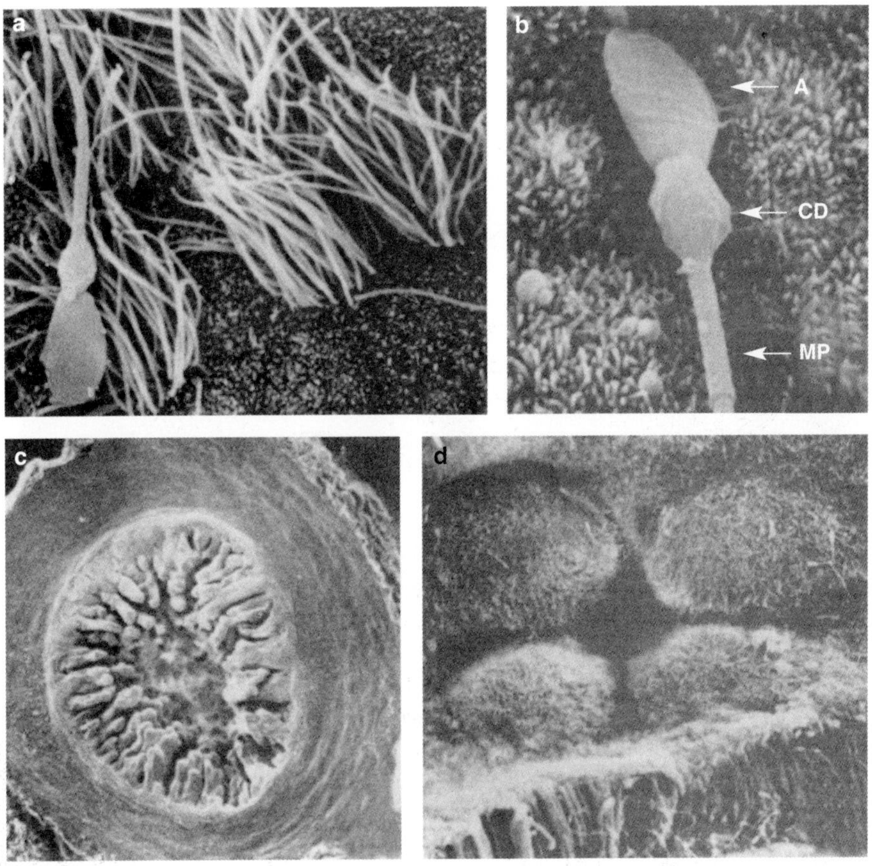

Figure 2.11 (**a**) Luminal surface of an efferent duct with ciliated and non-ciliated cells and a spermatozoon. (**b**) Short microvilli of the luminal surface of non-ciliated cells in the efferent ducts. The cytoplasm droplet (CD), acrosome (A) and middle piece (MP) of the spermatozoon are distinguishable by scanning electron microscopy (6500×). (**c**) Cross-section of the distal cauda epididymis. Thick layers of smooth muscle surround the highly infolded epithelium (25×). (**d**) Sagittal section of the corpus epididymis. Columnar cells covered with stereo cilia. Undulations are due to differences in cell height (276×). From Johnson (1991), with permission

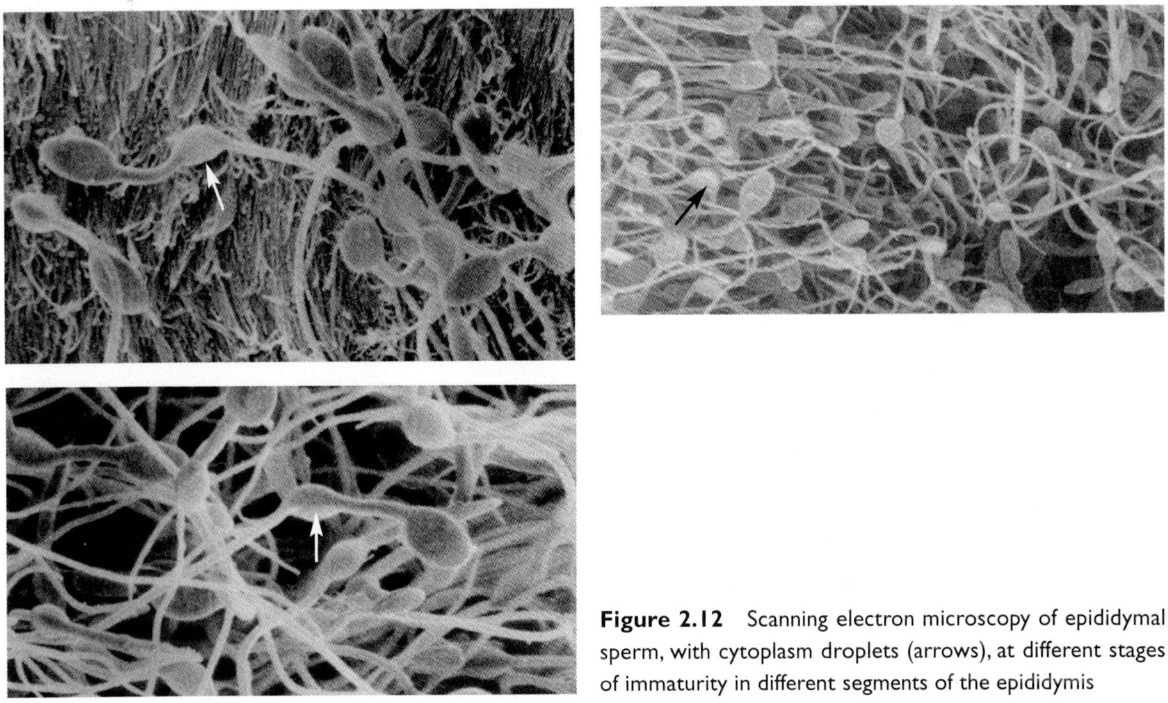

Figure 2.12 Scanning electron microscopy of epididymal sperm, with cytoplasm droplets (arrows), at different stages of immaturity in different segments of the epididymis

Sperm maturation in the epididymis is associated with complex biochemical, biophysical and ultrastructural molecular changes including loss of total protein, increase in cAMP, extensive modifications of energy metabolism, changes in lipoprotein content, changes in size, shape and internal structure of acrosome, variations in cohesiveness, migration of cytoplasm droplets from outer acrosomal membranes (Figures 2.11 and 2.12), increased disulfide bonds in the sperm tail with motility changes, alterations in antigenic properties of sperm surface and a net increase in negative surface charge, possibly due to addition of sialic acid groups.

3

Semen and the functional anatomy of sperm

ANATOMICAL PARAMETERS

Spermatozoa are elongated cells consisting of a flattened head containing the nucleus and a tail containing the apparatus necessary for cell motility. The entire spermatozoon is covered by the plasmalemma or plasma membrane. The acrosome or acrosomal cap is a double-walled structure situated between the plasma membrane and the anterior portion of the sperm head. A neck connects the sperm head with its tail (flagellum), which is subdivided into the middle, main and end pieces (Figures 3.1–3.3).

Sperm head

The sperm head contains an oval flattened nucleus containing highly compact chromatin. The condensed chromatin comprises deoxyribonucleic acid (DNA) complexed to a special class of basic proteins known as sperm protamines. The chromosome number and hence the DNA content of the sperm nucleus is haploid or half that of somatic cells of the same species. The haploid sperm cell results from the meiotic cell divisions that occur during formation of sperm with X or Y chromosomes. Several methods have been applied to separate X and Y chromosome-bearing sperm (Table 3.1).

The anterior end of the sperm nucleus is covered by the acrosome, a thin, double-layered membranous sac that is layered over the nucleus. This cap-like structure, which contains acrosin, hyaluronidase and other hydrolytic enzymes, is involved in the fertilization process. The equatorial segment of the acrosome is important because it is this part of the sperm, along with the anterior portion of the postacrosomal region, which initially fuses with the oocyte membrane during fertilization.

Sperm tail

The sperm tail is composed of the neck, middle, main and end pieces. The neck or connecting piece forms a basal plate that fits into a depression in the posterior aspect of the nucleus. The basal plate of the neck is continuous posteriorly, with nine outer coarse fibers that project throughout most of the tail. The region of the tail between the neck and the annulus is the middle piece. The central core of the middle piece together with the entire length of the tail constitutes the axoneme. The axoneme itself is composed of nine pairs of microtubules that are arranged radially around two central filaments. In the middle piece this 9+2 arrangement of microtubules is surrounded by the nine coarse or dense outer fibers that appear to be associated with the nine double fibers of the axoneme. The axoneme and associated dense fibers of the middle piece are covered peripherally by numerous mitochondria. The mitochondria are arranged in a helical pattern around the longitudinal fibers of the tail and supply the energy needed for sperm motility.

The main piece, which continues posteriorly from the annulus and extends to near to the end of the tail, is composed centrally of the axoneme and its associated coarse fibers. A fibrous sheath provides stability for the contractile elements of the tail.

The end piece, which is posterior to the termination of the fibrous sheath, contains only the central axoneme covered by the plasma membrane. The axoneme is responsible for sperm motility. The outer pairs of microtubules of the 9+2 pattern generate

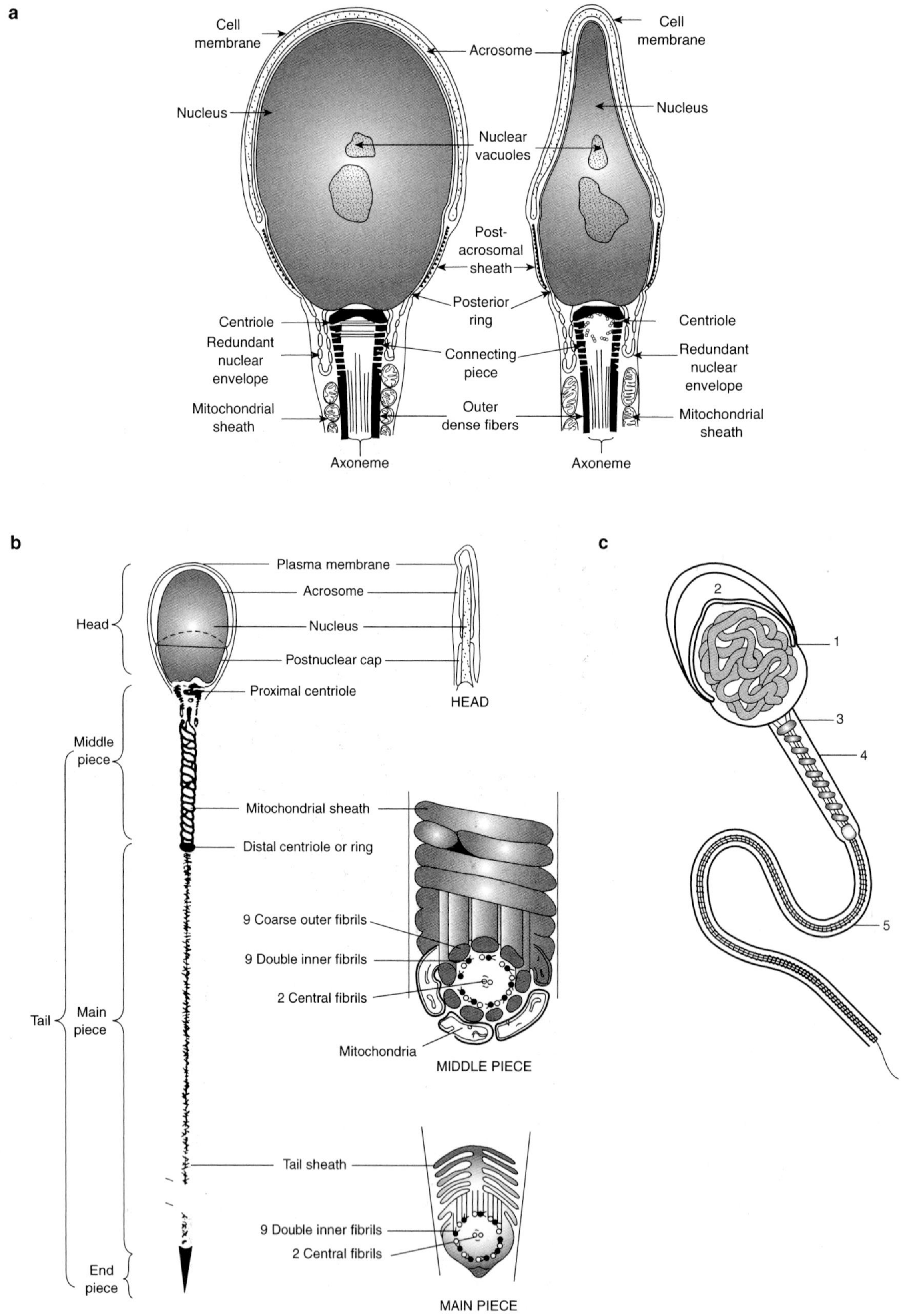

Figure 3.1 Human sperm functional anatomy. (**a**) Two cross-sections of sperm head and connecting piece (neck). (**b**) Cross-section of a spermatozoon showing the head, middle and main piece in detail. (**c**) The nucleus containing genetic material (1) fits inside the head cap (2) like an acorn in its cup. The neck (3) contains two thick bundles of fibers which continue through the body of the middle piece (4) and tail (5). Spiral structure like binding threads coils around middle piece and tail

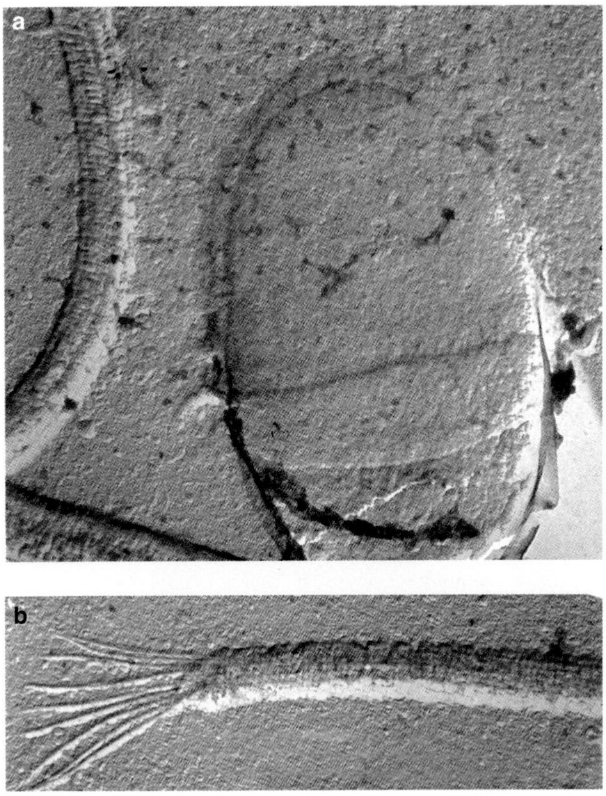

Figure 3.2 Functional ultrastructure of human sperm as shown by scanning electron microscopy after freeze drying. Note the characteristic pattern of the acrosome (**a**) and fibrils at the end of the tail (**b**). Courtesy of Zaneveld and Polakaski

the bending waves of the tail by a sliding movement between adjacent pairs. The protoplasmic or cytoplasmic droplet, which is usually detached from ejaculated sperm, is composed of residual cytoplasm. The principal chemical components of spermatozoa are nucleic acids, proteins and lipids.

Sperm morphology is examined by using eosin–nigrosin stain, and Wright's and Williams' stains. Stained slides are examined using a high microscopic magnification (400×). At least 150 spermatozoa are examined, with abnormal sperm being classified into five categories: tailless, abnormal heads, abnormal tail formations, abnormal tail formations with a proximal cytoplasm droplet, and abnormal tail formations with a distal droplet.

Globozoospermia

Globozoospermia is a unique condition in which sperm are abnormally shaped, have round-shaped nuclei, absence of an acrosome and aberrant structure of the middle piece. Intracytoplasmic sperm injection (ICSI) has been performed for individuals with this type of teratozoospermia. However, the egg activation rate after ICSI is very low and artificial activation is needed for successful fertilization. This fact suggests that lack of the acrosome or nuclear material might be the cause of low fertility in this type of infertility, as the sperm lacks the ability to initiate appropriate oocyte activation.

Sperm transport in female reproductive tract

Several endogenous and exogenous factors influence the pattern of sperm transport in the female reproductive tract from the site of ejaculation in the vagina to the site of fertilization in the oviduct (Figures 3.4–3.6). Sperm transport is under endocrine control, particularly during the early follicular, ovulatory and luteal phases (Figure 3.7).

Sperm–zona pellucida interaction

Capacitated sperm initially bind in a species-specific manner with the zona pellucida (ZP), an extracellular coat surrounding the egg. The sperm then undergo an exocytotic process, the acrosome reaction, because the sulfhydryl (SH) bonds are not oxidized until transit through the epididymis, testicular sperm DNA packaging is not complete, and their DNA may be more susceptible to assault. DNA integrity is determined by the modified alkaline single-cell gel electrophoresis (Comet) assay under yellow light to prevent further induced DNA damage. Fully frosted microscope slides are heated and covered with 100 µl of 1.0% normal melting point agarose in Ca^{2+}- and Mg^{2+}-free phosphate-buffered saline covered with a large coverslip. The slides are placed on a chilled metal tray and left at 4°C for ≥30 min to allow the agarose to solidify. The coverslips are removed and the slides immersed in a Coplin jar containing freshly prepared cold lysing solution. Testicular sperm from infertile men have more DNA fragmentation when incubated overnight after thawing than those assessed immediately after thawing. In contrast, DNA fragmentation in testicular sperm from fertile men is unaffected by the postcryopreservation incubation. The practice of incubating testicular sperm after cryopreservation damages their nuclear DNA, thus increasing the risk of selecting poor-quality sperm for ICSI (Dalzell *et al.*, 2003).

a

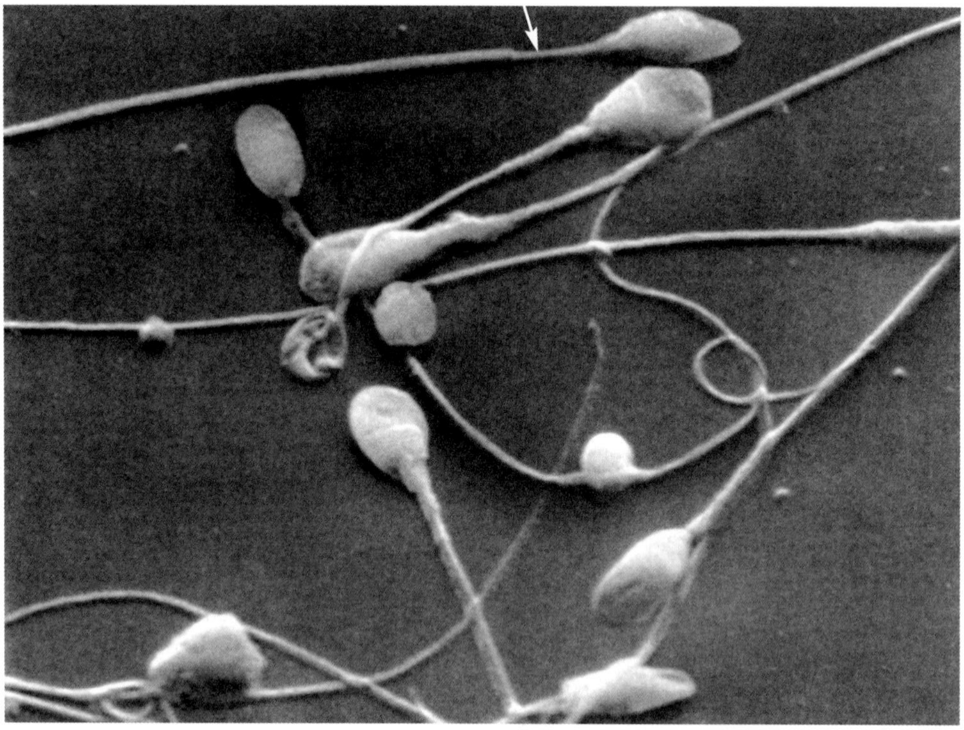

b

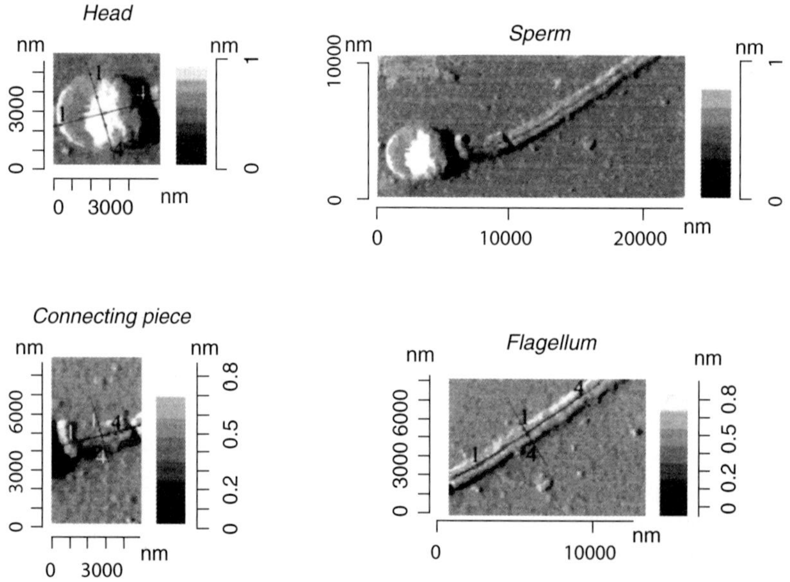

Figure 3.3 (**a**) Sperm from the ejaculate of a normal man showing the characteristic racket shape of the head and long tail reaching 60 µm. Five cytoplasmic beads are seen in top and side views. The anterior portion of the head has a thick hood called the acrosome, while the posterior tapering portion has a thinner sheath called postnuclear cap. A transverse furrow marks the space between them. The middle piece of the tail just behind the head shows an undulating relief. This corresponds to the mitochondria that spiral around this portion of the tail. (**b**) Dimensions of human sperm, head, connecting piece and flagellum as seen by atomic force microscopy. From Barboza *et al.*, 2004, with permission

BIOCHEMICAL PARAMETERS

Biochemical markers of sperm quality

Several biochemical markers have been used to evaluate human sperm maturity and function including sperm creatine-*N*-phosphotransferase or creatine kinase (CK), CK enzymatic active-site labeling and CK immunocytochemistry of individual sperm. Men with low sperm concentrations who have an increased incidence of infertility also show increased levels of sperm CK activity. This may be related to a

Table 3.1 Techniques employed to separate X and Y chromosome-bearing sperm

Technique	*Results*
Sedimentation of immobilized sperm on media	Insemination with sperm that had sedimented the greatest distance produced 70% females
Skimmed milk powder, glycine, sodium citrate, glycerol	Increase in number of male offspring when sperm from the top layers were used
Albumin column	Successful results with frozen bull sperm preselected on albumin column before cryopreservation
Velocity sedimentation	Sedimentation rates depend on size, density and shape of sperm. Cell size difference is predominant factor in separation of types; shape is usually the least important factor. Sperm heads have extremely aspherical shapes
Centrifugation through density gradients	Sperm separate according to their sedimentation rates by centrifugation through density gradients, provided the density of the gradient material is less than that of the sperm. The advantage is that the time required for separation is much shorter. Shorter time does not improve theoretical resolution of separation, because diffusion is insignificant
Motility and electrophoretic separation	Immotile sperm are electrophoretically attracted to the anode at neutral pH. When electrophoretic separation is under conditions consistent with sperm motility, sperm migrate to the cathode. Sperm are oriented by electric field and swim in the direction the head is facing. If negatively charged, sperm can be oriented so that the tail is facing the anode by virtue of its greater negative charge density, and their intrinsic motility is greater than the electrophoretic mobility
Isoelectric focusing	Separation performed in columns with the fluid stabilized using density gradients. Sperm layered on, or suspended in, this solution migrate electrophoretically until reaching an isoelectric point
H-Y antigens	Sperm treated with H-Y antisera. Insemination with mouse sperm treated with antisera to a Y-linked histocompatibility antigen produced 45% males compared with 53% for controls
Flow sorting by DNA content	Y chromosome-bearing sperm sorting is 72–80% successful. Disadvantages: low sorting rate and lack of sperm viability after sorting
Sephadex column	Approximately 70% (65–85%) of X chromosome-bearing sperm can be found in certain fractions of the filtrate when sperm are placed on top of a column of Sephadex

defect of sperm development in the last phase of spermatogenesis, when excess cytoplasm is normally extruded and left in the adluminal area as residual bodies. Thus, sperm with a high CK content, an indication of surplus cytoplasm, have not completed cellular maturation (Huszar *et al.*, 2003). There is also a second sperm maturation marker, which was initially thought to be a sperm-specific creatine kinase M-isoform and identified as the testis-expressed chaperone protein HspA2 (a member of the HSP70-2 family) that, along with the homologous hsc70, is synthesized in two waves of expression. The first wave occurs during meiosis, as HspA2 is part of the synaptonemal complex. The second wave of major expression occurs simultaneously with cytoplasm extrusion, in terminal spermatogenesis.

Seiwa (1993a, b, 1994, 1995a, b, 2000) conducted intensive investigations of *in vitro* sperm migration using various chemoattractants such as heparin, beta endorphin and sex steroids.

Sperm apoptosis

Degeneration of germ cells occurs via apoptosis. During apoptosis, an endogenous endonuclease is activated; this endoendonuclease cleaves DNA between nucleosides, fragmenting DNA into multiple 180–200 base-pair fragments that appear as a characteristic DNA ladder on agarose gel electorphoresis. Germ cell apoptosis occurs spontaneously and is induced by exposure to hypothermia (rats) and to chemotherapeutic agents and by reactive oxygen species (ROS). There is a significant difference between apoptotic cells after swim-up and Percoll™ gradient, with PureSperm at 24 hours of incubation.

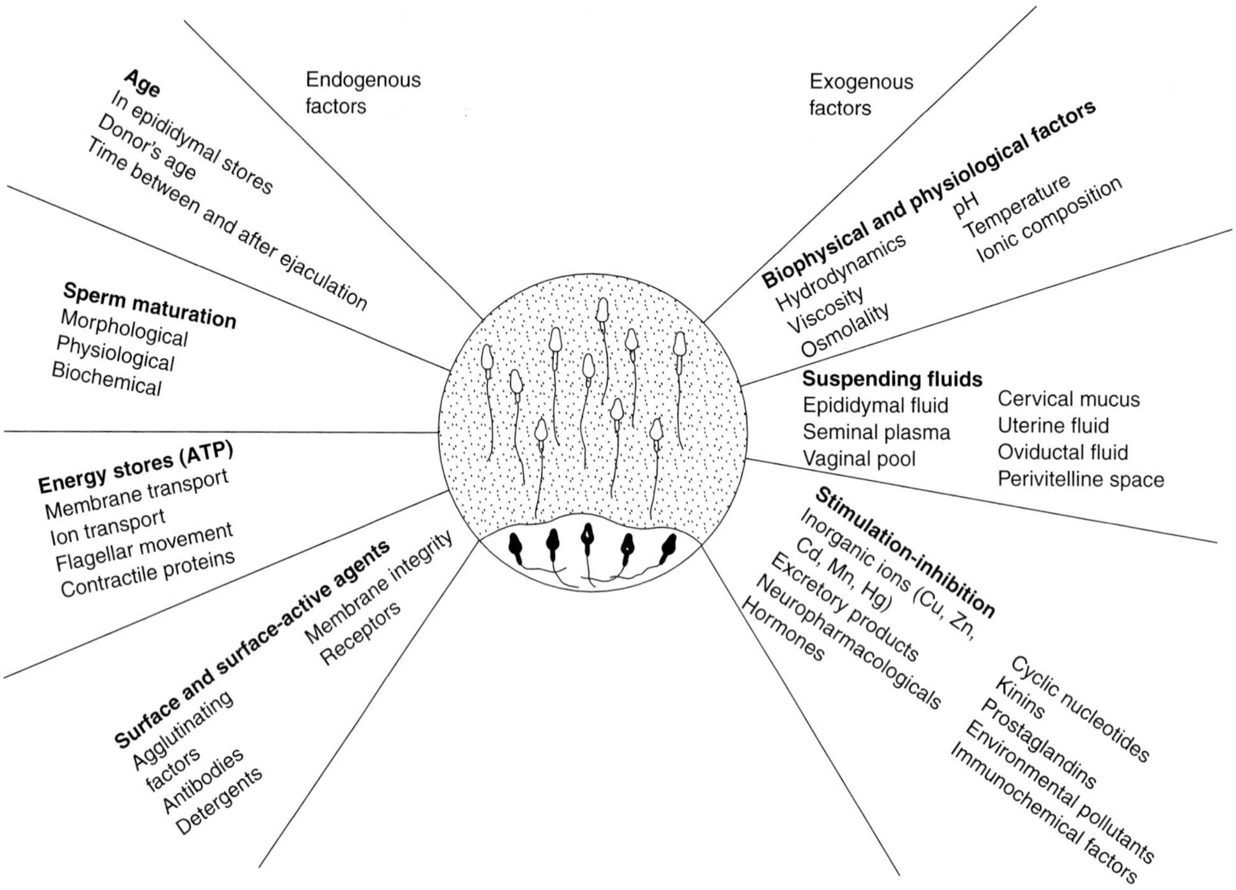

Figure 3.4 Endogenous and exogenous factors affecting sperm transport in female reproductive tract

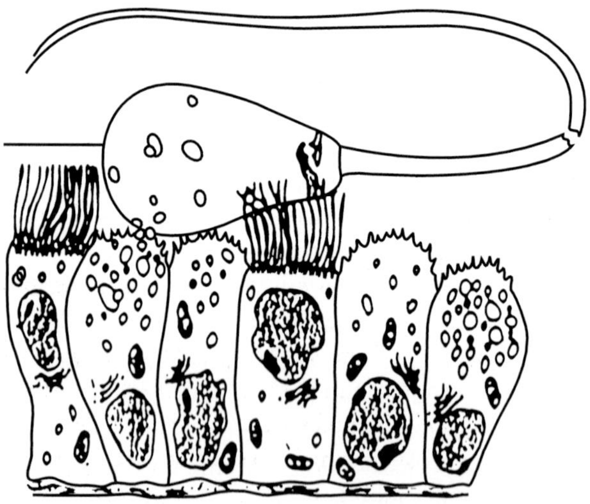

Figure 3.5 Secretory cells of the oviduct provide a physiological milieu for sperm capacitation and fertilization

Apoptosis is present in seminal samples. The percentage of apoptotic cells differs significantly between methods of purification, swim-up and Percoll gradient, with PureSperm. PureSperm has a significantly lower percentage of apoptotic cells. Further studies are necessary to determine the role of apoptotic cells and the mechanism by which different culture media affect sperm DNA integrity (Benitz *et al.*, 2002).

Sperm function test (Table 3.2)

Sperm penetration

Sperm films on microscopic slides are examined by phase-contrast microscopy at 400× magnification. The sperm penetration index is evaluated by counting the number of decondensed (swollen) sperm heads with an adjacent or closely associated sperm tail within the cytoplasm, as follows:

$$\text{Penetration percentage} = \frac{\text{number of oocytes penetrated by sperm}}{\text{total number of oocytes inseminated}} \times 100$$

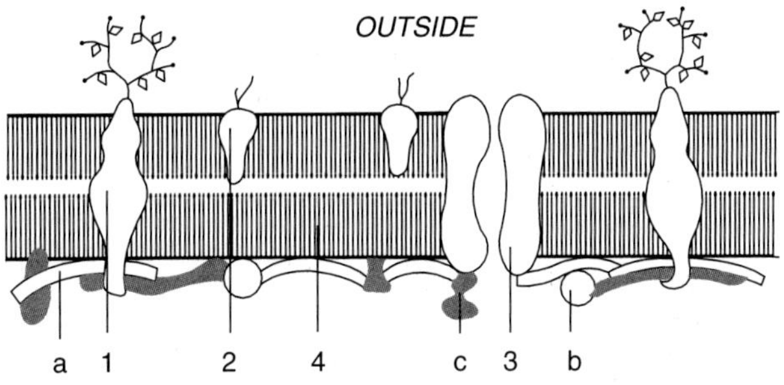

Figure 3.6 Sperm plasma membrane: (1) non-motile lipoproteins with oligosaccharide chains; (2) motile lipoproteins; (3) transmembrane proteins; (4) lipid bilayer; (a) spectrin; (b) actin; (c) binding protein. From Calamera (1998), with permission

$$\text{Penetration index} = \frac{\text{total number of sperm penetrated into oocytes}}{\text{total number of oocytes inseminated}}$$

Hemizona binding assay

Sperm are incubated with oviductal cells and conditioned at 37°C under 5% CO_2 in air for 24 h. The effect of the conditioned media on zona pellucida-binding capacity is evaluated as follows:

$$\text{Hemizona binding} = \frac{\text{number of sperm bound in test droplet}}{\text{number of sperm bound in a control droplet}} \times 100$$

MOLECULAR PARAMETERS

Sperm immobilizing proteins

Extensive investigations have been conducted to develop an effective non-invasive contraceptive agent that can block or retard sperm motility. Lysenin, a protein purified from the coelomic fluid (CF) of an earthworm, *Eisenia foetida*, immobilizes and kills the sperm of mammals including man. However, lysenin is not suitable because its addition to *ex vivo* blood destroys mammalian erythrocytes and its intravenous injection instantaneously kills rats/mice. Mukherjee *et al.* (2003) isolated a novel protein, immotilin, from CF of an earthworm, *Metaphire peguana*, that instantly immobilizes and kills human and other mammalian sperm without affecting other cells. Immotilin, a 47-KS protein, therefore, shows great promise as a non-invasive antifertilizing agent. Heat treatment of the CF destroys its sperm immobilizing activity, indicating that the active component may be a protein.

Based on its immobilizing activity, the bioactive molecule from the CF was purified to homogeneity by using gel-permeation chromatography and ion exchange chromatography on a high-pressure liquid chromatography (HPLC) Spherogel™ TSK DEAE column (Merck). Considering the remarkable sperm immobilizing activity of the purified protein, this protein has been called immotilin. Taking the crude extract as the initial step of purification, the purification was 106-fold.

A relationship between low acrosin activity and reduced fertilization rate has been demonstrated; the incidence of abnormal acrosin activity in male patients with unexplained infertility was 19%. The diminished activity apparently was not the result of a decrease in proacrosin/acrosin acrosomal levels, but rather of alterations in the proenzyme activation. By using polymerase chain reaction (PCR)-single-strand conformation polymorphism (SSCP) analysis, no changes were detected in the nucleotide sequence around the active site of the sample (Mukherjee *et al.*, 2003). Nucleotide sequence analysis on the sequence encoding human proacrosin and the 5'UTR region in genomic DNA from these patients may reveal alterations that could explain abnormal protein function.

$\alpha_6\beta_1$ Integrin as sperm quality marker

The sperm penetration assay with zona-free hamster eggs is often used as an *in vitro* prognostic test of male infertility. However, it is not known whether a low rate of binding and/or penetration is the result of poorly induced acrosomal reaction or impaired binding. Evaluation of the acrosomal status of sperm is an important task within the diagnostic work-up of male fertility to predict fertilizing potential. Expression of $\alpha_6\beta_1$ integrin was significantly reduced in sperm obtained from subfertile men. Only 35–40% of sperm from fertile men showed a positive reaction to $\alpha_6\beta_1$ antibody. Samples with a high rate of acrosomal reaction showed a high level of expression of $\alpha_6\beta_1$ and maximum binding to oocyte in an *in vitro* binding assay. $\alpha_6\beta_1$ Integrin may be used as a clinical marker to evaluate sperm quality.

Biochemistry of sperm flagellum

Several biochemical components have been identified in the flagellum of spermatids and spermatozoa

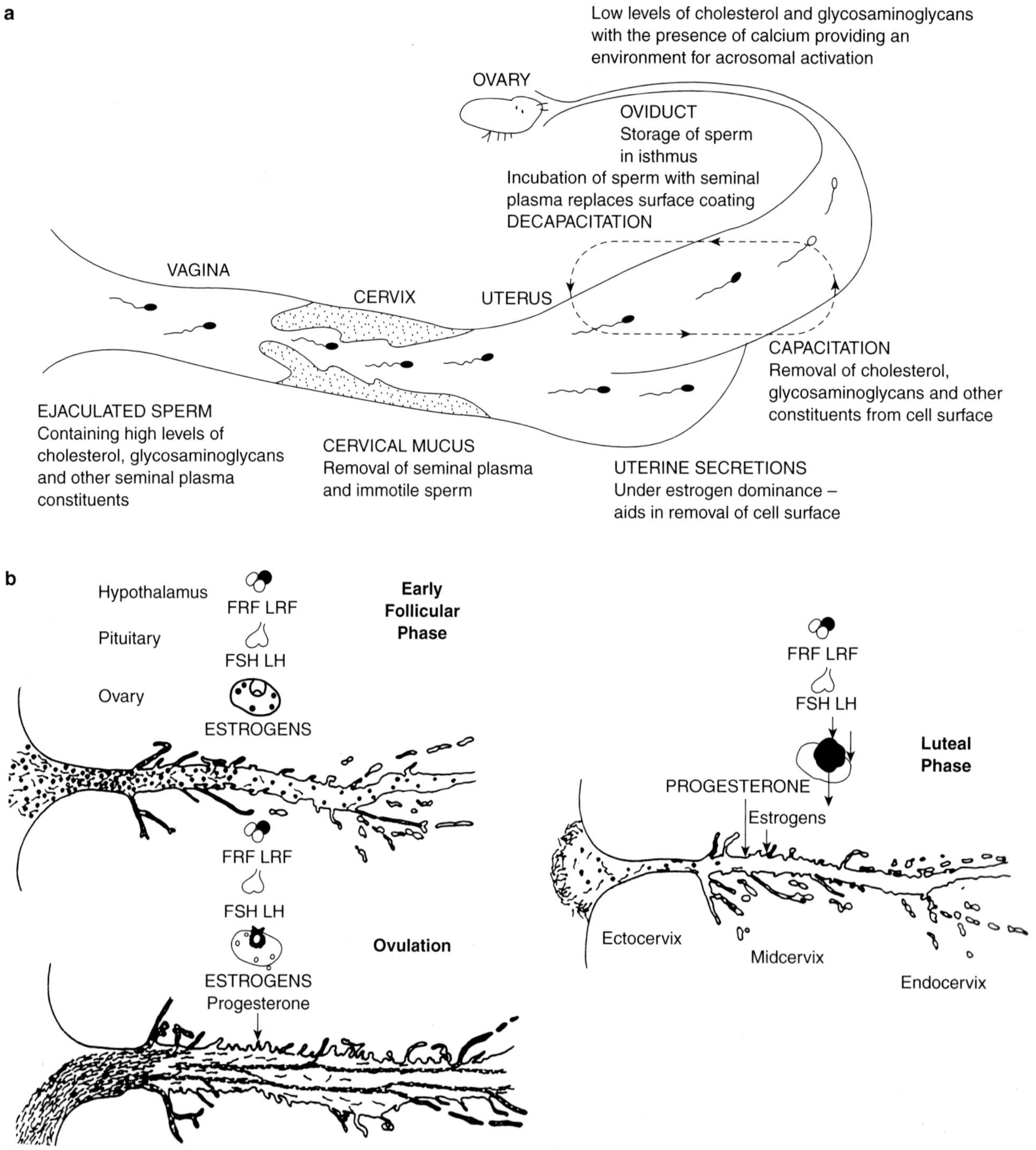

Figure 3.7 (**a**) Endocrine control of sperm transport in various segments of female reproductive tract. (**b**) Pattern of sperm transport during early follicular, ovulatory and luteal phases of the menstrual cycle. FSH, follicle stimulating hormone; FRF, FSH-releasing factor; LH, luteinizing hormone; LRF, LH-releasing factor

in mammals. They increase the future probability of determining the genetic pathways controlling flagellar morphogenesis (Figures 3.8 and 3.9). The recent findings of flagellar anomalies in Ube2b-deficient mice, associated with a better understanding of flagellar elements, could help to identify candidate flagellar proteins as targets of UBE2B. Additionally, Ube2b-null mice are an unexpected and precious murine model for a similar human sperm pathology.

Reactive oxygen species

Sperm generate reactive oxygen species (ROS), which play a physiological role in signaling the events

Table 3.2 Assays and markers of sperm function, acrosome reaction and secretory products of accessory sex glands

Sperm function
Acrosin content
Adenosine triphosphate (ATP)
Reactive oxygen species (ROS)
Cervical mucus penetration
Evaluation of acrosome status
Triple staining
Ligands
Immunological
Hypo-osmotic swelling test
Hamster zona-free oocyte
Hemizona assay
Acrosome reaction
Triple staining (trypan blue rose Bengal–Bismarck brown)
Fluorescein isocyanate (FITC) conjugated lectins
Soybean agglutinin
Concanavalin A
Pisum sativum agglutinin (PSA)
Ricinus communis agglutinin (RCA)
Hoechst 33258 (supravital stain)
Wheat sperm agglutinin
Electron microscopy
Indirect immunofluorescence assay
Monoclonal antibodies
TG (keratin-like protein)
Chlortetracycline fluorescence assay
Accessory sex gland secretions
Epididymis
neutral α-glucosidase
free L-carnitine
Seminal vesicles
glycerylphosphorylcholine
fructose
fluid volume
Prostate
prostaglandins
citric acid; acid phosphatase
γ-glutamyl transpeptidase
zinc, calcium
semen liquefaction

controlling sperm capacitation, sperm hyperactivation, acrosome reaction and sperm–egg fusion. However, excessive generation of ROS by defective sperm or contaminating leukocytes exerts a detrimental effect on sperm function. Hydrogen peroxide is the primary ROS responsible for such molecular changes and membrane lipid peroxidation is an important mechanism of action. Semen contains antioxidants, including ascorbic acid, tocopherol, β-carotene, catalase, glutathione peroxides and superoxide dismutase, that balance lipid peroxidation and prevent excessive peroxide formation (Aitken *et al.*, 1998a; Aurech *et al.*, 1997). Glutathione peroxide functions in the aqueous phase of cells and vitamin E is stored and functions in the lipid portions of cell membrane parts. A possible relationship exists between the intoxicative function of selenium and cytochromes and oxygen metabolism. Selenium also has a role in electron transfer in the cytochrome system.

DYNAMICS OF SPERM MOTILITY

Initiation of sperm motility has been associated with protein phosphorylation as well as with changes in intracellular calcium and pH. Several proteins become phosphorylated at the time when sperm start moving actively. The majority of these proteins are phosphorylated on serine or threonine residues and their phosphorylation is cAMP dependent. Most studies have focused on the initiation and activation of sperm motility. Motility assessment involves subjective estimation of the viability of sperm and the quality of the motility. Light microscopic analysis of sperm is most commonly used. Evaluation of sperm motility is conducted with raw and diluted semen. Evaluation of raw semen is an indicator of sperm performance in their own accessory gland fluid. Measuring motility in the raw form can be hampered by higher sperm concentrations, making it difficult to discern individual motility patterns. To overcome this limitation, an aliquot of semen should be diluted to a concentration of 25×10^6 sperm/ml) in a good-quality diluent.

Sperm motility is extremely susceptible to environmental conditions (such as excessive heat or cold), so it is necessary to protect the semen from injurious agents or conditions prior to analysis. To further enhance the reliability of motility estimation, experienced personnel and a properly equipped microscope are required. A drop of diluted semen is placed on a glass slide and covered with another slide; it is then observed using a microscope with a built-in stage warmer and phase-contrast optics. Magnification of 200–400× is generally used to estimate sperm motility.

Various patterns of sperm motility have been established by the World Health Organization (WHO) and different governmental agencies (Tables 3.3 and 3.4).

Sperm hyperactivated motility

Hyperactivated motility is characterized by vigorous, large-amplitude, whiplash-like flagellar beats with the

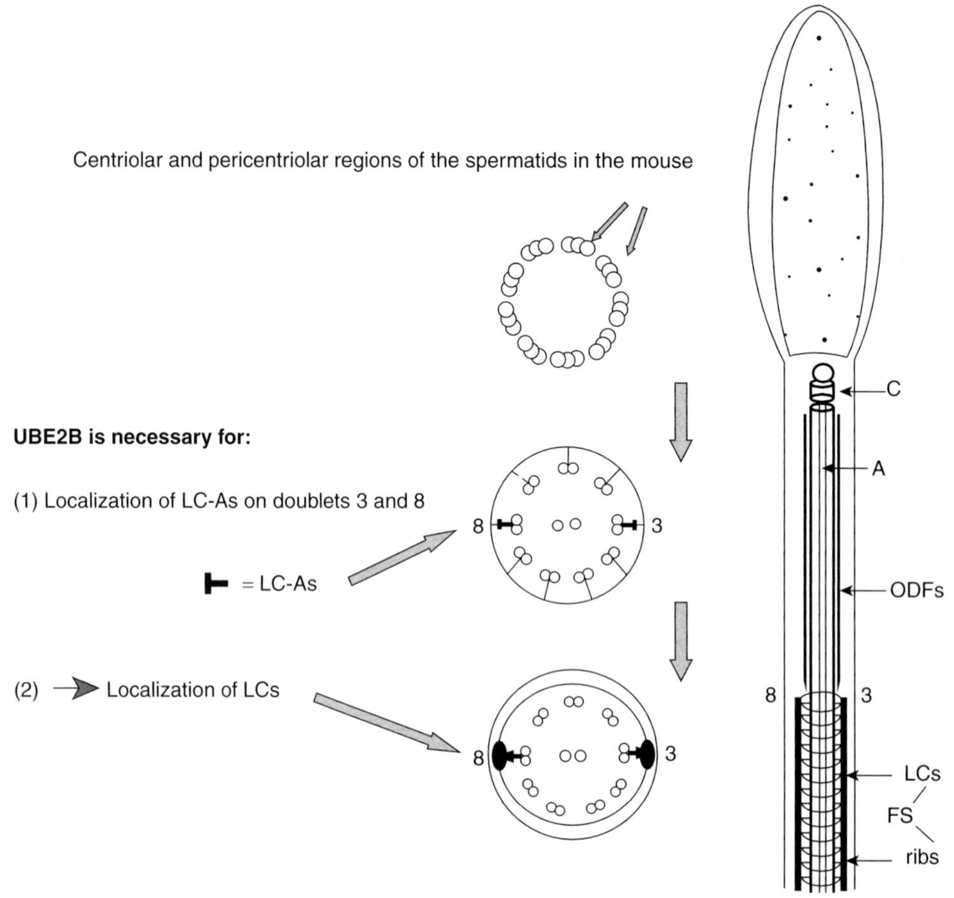

Figure 3.8 UBE2B and mammalian flagellum morphogenesis. Possible involvement of UBE2B in the assembly of flagellar cytoskeletal structures, as suggested by the murine Ube2b phenotype, is shown. The gray arrows represent the stages of assembly of flagellar structures. First, the distal centriole gives rise to the axoneme (black), and then the structure of the longitudinal column (LC) appears on double fibers 3 and 8 (white circles), where the LCs of the fibrous sheath (FS) are finally assembled. A, axoneme; C, centrosome; As, anchorage structures; ODFs, outer dense fibers. From Escalier, 2003, with permission

sperm heads tracing erratic trajectories (Figure 3.10). Sperm hyperactivity is critical for binding with the oocyte and subsequent fertilization. Hyperactivity can be assessed in a computer-assisted motion analyzer (Hamilton–Thorn v. 10.8, Beverly, MA) using a 20-µm chamber at 37°C. The required settings are frames, 30; frame rate, 60 Hz; minimum contrast, 85; minimum cell size, 2 pixels; and minimum static contrast, 30. The following parameters are used to define hyperactivation: curvilinear velocity (VCL) >100 µm/s, linearity of forward progression (LIN) <65% and amplitude of lateral head displacement (ALH) >7.5 µm.

VCL is the rate of travel of the centroid of the sperm head over a given period of time. Straight-line velocity (VSL) is the straight-line distance between the first and the last centroid positions for a given period of time. Average path velocity (VAP) is the spatial average path that eliminates the wobble of the sperm head. LIN is the ratio of VSL to VCL.

Inhibitors of sperm motility

Inhibitors of sperm motility are of great clinical significance in the development of male contraceptives. Among the selective protein tyrosine kinase inhibitors, genistein is the most active and consistent, inhibiting sperm tyrosine kinase activity. This involves inhibition of sperm mobility/motility patterns such as VCL, ALH and hyperactivation motility patterns. Other kinase inhibitors decrease motility characteristics to a variable extent and have different effects on phosphorylation parameters (Figure 3.11). In general, they decreased phosphorylation of two proteins (83 and 54 kDa) present in whole sperm extracts, and two sets of proteins of low (39–49 kDa) and medium (55–87 kDa) molecular weight present in the Triton X-100-solubilized sperm protein fraction (Bajpai *et al.*, 2003).

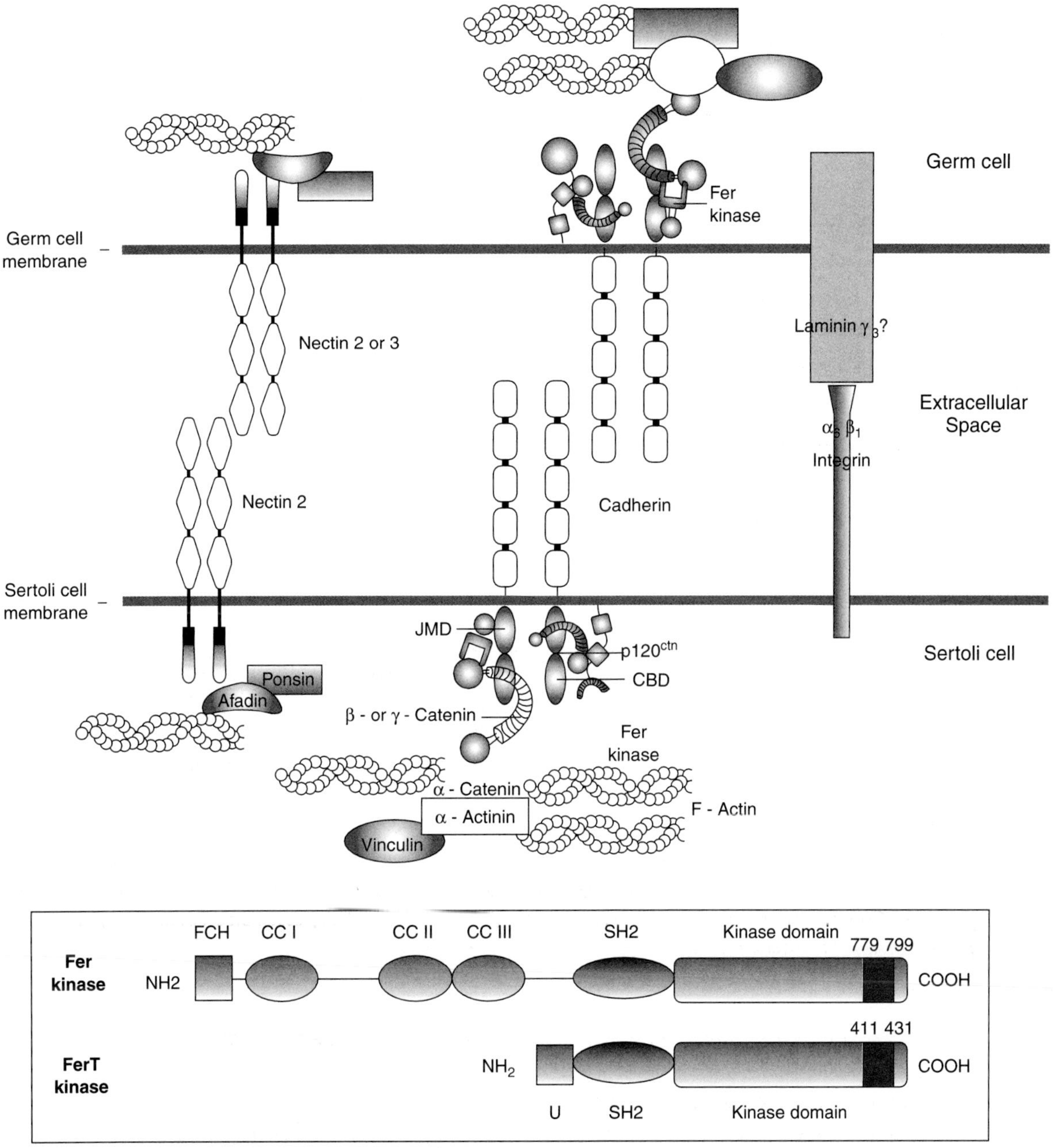

Figure 3.9 A molecular model illustrating the structural association of Fer kinase with the known adherens junction (AJ) structures at the site of ectoplasmic specialization. The three known AJ structural protein complexes at the site of ectoplasmic specialization in the testis are the cadherin–catenin complex, nectin–afadin–ponsin complex and $\alpha_6\beta_1$ integrin–laminin complex. The functional laminin, the receptor for $\alpha_6\beta_1$ integrin, consists of three chains, yet laminin γ_3 is the only known non-basement-membrane laminin in the testis; the other two chains remain to be identified. Based on the results presented by Chen *et al.* (2003), it is apparent that Fer kinase is associated with the *N*-cadherin-based cadherin–catenin complex and interacts with other AJ-associated signaling molecules. Also shown (lower panel) are the structural similarities between Fer kinase and Fer T kinase. CBD, catenin-binding domain; CC, coiled-coil domain; FCH, Fps/Fes/Fer/CIP4 homology; JMD, juxta membrane domain; SH2, Src homology 2 domain; U, unique Fer T sequence, 44 amino acids. From Chen *et al.*, 2003, with permission

Sperm motility and metal chelators

The kinetic energy required for sperm motility is generated in the axoneme. The outer dense fibers extend along 60% of the length of the main piece of the sperm tail, consist of a few structural proteins and comprise medulla and cortex. Immunoelectron microscopic studies in the bull have shown an 84-kDa protein to be localized over the whole structure. This protein is apparently a basic structural

Table 3.3 Parameters of sperm motility patterns (World Health Organization)

Grades of sperm motility (100 sperm are evaluated twice in 2 drops)

Grade a: rapid progressive motility
Grade b: slow or sluggish progressive motility
Grade c: non-progressive motility
Grade d: immotile

Duration of motility

Artifacts
- caused by incorrect method of collection (e.g. use of a condom, which may be sperm toxic)
- sample contaminated by vaginal secretions
- use of lubricants, an incomplete sample
- long delay in transferring the sample to laboratory or exposure to extreme temperatures
- technical factors
  - cold shock as a result of use of cold containers in laboratory
  - use of unsuitable, contaminated or wet slides, pipettes, containers, etc.
  - storage of sample at adverse temperature
  - incorrect temperature, thickness of wet preparations

Morpohological
- structural abnormalities of the middle piece
- immotile cilia or Kartagener syndromes
- inherent factors
  - fault during formation/maturation of sperm before released from Sertoli cells
  - fault during transport through epididymis and ductal system
  - abnormal functions of prostate or seminal vesicle
- other factors
  - hematospermia, a varicocele, chromosomal aberrations
  - bacterial infection
  - presence of certain metals or metal ions

Motility forward progression

Type/aggressiveness of movement or qualitative motility (speed of forward progression)
Quantitative motility expressing percentage of (un)active sperm (% motile)
Duration of motility (*in vitro*)

Forward progression

0	no movement
1	movement – none forward
1+	movement – a few now and then
2	movement – undirected, slow
2+	movement – slowly but directly forward
3–	movement – fast but undirected
3	movement – fast and directly forward
3+	movement – very fast and directly forward
4	movement – extremely fast and directly forward (wave-like)

element of the outer dense fibers. The results imply that chelators can eliminate at least some part of the zinc from the flagellum. This zinc elimination appears to lead to comparable changes of the outer dense fibers as seen *in vivo* during epididymal maturation, finally resulting in improved motility (Wroblewski *et al.*, 2003).

SEMEN TECHNOLOGY

Semen analysis

Assisted reproductive technology (ART) requires semen to be processed to obtain a sample with progressively motile (types A and B) and morphologically

Table 3.4 Functional patterns of sperm motility

Wobble (WOB) (curvilinear progressiveness ratio)	Ratio of VAP to VCL. This measures the wobble of sperm head about average path
Straightness (STR) linear index	Ratio of VAP to VSL. This measures the straightness of the average path
Maximum amplitude lateral head displacement (max ALH)	Centroid positions are recorded and a mean trajectory, based on each of these positions, is generated. For each point, the two adjacent points on either side (total of five points) are averaged and a least-square curve fit is applied. Values for max ALH, calculated from the computer-generated mean trajectory, are multiplied by 2 and expressed in µm
Beat cross frequency (BCF)	Number of times the centroid of sperm head crosses the computer-generated mean trajectory for that frequency (beats/s). This parameter provides an estimate of flagellar beat frequency based on movement of sperm head
Dance	Product of VCL and mean ALH expressed in $\mu m^2/s$
Dance mean	Product of mean ALH and the ratio of VCL and VSL expressed in µm
Mean angle of deviation (MAD)	Time average of absolute values of instantaneous turning angle of sperm head along its curvilinear trajectory. MAD is a measure of curvature of sperm track
Curvature (CURV) riser displacement (RIS)	Curvature of sperm path based on a scale of 0–1. Point-to-point distance of actual sperm-head trajectory to its average path
Frequency of fundamental harmonic (HAR)	Fundamental frequency of oscillation of curvilinear trajectory around its average path
Magnitude of fundamental harmonic (MAG)	Measurement of peak-to-peak dispersion of curvilinear trajectory about its average path at fundamental frequency (amplitude squared height of HAR)
Area of fundamental harmonic (PBW)	Area under fundamental harmonic peak in magnitude spectrum. This parameter is a measurement of power bandwidth of the signal
Circular high curvature	Wide amplitude, relative planar beating of high flagellum. Marked side-to-side head movements, beat envelope of $>19\mu m^2$
Thrashing	Extremely erratic trajectory, at least three rapid U-shaped flexions, change in the plane of flagellar beat with each flexion
Star-spin	Rapidly spinning in one place, with no forward progression
Helical	Highly three-dimensional trajectory with regular repeats
Non-hyperactivated	Fairly straight trajectory, an even roll of the head about central axis, minimal curvature of the flagellum

VAP, average path velocity; VCL, curvilinear velocity

normal sperm (strict morphology), after the elimination of undesired elements (i.e. round cells, morphologically abnormal sperm and sperm with abnormal or no motility (types C and D)) and prostaglandin. Three main techniques are used to process semen samples in the laboratory: gradients, migration and filtration. These procedures are applied to generate post-processing samples containing a high

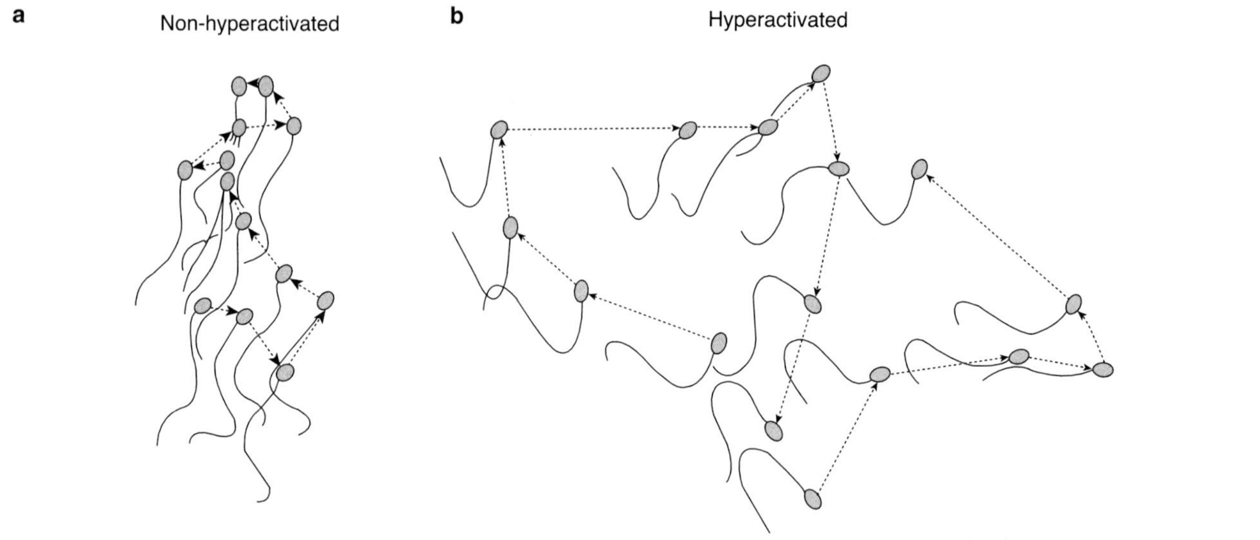

Figure 3.10 Different patterns of sperm motility, sperm tail beating and head-centroid trajectories: (**a**) non-hyperactivated; (**b**) hyperactivated. This is a method of discriminating between non-hyperactivated and classical hyperactivated motility patterns in sperm using computerized analysis of sperm motility and kinematics

concentration of morphologically normal sperm with good progressive motility. There is positive correlation between these parameters and the rate of clinical pregnancy obtained by intrauterine insemination (IUI) and *in vitro* fertilization (IVF).

The sperm recovering efficiency (SRE) model is an equation that can be used to quantify objectively the technical skill of individual operators processing semen specimens in an andrology laboratory. Additionally, this equation can be used to compare different semen processing methods and protocols. The model integrates the semen parameters of initial sperm concentration, motility and morphology, with final sperm recovery to produce a unique number that can be used to compare results.

Semen analysis technology

The value of sperm morphology as a predictor of a man's fertilizing potential is challenged because of the use of different classification systems and numerous technical variations, including differences in the methods used to prepare and stain specimens, differences in proficiency among technicians and inherent differences in classification criteria and methods. Careful determination of sperm concentration, movement and morphology requires a great deal of technical expertise and procedural care in semen handling and evaluation, e.g. the installation of meticulous quality control (QC) programs and technician proficiency testing (PT) systems. A continuous QC program can be initiated only after intensive training, because baseline values at the onset of the QC program serve as an internal reference value (Franken *et al.*, 2003).

Leukospermia

Routine application of antibiotics for leukospermia may have a negative impact on semen parameters as well as increasing the possibility of inoculating the reproductive tract of the female partner with antibiotic-resistant bacteria. The presence or absence of bacteriospermia or leukospermia do not correlate with each other. Leukospermia has been shown not to correlate with semen parameters. Staphylococcus species were the most common isolates and did not correlate with semen parameters or leukospermia. *Streptococcus viridians* and *Enterococcus faecalis* were the next most common isolates and were associated with statistically significantly poorer semen quality (Rodin *et al.*, 2003). Leukospermia is a poor marker for either bacteriospermia or impaired semen quality. Staphylococcus species are commonly isolated but appear to be innocuous. *Streptococcus viridians* and *Enterococcus faecalis* are associated with poorer semen quality and may warrant treatment.

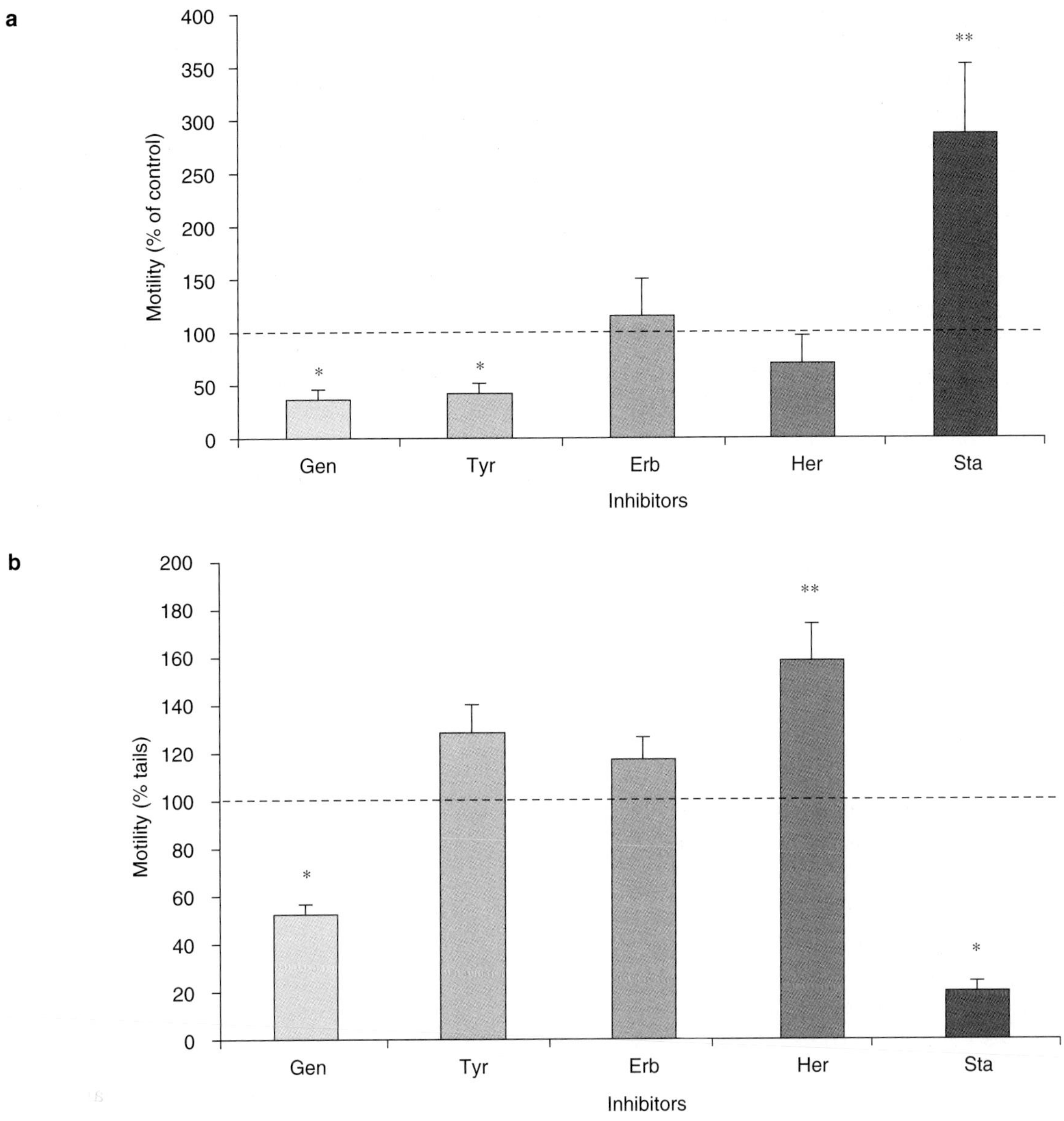

Figure 3.11 (**a**) Effect of kinase inhibitors on hyperactivated sperm motility. Washed sperm were incubated with or without kinase inhibitors for 6 h in Ham's solution at 37°C in 5% CO_2. Motion parameters were assessed using the Hamilton–Thorn Motion Analyzer (v. 10.8). Data are expressed as percentages of the control (without inhibitors) indicated by the dashed line. (**b**) Effect of kinase inhibitors on the incidence of immunoreactive sperm tails after a 6-h incubation in Ham's solution at 37°C in 5% CO_2. Sperm were fixed and permeated with methanol and labeled with phosphotyrosine monoclonal antibody and fluorescein isothiocyanate (FITC)-conjugated anti-mouse IgG (Bajpai *et al.*, 2003). Wilcoxon's signed rank test was used to analyze the data (vs. control). $^*p < 0.0001$; $^{**}p < 0.05$; Gen, genistein; Tyr, tyrphostin, Erb, erbstatin; Her, herbimycin A; Sta, staurosporin

Azoospermia and oligozoospermia

Azoospermia and oligozoospermia are associated with a wide variety of genetic anomalies. Chromosomal anomalies are more frequent in infertile men compared with fertile men, with a frequency of 2% of all men attending infertility clinics. In azoospermia, the frequency rises to 15%, including about 13% with a 47,XXY chromosome constitution. The remaining azoospermic cases are characterized by specific anomalies which include other numerical structural anomalies, such as reciprocal and Robertsonian translocations, inversions, ring chromosomes, aneuploidies and supernumerary chromosomes. Congenital bilateral absence of the vas deferens (CBAVD) leading to obstructive zoospermia in healthy males is a relatively frequent cause of male infertility, occurring at the rate of 1–2% of cases with male sterility and ≥6% of cases with obstructive zoospermia. Most men with CBAVD have mutations in the cystic fibrosis transmembrane conductance regulator (CFTR) gene, with an increased risk of carrying the 5T variant.

Sperm chromosome aneuploidy/globozoospermia

Globozoospermia (round-headed sperm) is a very rare condition observed in < 1% of infertility patients. The sperm lack an acrosomal cap. Pregnancy is rare even with application of ICSI. It would appear that other abnormalities may coexist with the lack of an acrosome. An increased frequency of sperm chromosome aneuploidy might be associated with globozoospermia and, therefore, might be responsible for the poor pregnancy prognosis. Aneuploidy for chromosome 15 has been implicated. There is a remarkable increase in the frequency of chromosome 15 aneuploidy in globozoospermia patients who have subsequently fathered a trisomy 15 conceptus. Little is known about the frequency of chromosome 15 aneuploidy in these infertile men. An increased frequency of XY disomy, which is the most common type of chromosome abnormality, has been observed in the sperm of infertile men (Martin *et al.*, 2003).

4

Capacitation, acrosome reaction and fertilization

After ejaculation, sperm are transported through the female reproductive tract. Most sperm cells are completely matured in the epididymis, while a few may still have a cytoplasmic droplet, particularly in subfertile men (Figures 4.1–4.3).

Sperm undergo the acrosome reaction before fertilization in order to penetrate the zona pellucida (ZP) of the oocyte. This process occurs following binding to the ZP only if the sperm have previously undergone a maturation process called capacitation. Binding of the capacitated sperm to the oocyte ZP activates a low-voltage Ca^{2+} channel and a store-operated Ca^{2+} channel, which causes a sustained elevation in the concentration of intracellular Ca^{2+} leading to the acrosome reaction (Tables 4.1 and 4.2). The priming of sperm to such calcium signals during capacitation involves many changes, including cholesterol efflux from the plasma membrane and increases in intracellular free Ca^{2+} cyclic adenosine monophosphate (cAMP), pH, protein tyrosine phosphorylation and actin polymerization (Aitken *et al.*, 1998; Arnoult *et al.*, 1999; de Lamirande *et al.*, 1997; Galantino-Homer *et al.*, 1997; Yanagamachi, 1994).

Reactive oxygen species (ROS) such as hydrogen peroxide and superoxide anions are involved in the regulation of sperm capacitation and protein tyrosine phosphorylation. Hydrogen peroxide is also involved in actin polymerization in bovine sperm and in the elevation of intracellular Ca^{2+} levels and fertilizing potential of sperm. cAMP and protein kinase A are regulators of protein tyrosine phosphorylation. ROS generation must lie upstream from cAMP in the reaction cascade, because ROS are located downstream from cAMP in the reaction sequence. The soluble adenylyl cyclase (AC) present in sperm is activated by HCO_3. Relatively low concentrations of hydrogen

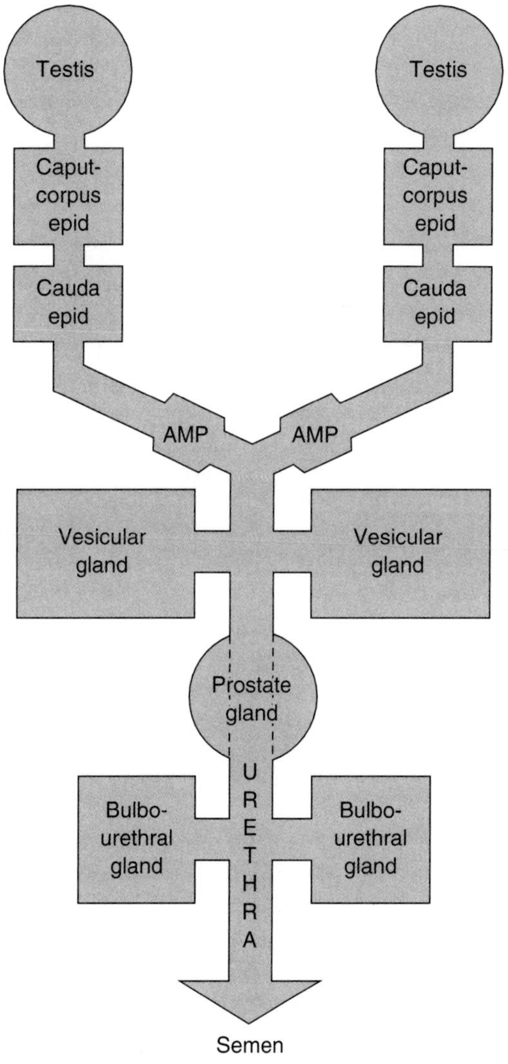

Figure 4.1 Ejaculated semen is composed of, in addition to a small amount of testicular fluid, contributions from several accessory organs including the epididymis (Caput-corpus epid and Cauda epid), ampullary glands (AMP), vesicular glands, prostate and bulbourethral glands

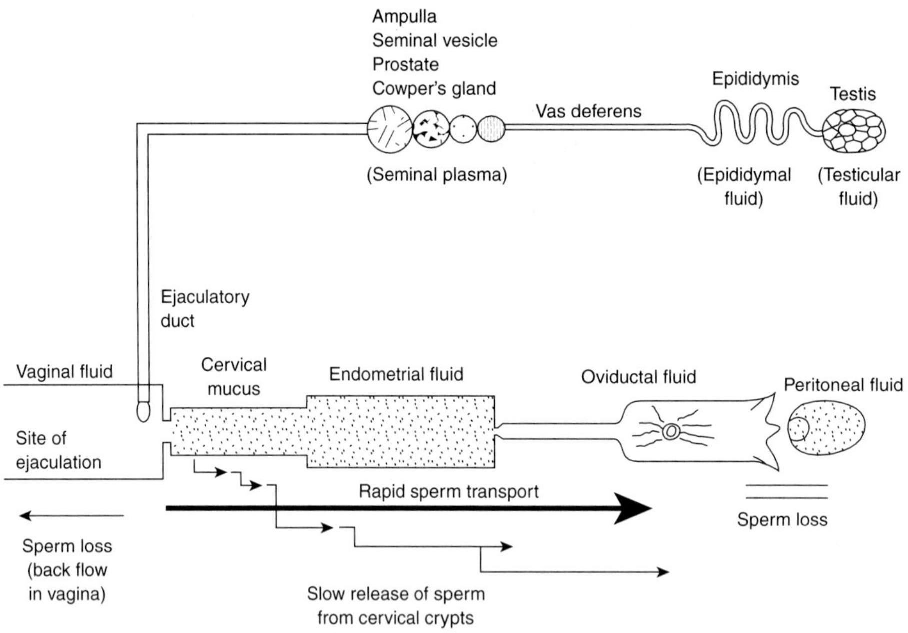

Figure 4.2 Sperm are suspended in various luminal fluids from the time of sperm production in the seminiferous tubules until fertilization in the oviduct

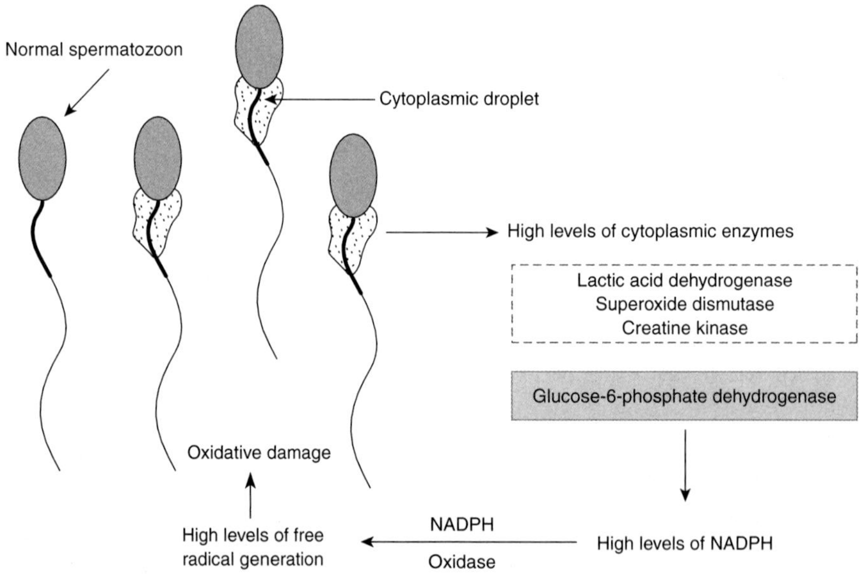

Figure 4.3 Relationships between the retention of excess residual cytoplasm, oxidative stress and defective sperm function are shown. The presence of glucose-6-phosphate dehydrogenase in excess cytoplasm generates NADPH, which acts as a substrate to produce superoxide anions, which dismutate to hydrogen peroxide causing cell damage. From Aitken *et al.*, 1994, with permission

peroxide are beneficial for sperm capacitation; however, too high a concentration inhibits the process. Hydrogen peroxide activates adenylyl cyclase to produce cAMP, leading to protein kinase A-dependent protein tyrosine phosphorylation (Aitken *et al.*, 1998; Chen *et al.*, 2000; Lecleere *et al.*, 1998; O'Toole *et al.*, 2000; Pariaud and Milhet, 1996; Rivlin *et al.*, 2004).

Sperm capacitation

Sperm acquire fertilizability after residing in the female tract for some time. Capacitation involves several physiological, biochemical and molecular changes involved in the removal or alteration of a stabilizer or protective coat from the sperm plasma

Table 4.1 Capacitation and acrosome reaction: major biochemical and biophysical changes in the membrane complex, energy metabolism and ion permeability

Major components of sperm head
Plasma membrane
Outer acrosomal membrane
Acrosomal matrix
Inner acrosomal membrane
Equatorial segment
Major biochemical parameters
Activation of many enzymes (acrosin, hyaluronidase, phospholipase A_2)
Enzyme systems (adenylate cyclase)
Neutralization of the net negative charge
Induction of hyperactivated motility
Sperm capacitation
Modification, redistribution and/or loss of the epididymal seminal plasma and cervical decapacitation factors by exogenous or endogenous proteases specifically activated (plasmin, kallikrein and acrosin)
The net negative charge is decreased by endogenous hydrolases (sterol sulfatase)
The fluidity is increased by the efflux of cholesterol, altering the cholesterol phospholipid ratio and the influx of unsaturated fatty acids. These changes are thought to be serum albumin-mediated
The altered permeability allows the increased uptake of calcium ions, glucose and oxygen, resulting in an elevated state, inducing hyperactivated motility and the ability to undergo acrosome reaction
Acrosome reaction
Decondensation of the acrosomal matrix
Fenestration and vesiculation of the plasma membrane and outer acrosomal membrane
Dispersion of the vesicles
Release of the acrosomal content

Table 4.2 Sperm–egg fusion: cortical reaction, polyspermy block, sperm decondensation and pronuclei development

Cortical reaction
Sperm–egg fusion does not involve the inner acrosomal membrane of anterior region, involves the plasma membrane equatorial segment/postacrosomal region of sperm head
Surface of equatorial region of sperm is incorporated into plasma membrane of ovum
Equatorial region of sperm plasma membrane is intermixed with ovum plasma membrane and is identified in egg membrane as late as the eight-cell stage
Polyspermy block
Block to polyspermy is at zona pellucida
Initiation of block is at sperm penetration of ovum when cortical granules are released into perivitelline space
Release of content of these granules causes extensive reorganization of zona pellucida and/or vitelline surface, the 'cortical reaction'
Cortical reaction results in release of enzymes which cause hardening of zona pellucida/inactivation of sperm captors (ZP3)
Enzymatic digestion of O-linked oligosaccharides on ZP3 removes specific carbohydrates involved in zona binding of sperm
Proteolysis of ZP2 may also alter physical characteristics of the zona to prevent further penetration of unwanted accessory sperm
Decondensation of nucleus in ooplasm
After fusion with egg plasma membrane, sperm nuclear envelope disintegrates, released chromatin material undergoes condensation
Sperm nuclear envelope is rapidly replaced by a new envelope within the ovum cytoplasm, forming male pronucleus
Decondensation of sperm nuclear envelope requires special components in cytoplasm of ovum
Completion of meiosis, pronuclei development
Once the male/female pronuclei are in close proximity, the nuclear envelopes disperse, allowing intermixing of chromosomes
Associated with these events is the initiation of DNA synthesis from cytoplasm precursors
The chromosomes then aggregate in prophase of first cleavage division forming a zygote restoration diploid state
Process of fertilization allows combining of maternal/paternal hereditary elements
During fusion of sperm–egg, sperm constituents from cell membranes/sperm head are released into ooplasm

membrane; this is under autonomic nerve and hormonal controls. Capacitation involves various parameters:

(1) Sperm are found in close contact with epithelial cells of the isthmus and uterotubal junction.

(2) Most capacitation occurs in the lower segment of the isthmus where fertilizing sperm are stored; capacitation within the isthmus progresses faster when females mate after ovulation rather than before ovulation.

(3) Capacitation is facilitated by 'rubbing off' sperm surface-absorbed materials (including seminal plasma proteins) against cervical mucus.

(4) Specificity/specialty of female tract: sperm are fully capacitated in the uterus without ascending the oviduct. Successful pregnancies occur following gamete intrafallopian transfer (GIFT) or direct intraperitoneal insemination (DIPI); capacitation is possible in the peritoneal cavity and/or ampulla. Capacitation is not strictly organ specific. Sperm adhering to the epithelium of the isthmus undergo capacitation slowly.

(5) *In vitro* sperm capacitation (IVC) and *in vitro* fertilization (IVF) are routinely applied using several commercially available tissue culture media or in modified Tyrode's/Krebs–Ringer solutions supplemented with energy sources (e.g. glucose, lactate and pyruvate) and albumin (e.g. Ham's F10) supplemented with blood serum. Serum is also commonly used, particularly for human IVF.

Sperm capacitation is associated with modifications in plasma membrane composition and fluidity, changes in intracellular ion concentrations, an increase in protein tyrosine phosphorylation and alterations in the oxidative metabolism. Changes at the flagellum enable sperm to develop hyperactivated motility. Modifications on the sperm head allow the initiation of the acrosome reaction (AR) in response to adequate stimuli such as the ZP or follicular fluid components. Different steps of the fertilization process have distinctive Ca^{2+} requirements. Whereas 0.22 mmol/l of Ca^{2+} is sufficient for the development of some capacitation-related events, human follicular fluid-induced AR and sperm–ZP interaction require 0.58 mmol/l of this cation (Marin-Briggiler *et al.*, 2003).

Ultrastructural and biochemical parameters

Several ultrastructural and biochemical changes occur during capacitation of mammalian sperm:

(1) Antigens change their distribution, particularly fibronectin-like molecules, on the sperm surface;

(2) Some glycoproteins or proteins are released from sperm surfaces;

(3) Changes occur in the lectin-binding ability of the sperm plasma membrane;

(4) Intramembranous particles (IMPs), intrinsic proteins within lipid bilayers, change their distribution in both the head and tail regions. IMPs are evenly distributed in the plasma membrane over the acrosome. The membrane of capacitated sperm has many small patches free of IMPs.

Uncapacitated sperm treated with filipin contain densely and evenly distributed complexes in the plasma membranes of the acrosomal region. The sperm plasma membrane undergoes several complex changes in preparation for fertilization. Sperm plasma membrane is 'biologically frozen' when sperm leave the male's body and its 'defrosting' represents capacitation.

Sperm hyperactivation

Sperm hyperactivation is a necessary step in the capacitation sequence. Sperm motility is measured by videotape to evaluate the straight line velocity (μm/s) (VSL). Fertilization, and subsequent embryonic development, result from single-sperm transfer (S-MIST) and multiple-sperm transfer.

Fertilization, and subsequent embryo development, is achieved by injection of immotile sperm into the perivitelline space. To assess sperm viability, a survival stain suitable for use in combination with immunofluorescent assay, Hoechst 33258, is used. The dye fluoresces an intense blue when bound to DNA. To assess sperm plasma membrane integrity, a hypo-osmotic swelling test (HOST) is performed, using fluoresceinated D-mannose-enriched albumin (FITC-DMA). The ability of sperm to swell under hypo-osmotic conditions indicates an intact membrane.

Biochemical markers of sperm quality

Several biochemical markers have been used to evaluate human sperm maturity and function including sperm creatine-*N*-phosphotransferase or creatine kinase (CK), CK enzymatic active-site labeling and CK immunocytochemistry of individual sperm; men with low sperm concentrations who have increased numbers of individual sperm, and men with low sperm concentrations who have increased incidence of infertility, also show increased levels of sperm CK activity. This may be related to a defect of sperm development in the last phase of spermatogenesis, when excess cytoplasm is normally extruded and left in the adluminal area as residual bodies. Thus, sperm with a high CK content, an indication of surplus cytoplasm, have not completed cellular maturation (Huszar *et al.*, 2003). There is also a second sperm maturation marker, which was initially thought to be a sperm-specific creatine kinase M-isoform and identified as the testis-expressed chaperone protein HspA2 (a member of the HSP70-2 family), that, along with the homologous hsc70, is synthesized in two waves of expression. The first wave occurs during meiosis, as HspA2 is part of the synaptonemal complex. The second wave of major expression occurs simultaneously with cytoplasm extrusion, in terminal spermatogenesis.

THE ACROSOME AND ACROSOME REACTION

The acrosome consists of an anteriorly located acrosomal cap and posteriorly located equatorial segment. The acrosomal cap is endowed with a variety of hydrolyzing enzymes, whereas the equatorial segment is enzymatically 'empty'. Hyaluronidase and acrosin are acrosomal enzymes that have been extensively studied and characterized. The acrosome contains several powerful hydrolyzing enzymes. Structural proteins maintain acrosome shape and the positioning of different functional components within the acrosomal matrix; acrosome organization is required to ensure release of acrosome components in a precise sequence so that sperm can traverse the egg vestments (Figures 4.4–4.12).

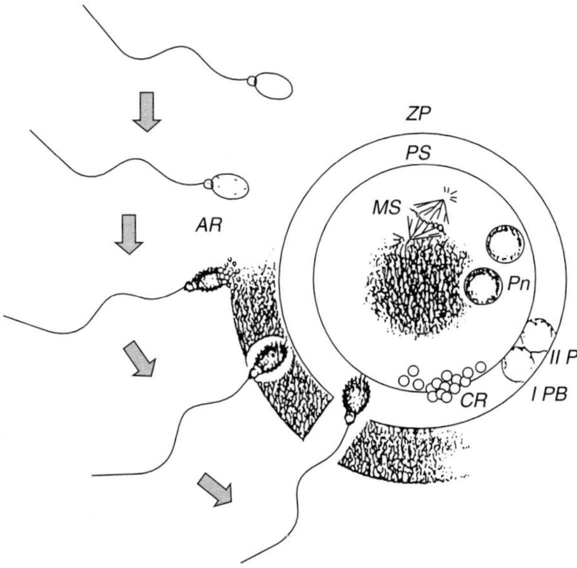

Figure 4.4 Fertilization sequence: interaction of the zona pellucida (ZP) and its receptor on the sperm head leads to the acrosomal reaction (AR) and to the subsequent enzymatic attack of the ZP. The sperm penetrates the ZP and reaches the perivitelline space (PS). The oocyte and sperm membranes fuse and fertilization takes place. The cortical reaction (CR) prevents polyspermia. The second meiotic division of the oocyte is completed and the second polar body (II PB) is extruded. Upon fusion, the two pronuclei (Pn) give rise to the formation of the mitotic spindle (MS) and to the first cleavage. I PB, first polar body

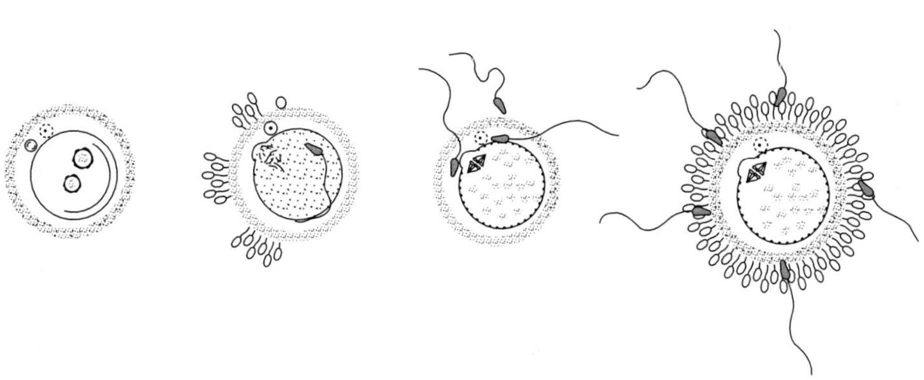

Figure 4.5 Sperm–egg interaction

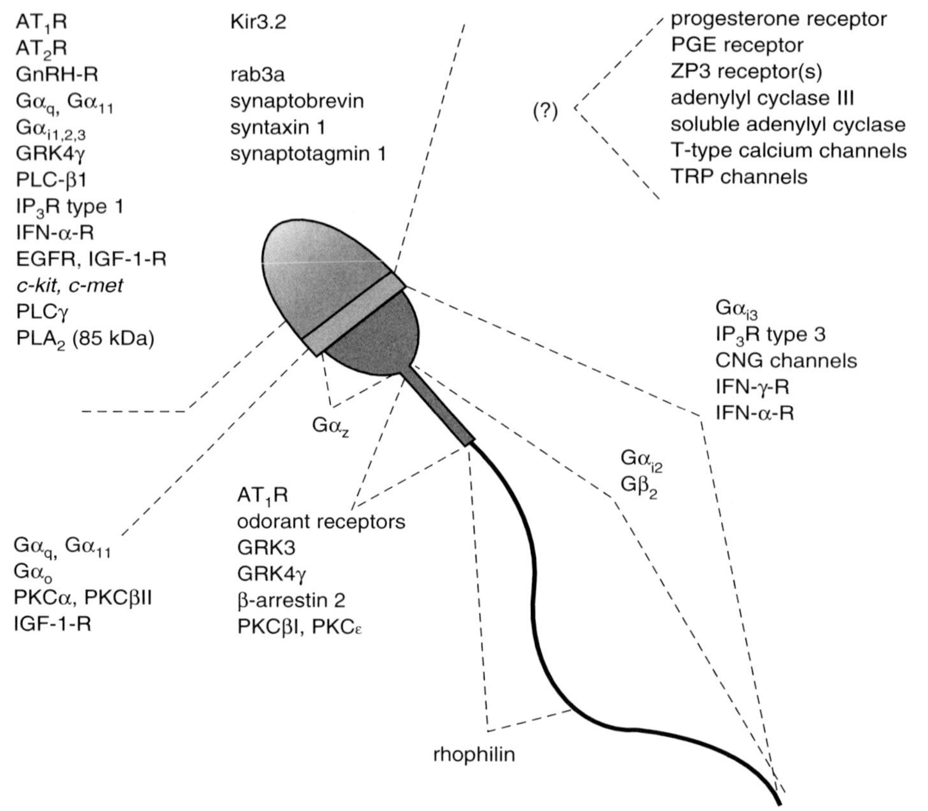

Figure 4.6 Signaling proteins expressed in sperm. Several proteins involved in signal transduction processes in somatic cells are also expressed in sperm. Their differential expression in the acrosomal compartment, equatorial region, postacrosomal region, and middle, main and end pieces of the sperm tail is shown. Those signaling components the expression of which is postulated but not proven or the exact localization of which is not known are labeled by a question mark. AT$_1$R, AT$_1$ angiotensin receptor; AT$_2$R, AT$_2$ angiotensin receptor; CNG channels, cyclic nucleotide-gated channels; EGFR, epidermal growth factor receptor; Gα, α subunit of heterotrimeric guanine nucleotide-binding protein; Gβ, β subunit of heterotrimeric guanine nucleotide-binding protein; GnRH-R, gonadotropin-releasing hormone receptor; GRK, G-protein-coupled receptor kinase; IFN-γ-R, interferon-γ-receptor; IGF-1-R, insulin-like growth factor-1 receptor; IP$_3$R, inositol triphosphate receptor; Kir3.2, a G-protein-gated inwardly rectifying K^+ channel subunit; PGE, prostaglandin E; PKC, protein kinase C; PLA$_2$, phospholipase A$_2$; PLC, phospholipase C; TRP channels, transient receptor potential channels; ZP3, zona pellucida protein 3

The acrosome reaction involves the following parameters:

(1) To fertilize eggs, sperm must be highly motile as well as capable of undergoing the acrosome reaction (AR), penetrating through egg investments and fusing with the egg.

(2) AR acts as in indicator of completed capacitation because sperm do not undergo AR either spontaneously or mediated by ligands (e.g. zona pellucida) unless they become capacitated.

(3) Massive influx of Ca^{2+} occurs during AR. Concentration of intracellular CA^{2+} in sperm is low, in both head and tail regions, because of the presence of ATPase-mediated Ca^{2+} antiporter, and a Ca^{2+}/H^+ exchange system in plasma membrane.

(4) Carbohydrate is a distinct component of the acrosomal matrix. A glycoprotein layer covering the inner surface of the outer acrosomal membrane holds vesiculated (fenestrated) plasma and outer acrosomal membranes together during the acrosome reaction.

(5) The form of acrosome does not change during capacitation; enzymatically inactive proacrosin in the sperm acrosome is converted to enzymatically active acrosin by glycosaminoglycans in uterine fluid.

(6) Function of AR: eggs are surrounded by lipoprotein coats through which sperm must

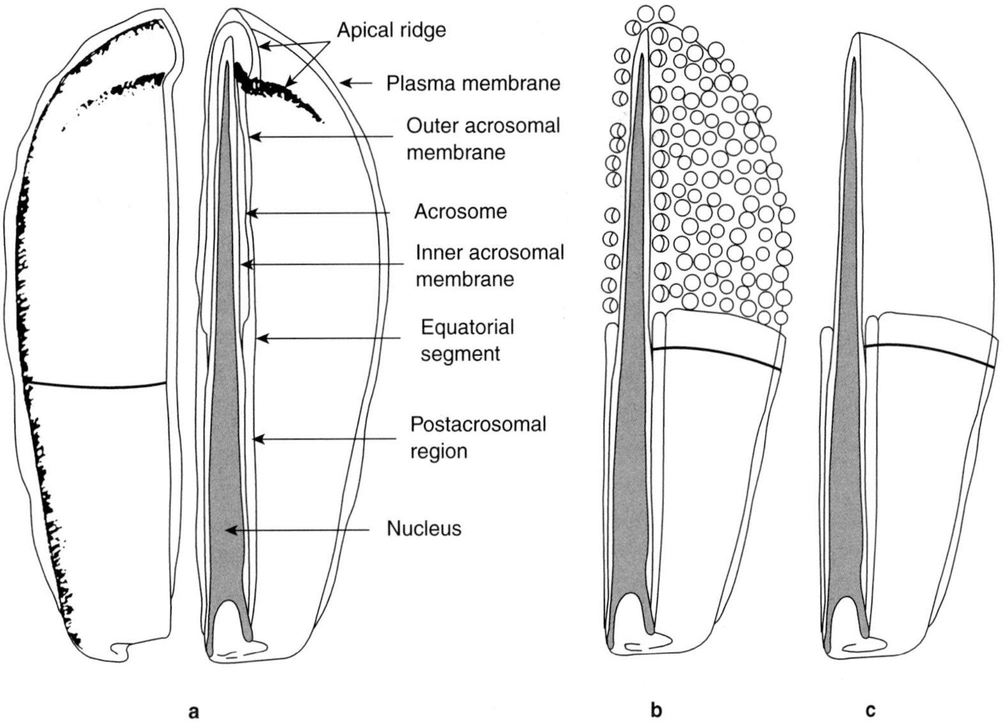

Figure 4.7 Acrosome reaction in mammalian sperm. (**a**) Intact plasma and acrosomal membrane of an unreacted spermatozoon. (**b**) Initiation of the acrosome reaction showing multiple fusion points between the plasma membrane and outer acrosomal membrane. Fusion leaves the appearance of numerous vesicles over the cell surface. Note that fusion is absent in the equatorial and postacrosomal regions. Acrosomal enzymes involved with ovum penetration are released and exposed on the inner acrosomal membrane. (**c**) The acrosome swells and is eventually lost during penetration of the zona pellucida, leaving only the inner acrosomal membrane exposed on the upper portion of the sperm head. From Saacke and White (1972), with permission

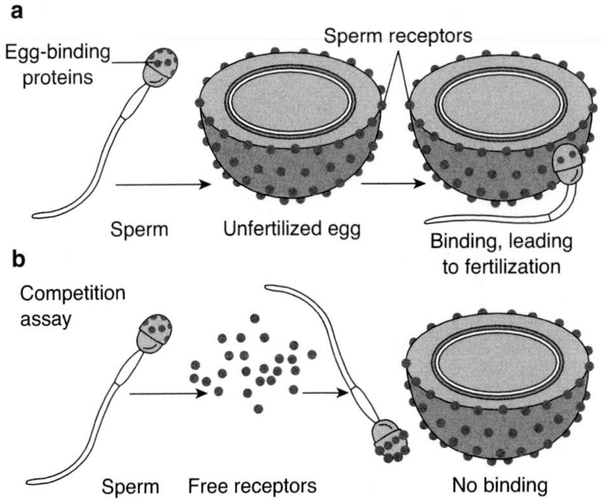

Figure 4.8 The protein ZP3 in the zona pellucida is the sperm receptor. Exposure of sperm to unfertilized ova results in sperm binding to ZP3 (**a**). In the competition assay (**b**), sperm are incubated with ZP3 first and then exposed to ova; however, the sperm are unable to bind to the ZP3 proteins on the zona pellucida because their P3 binding proteins are already occupied (blocked) by the free ZP3 to which the sperm were exposed before introduction of ova. From Wassarman (1988), with permission

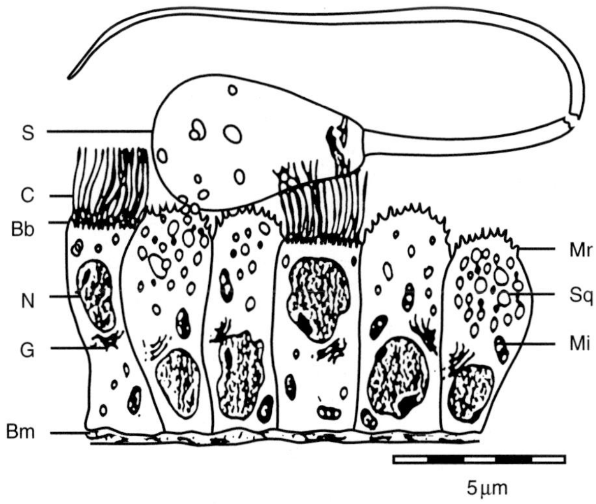

Figure 4.9 Interaction between sperm receptors and metabolite from oviduct epithelium during fertilization. S, sperm; C, kinocilia which mix sperm with oviduct secretions; Bb, basal bodies of kinocilia for locomotion; N, nucleus; G, Golgi apparatus; Bm, basal membrane of epithelium; Mr, microvilli; Sq, secretory granules; Mi, mitochondria

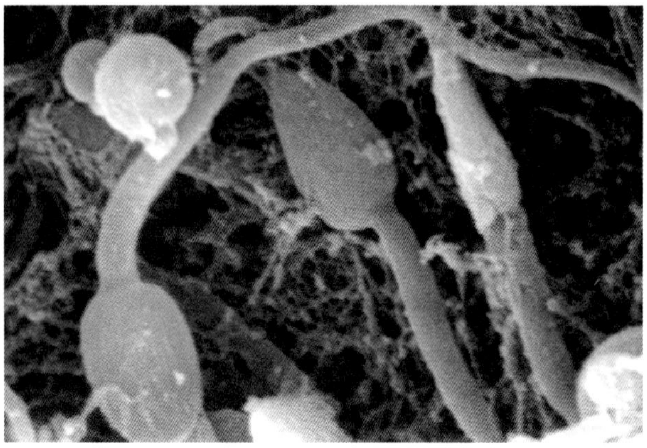

Figure 4.10 Scanning electron microscopy of capacitated sperm at site of fertilization

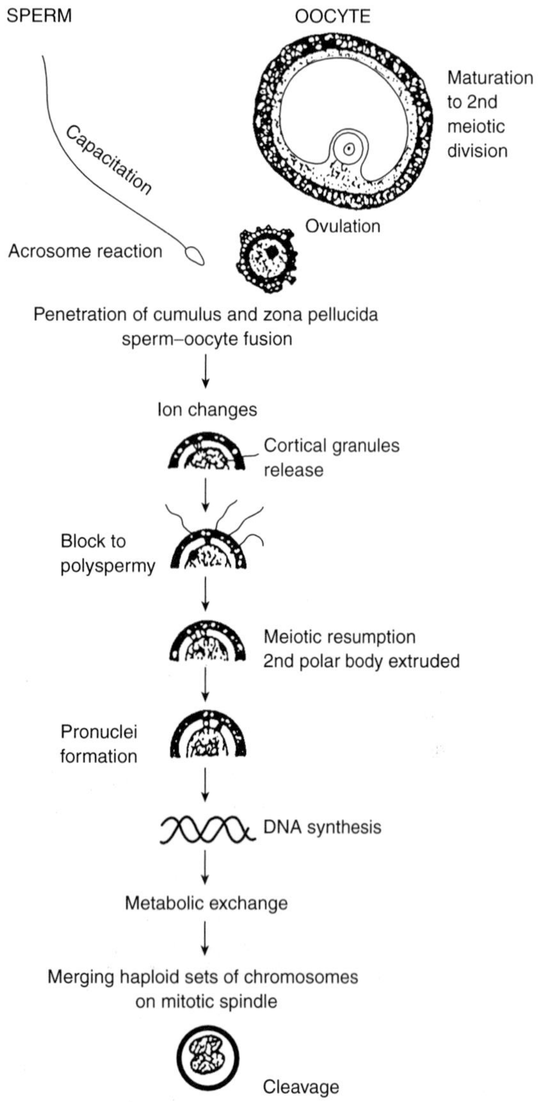

Figure 4.11 Sequence of events of sperm–oocyte interaction: penetration of cumulus and zona pellucida, ion exchange, pronuclei formation, DNA synthesis, merging haploid sets of chrosomes and cleavage

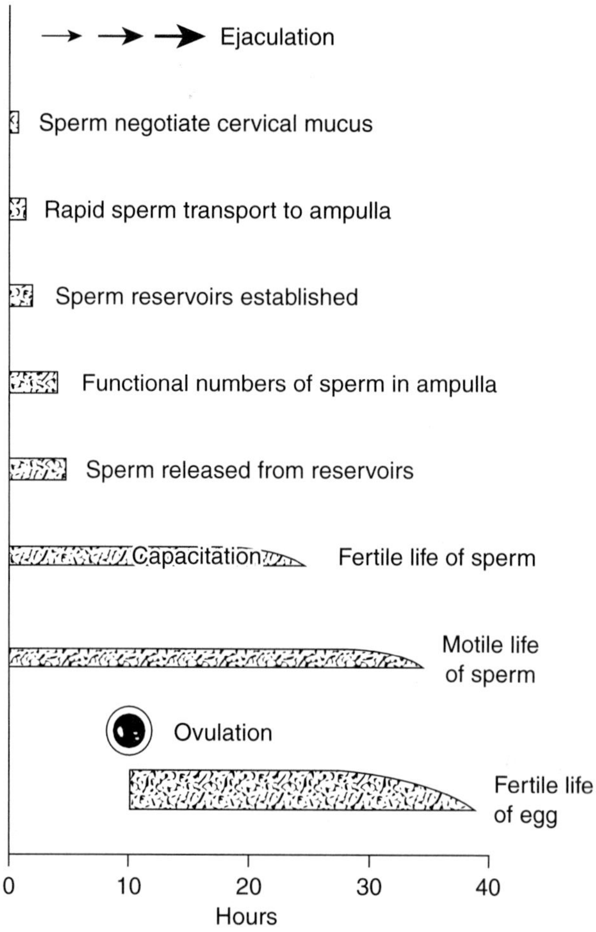

Figure 4.12 Time sequence of ejaculation, sperm migration, sperm release from reservoirs, penetration of zona pellucida and fertile lives of sperm and egg

pass before reaching the egg plasma membrane. Acrosome-reacted sperm dissolve the coat locally to produce a 'hole' through which the sperm swim. The outer acrosomal membrane overlying the plasma membrane is partially or totally destroyed, or becomes detached from the main body of the sperm.

Oocyte–cumulus complex

The oocyte–cumulus complex (OCC) in the mature, ovulated oocyte is made up of corona cells loosely attached to each other around the zona pellucida, and radially expanded cumulus cells with an extracellular matrix of glycosaminoglycans. This extracellular matrix is composed of granules that are trypsin sensitive and filaments of mostly hyaluronic acid (Acosta, 1996).

Table 4.3 Sperm and egg physiology related to fertilization

Parameter	*Oogenesis and characteristics of ova*	*Spermatogenesis and characteristics of sperm*
First maturational division in gamete	First maturational division is completed in preovulatory follicle	First meiotic division results in two cells of equal size
Second maturational division	Second maturational division is completed only when the egg is penetrated by sperm	Not comparable
Number of gametes produced during reproductive life	Thousands of oogonia are found in the neonatal ovary	Millions of sperm are produced in each ejaculate from puberty, with reduced numbers during senility
Sex chromosome in gamete	X	X or Y
Amount of cytoplasm in gamete	As oocyte matures, the amount of its cytoplasm increases	As spermatid develops into sperm, the amount of cytoplasm decreases, acrosome and tail develop in late spermatid
Motility of gamete	Oocytes, surrounded by follicular cells, are immotile	Sperm motility develops gradually in various parts of epididymis and increases at ejaculation
Plasma membrane at fertilization	Egg acquires plasma membranes from sperm	Sperm loses its plasma membranes to egg
Survival in female reproductive tract	12–24 h after ovulation	Fertilizability is maintained 24 h after ejaculation

Table 4.4 Sperm–zona attachment and interaction during fertilization

Sperm attachment to zona

Specific sperm receptor in the zona pellucida is one of three major glycoproteins that form extracellular matrix of zona pellucida

Three glycoproteins, ZP1, ZP2 and ZP3, are synthesized by maturing oocytes. These are present in all mammals but with variations in these proteins

ZP3 functions as sperm receptor to which only sperm with an intact acrosome can bind

Binding of sperm to sperm receptors occurs through an interaction with O-linked oligosaccharides on ZP3

Cumulus and sperm attachment

Role of cumulus cells in sperm attachment is debated in domestic animals (especially the cow), since they are usually absent 3–4 h after ovulation

Hyaluronidase in bull acrosome allows penetration of cumulus oophorus

Arylsulfatase from boar acrosome causes cells of the cumulus oophorus to disperse. Enzymes necessary for cumulus penetration or dispersion are present in these species

Sperm interaction with cumulus oophorus

Properties of cumulus oophorus

Sperm entry into cumulus

Inhibition of sperm penetration in cumulus

Role of cumulus

Acrosome hyaluronidase

- acrosome reaction allows release of zona lysin by which sperm digest a path through the zona pellucida to the vitelline membrane
- acrosome contains several enzymes: hyaluronidase, acrosin, proacrosin (inactive form of acrosin), esterase, phospholipase A_2, acid phosphatases, aryl sulfatase, β-*N*-acetyl glucosaminidase, aryl amidase and non-specific acid proteinases; with quantitative/qualitative species differences

Sperm–zona pellucida interaction

Function of zona

Properties of zona

Sperm binding/penetration through zona

- acrosome is activated by the time of sperm attachment and penetration of zona. Once sperm has traversed the zona pellucida, the head moves into vitelline space and contacts vitelline membrane

Table 4.5 Chromosomal abnormalities and different developmental stages (Rosnina *et al.*, 2000)

Stage	*Cytogenetic anomalies*
Maternal gametogenesis	Somatic division of oogonia before onset of meiosis or during first or second meiotic division
Paternal gametogenesis	Mitotic divisions while male is *in utero*, or during post-puberty first or second meiotic division after puberty
Fertilization	Normal chromosomes with errors during fertilization; fertilization of a normal egg by two normal sperm
Zygote	Improper division of one or more chromosomes, anaphase lag or no disjunction; failure of cleavage of blastomeres or mosaic embryo

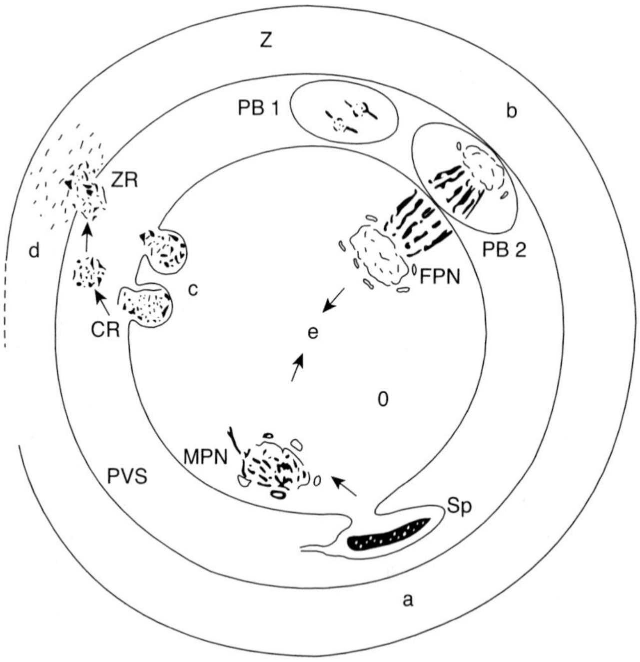

Figure 4.13 Physiological processes of human fertilization. (a) Sperm (Sp)–oocyte (O) membrane fusion: plasma membrane (PM) of midsegment of sperm head fuses. (b) Sperm–egg fusion: the second polar body (PB2) is extruded into the perivitelline space (PVS) and the fertilized ovum completes the second meiotic maturation division (the anaphase 2 spindle). (c) Cortical reaction (CR): sperm fuses with egg cortical granules (CG) beneath oolemma and they release their contents into PVS by exocytosis. (d) Zona reaction (ZR): interaction of CG contents with lipoproteins of the zona pellucida (ZP) establishes a primary block to polyspermy at the level of the ZP. (Chemical hardening prevents supernumerary sperm from entering PVS after fertilization.) (e) Female and male pronuclei (FPN and MPN) migrate to the center of egg and become closely associated with one another but do not fuse

Gamete interaction

The bulk of semen enters the uterus directly or is forced through the cervical canal during momentary relaxation of the cervix assisted by the vaginal contraction resulting from copulatory stimuli. Most sperm are eliminated from the female reproductive tract, leaving a few sperm to be transported to the site of fertilization in the ampulla and/or ampulla–isthmic junction (Tables 4.2–4.4).

The sperm-to-egg ratio in the ampulla during fertilization is 1 : 1 or less. The female reproductive tract prevents morphologically abnormal sperm from reaching the site of fertilization. Not all fertilizing sperm are genetically normal. Normal embryonic development is maximal when eggs in the oviduct are fertilized soon after ovulation.

The gametes undergo a complex ultrastructural process of proliferation, chromosomal exchange and reduction at meiosis, differentiation,

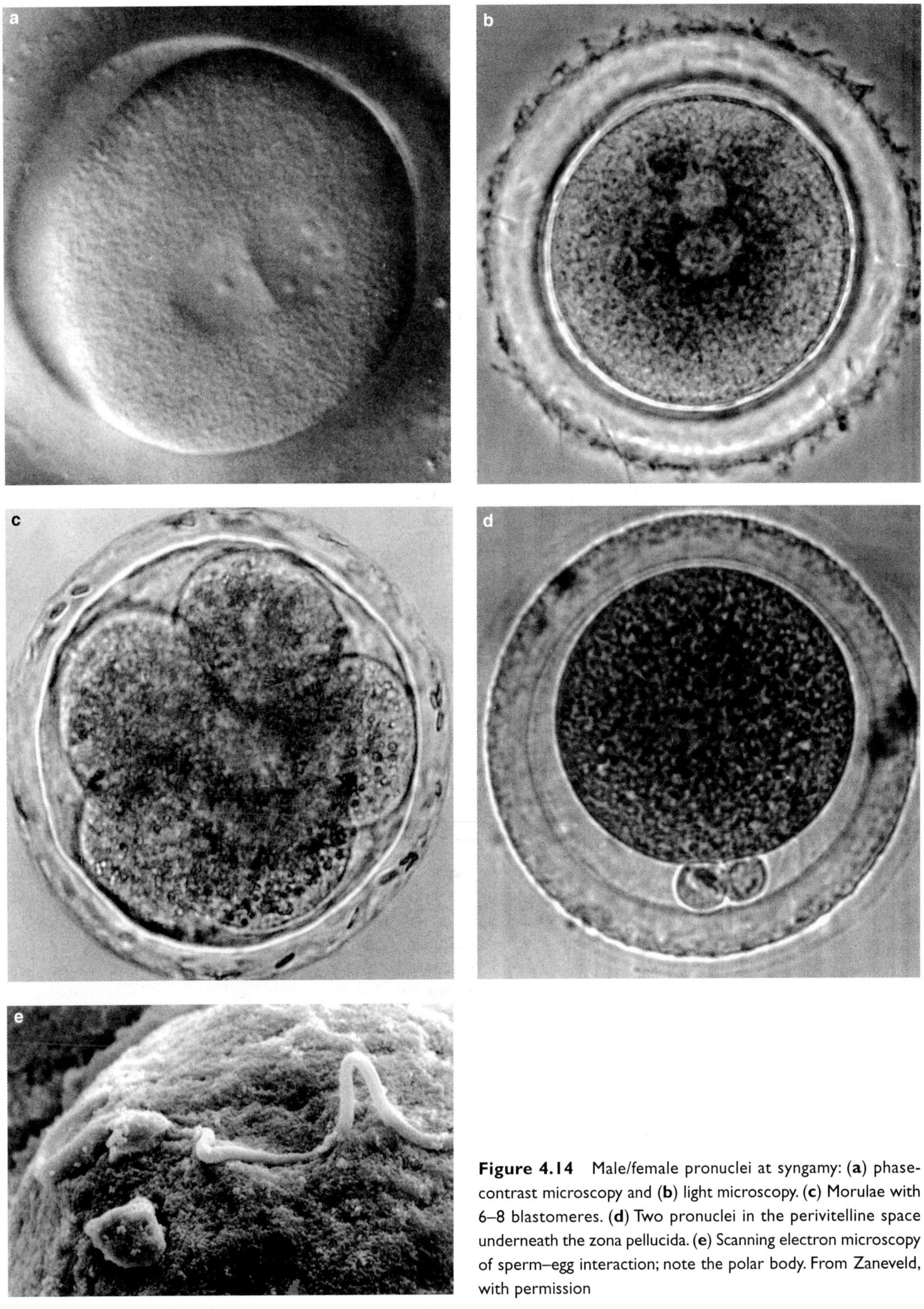

Figure 4.14 Male/female pronuclei at syngamy: (**a**) phase-contrast microscopy and (**b**) light microscopy. (**c**) Morulae with 6–8 blastomeres. (**d**) Two pronuclei in the perivitelline space underneath the zona pellucida. (**e**) Scanning electron microscopy of sperm–egg interaction; note the polar body. From Zaneveld, with permission

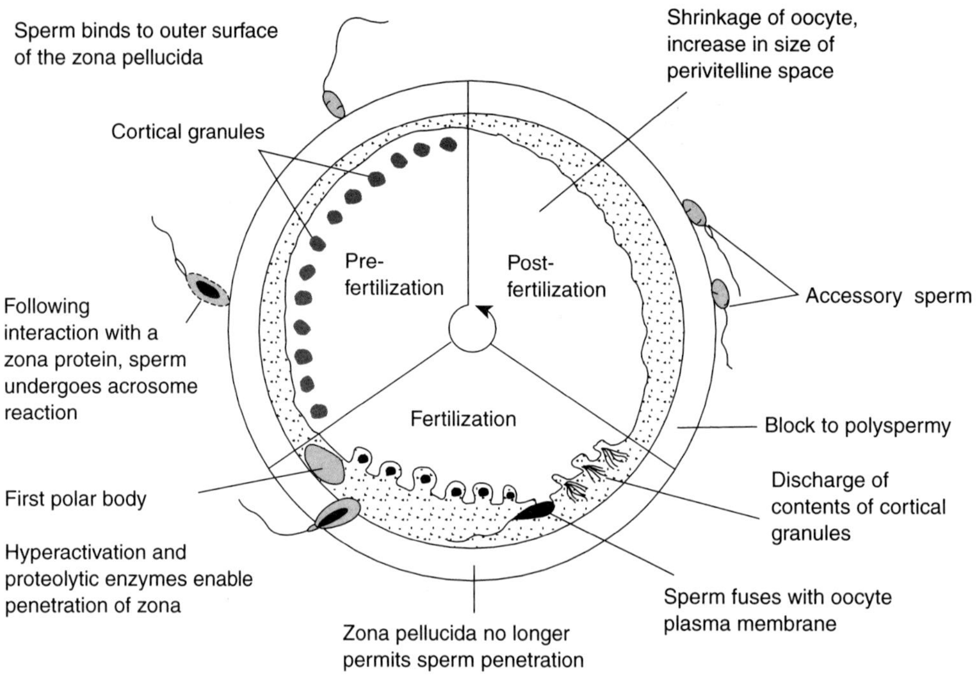

Figure 4.15 Prefertilization, fertilization and postfertilization in farm animals

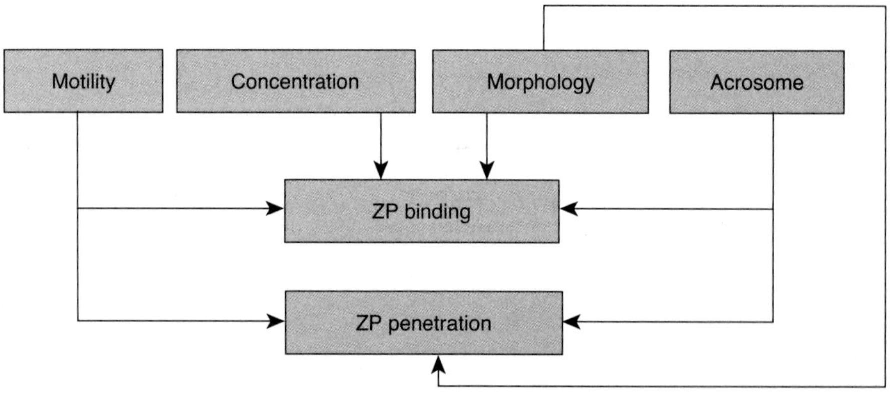

Figure 4.16 Relationship between sperm characteristics and sperm–zona pellucida (ZP) binding and penetration

maturation and transport. Membrane fusion occurs between the sperm and oocyte. Chromosomal abnormalities occur at different developmental stages (Table 4.5).

FERTILIZATION

The interaction between the protein ZP3 of the zona pellucida (ZP) and its receptor on the sperm head leads to the AR and to the subsequent enzymatic attack of the ZP (Figures 4.4 and 4.13–4.17). The sperm penetrates the ZP and reaches the perivitelline space. The oocyte and sperm membranes fuse and fertilization takes place. The cortical reaction prevents polyspermia. The second meiotic division of the oocyte is completed and the second polar body is extruded. Upon fusion, the two pronuclei give rise to the formation of the mitotic spindle and to the first cleavage (Revelli *et al.*, 2003a).

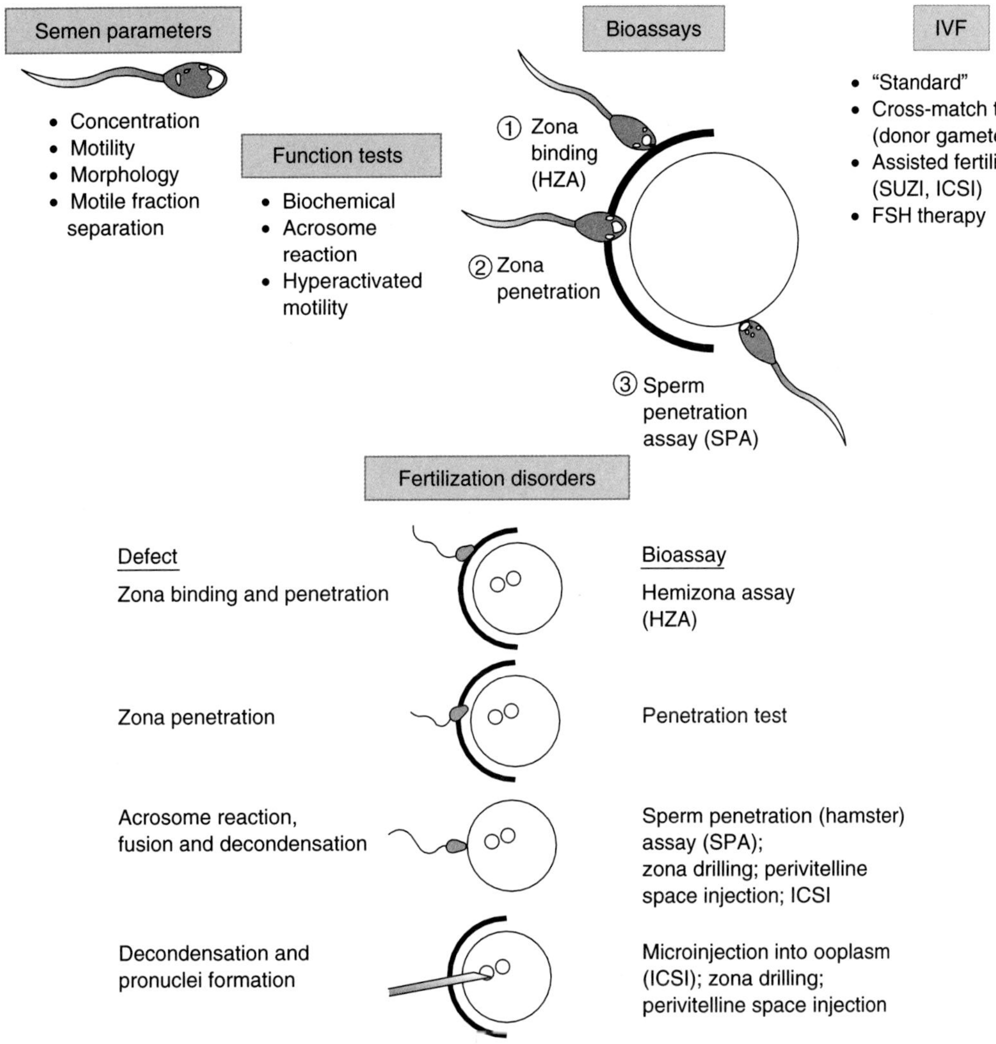

Figure 4.17 Stepwise progressive diagnosis in cases of recurrent failed *in vitro* fertilization (IVF). Sequential analysis of specific sperm defects in cases of recurrent failed fertilization. FSH, follicle stimulating hormone; ICSI, intracytoplasmic sperm injection; SUZI, subzonal insemination

IMPLANTATION

The uterine endometrium is an extremely dynamic tissue, undergoing sequential developmental changes in preparation for implantation during each estrous cycle. Successful implantation of the blastocyst requires successful development of uterine endometrial receptivity. Cyclic endometrial development in the adult can be considered to be analogous to embryonic development.

Section II Reproductive Pathology

5

Testicular dysfunction and male infertility

There are various anatomical syndromes of male infertility which include those due to absence of the vas deferens, one testis being non-palpable, spermatocele, absence of epididymis, failure of union of epididymis–testis and other related anomalies. These anomalies are associated with testicular feminization syndrome or male hermaphroditism (Figures 5.1 and 5.2). Testicular dysfunction is due to spermatogenesis anomalies, anatomical/ultrastructural parameters, genetic factors and testicular tumors.

ANATOMICAL/ULTRASTRUCTURAL PARAMETERS

Cryptorchidism

Exposure to compounds with estrogenic or anti-androgenic activities may cause deleterious effects on male reproduction, a decrease in sperm production and an increased incidence of testicular carcinoma and/or increased cryptorchidism (Table 5.1). Any form of cryptorchidism at birth, regardless of the outcome, should be considered to be a risk factor for testicular cancer and/or male infertility. Most cases of cryptorchidism diagnosed at birth resolve spontaneously during the first years of life (natural course of cryptorchid testes). The risk of cryptorchidism is higher for boys born to young mothers (<20 years). The risk also increases with the first birth, Cesarean section or toxemia, infants small for gestational age and in boys with low birth weight and when estrogens (estradiol, diethylstilbestrol (DES) and estrone) have been administered during gestation (Thonneau *et al.*, 2003).

Cryptorchidism is associated with an increased risk of developing testicular cancer, decreased sperm count and infertility. Infertility occurs in 60% of men with bilateral, and in 35% of men with unilateral, cryptorchidism. Cryptorchidism is caused by interaction of endocrine disorders, anatomical abnormalities, and environmental and genetic factors. Genes in the achromatic region of the long arm of the Y chromosome (Yq11) are required for normal spermatogenesis. Y-chromosome microdeletions are an important genetic cause of primary testiculopathies (Kunej *et al.*, 2003).

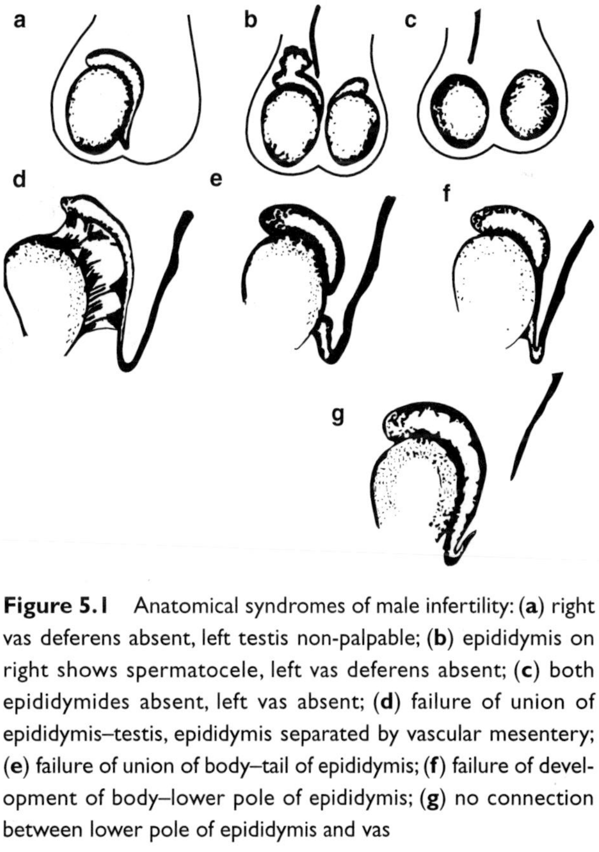

Figure 5.1 Anatomical syndromes of male infertility: (**a**) right vas deferens absent, left testis non-palpable; (**b**) epididymis on right shows spermatocele, left vas deferens absent; (**c**) both epididymides absent, left vas absent; (**d**) failure of union of epididymis–testis, epididymis separated by vascular mesentery; (**e**) failure of union of body–tail of epididymis; (**f**) failure of development of body–lower pole of epididymis; (**g**) no connection between lower pole of epididymis and vas

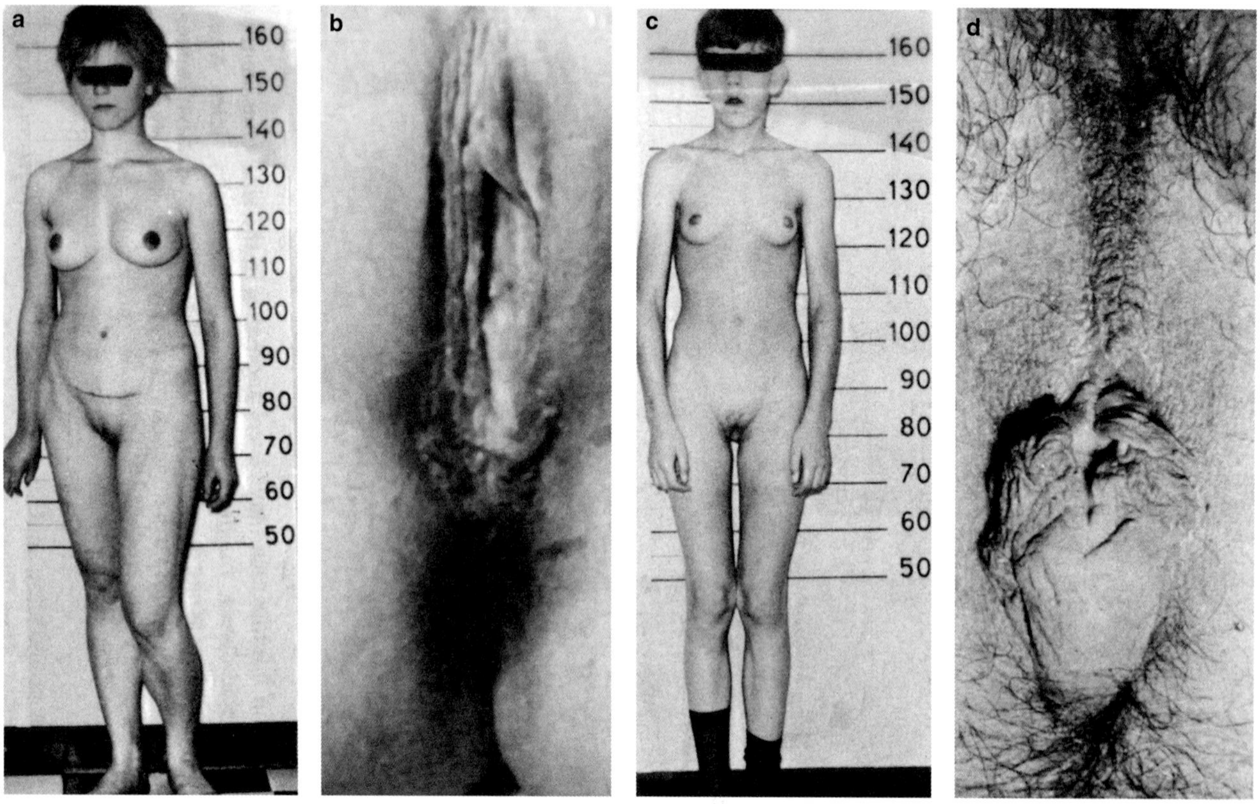

Figure 5.2 Testicular feminization syndrome: (**a**) female habitus with significant breast development; (**b**) female external genitals without pubic hair. Male hermaphrodite: (**c**) male legal sex, male psychosexual orientation, female habitus; (**d**) external genitals

Hydrocele

The description, symptoms, causes, risk factors, diagnosis and surgical approaches to hydrocele are summarized in Table 5.2.

Varicocele

Varicocele, a dilatation of the pampiniform plexus of the spermatic cord, is a treatable cause of male infertility (Figures 5.3–5.7). While the incidence of varicocele in the general population is estimated to be 15%, the incidence in men with subfertility increases to approximately 30%. With the advent of new microsurgical techniques for varicocele ligation, it is assumed that the complication rate following this procedure will be diminished compared to historic norms. In particular, since magnification allows identification and preservation of lymphatic vessels, it is thought that microsurgical varicocele ligation will lead to a lower rate of hydrocele formation than non-microsurgical techniques.

Varicoceles are associated with a time-dependent decline in testicular function in animals and man. Approximately 15% of all adult men have a varicocele. One-third of all males evaluated for infertility have a varicocele, demonstrating the negative impact of varicoceles on testicular function. Significant volume loss occurs in 77% of adolescent boys with a varicocele, with 10% having a left testis one-quarter the size of the right testis. The loss of testicular volume in adolescents with left testicular varicocele is accompanied by a decrease in sperm count. The growth arrest associated with the adolescent varicocele is reversible in most patients.

Varicocele may be associated with poor semen and hormonal parameters, with increased follicle stimulating hormone (FSH) levels indicating damage to the germinal epithelium and a poor prognosis. Studies have reported a lower mean serum testosterone level in patients with varicocele and sexual dysfunction. Varicocele is also associated with decreased testicular size and impaired sex accessory gland secretion with lower semen quality. Thus,

Table 5.1 Cryptorchidism

Description
Incomplete or improper descent of one or both testicles. Normally, descent occurs in the 7th or 8th month of gestation. Cryptorchid testes may be palpable or non-palpable
abdominal – located inside the internal ring
canalicular – located between the internal and external ring
ectopic – located outside the normal path of testicular descent from abdominal cavity to scrotum – may be ectopic to perineum, femoral canal, superficial inguinal pouch (most common), suprapubic area/opposite hemiscrotum
retractile – fully descended testis that moves freely between scrotum and groin
iatrogenic – previously descended testis becomes undecided secondary to scar tissue after inguinal surgery, such as an inguinal hernia repair or hydrocelectomy
Causes
May involve alterations in mechanical factors (gubernaculum, length of vas deferens/testicular vessels, groin anatomy, epididymis, cremasteric muscles or abdominal pressure), hormonal factors (gonadotropin, testosterone, dihydrotestosterone, Müllerian inhibiting substance), neutral factors (ilioinguinal nerve or genitofemoral nerve)
Medication
hCG therapy is biweekly injections of 250 IU for infants, 500 IU for children up to 6 years of age and 1000 IU for those 6 years of age and older, for a total of 5 weeks
Imaging
MRI (even if prolactin minimally elevated, to rule out hypothalamic tumors which may compress the pituitary stalk thereby decreasing delivery of prolactin inhibitory hormone with subsequent rise in prolactin)
CT if MRI not available
avoid 'coned-down' or plain tomograms of pituitary as they are relatively insensitive/will not rule out presence of hypothalamic lesions compressing pituitary stalk
bromocriptine (Parlodel). Start with low dose of 1.25 mg or 2.5 mg daily, then increase as tolerated over several weeks for 2.5 mg tid
Medication
Doses up to 30 mg daily are occasionally required for prolactinoma regression, after which lower doses can be used for maintenance. First dose should be taken with evening meal

varicocele repair should be performed to prevent infertility and subsequent testosterone deficiency. Successful venous occlusion will relieve pain, if present, and will reduce the size of large varicoceles. Surgical treatment of varicocele produces a significant improvement in semen analysis in 60–80% of patients affected by testicular dysfunction, with pregnancy rates of 35% after varicocelectomy. In patients who have undergone varicocele repair, there is a preoperative correlation between semen analysis and varicocele size. Postoperatively, all semen parameters improve with increased left testicular volume varicocele repair, leading to an increase in pregnancy rate.

Peyronie's disease

Peyronie's disease is a connective tissue disorder affecting the tunica albuginea and adjacent corpus cavernous tissue. There are two phases of the disease. The early phase consists of a vascular inflammatory reaction. This period usually lasts 2–10 months and symptoms consist primarily of pain during erection. The disease either regresses or continues to the second phase.

In the second or late phase of the disease, the initial inflammatory reaction progresses to form a fibrotic calcified and palpable plaque. Consequences of this plaque include symptoms associated with

Table 5.2 Hydrocele

Description

Hydrocele is a collection of fluid within scrotum

Communicating hydrocele

associated with a patent processus vaginalis, has associated indirect inguinal hernia

Non-communicating hydrocele

infantile type – no communication, frequent spontaneous resolution

adult type – no communication, infrequent resolution

Hydrocele of the cord

distal portion of processus vaginalis has closed, mid-portion patent and fluid-filled, proximal portion may be open or closed

Acute hydrocele

acute fluid collection resulting from an acute process within tunica vaginalis

Symptoms

Swelling in scrotum or inguinal canal; demonstrated fluctuation in size (communicating hydrocele); pain radiating to back (occasionally); sensation of heaviness in scrotum; fluid collection in scrotum that transilluminates; usually not painful

Causes

Closure of processus vaginalis trapping peritoneal fluid (non-communicating)

Closure of distal processus, trapping fluid in mid-portion of processus vaginalis (hydrocele of cord)

Failure of closure of processus vaginalis (communicating hydrocele)

Ipsilateral renal transplantation

Trauma

Tumors

Infection

Risk factors

Ventriculoperitoneal shunt

Exstrophy of the bladder

Ehlers–Danlos syndrome

Peritoneal dialysis

Diagnosis

Indirect inguinal hernia

Traumatic injury to testicle

Torsion of testicle or torsion of appendix testes

Orchtis

Epididymitis

Surgery

Inguinal approach with ligation of processus vaginalis, drainage of hydrocele sac in children. (In hydrocele of cord, sac can be completely removed)

Scrotal approach with drainage of hydrocele/resection of tunica vaginalis in adults

In adults no therapy is needed unless hydrocele causes discomfort or unless there is a significant underlying cause such as tumor

Jaboulay–Winkelmann procedure (for thick hydrocele sac) hydrocele sac wrapped posteriorly around cord structures

Lord procedure (for thin hydrocele sac) – radial sutures used to gather hydrocele sac posterior to testis/epididymis

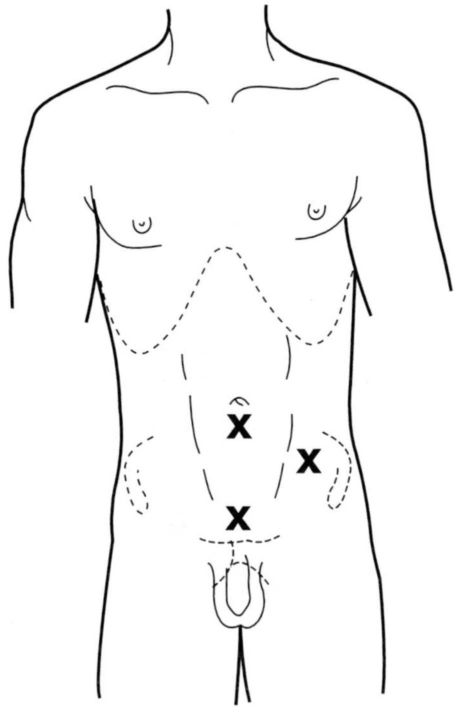

Figure 5.3 Laparoscopic Palomo varicocelectomy by transabdominal approach

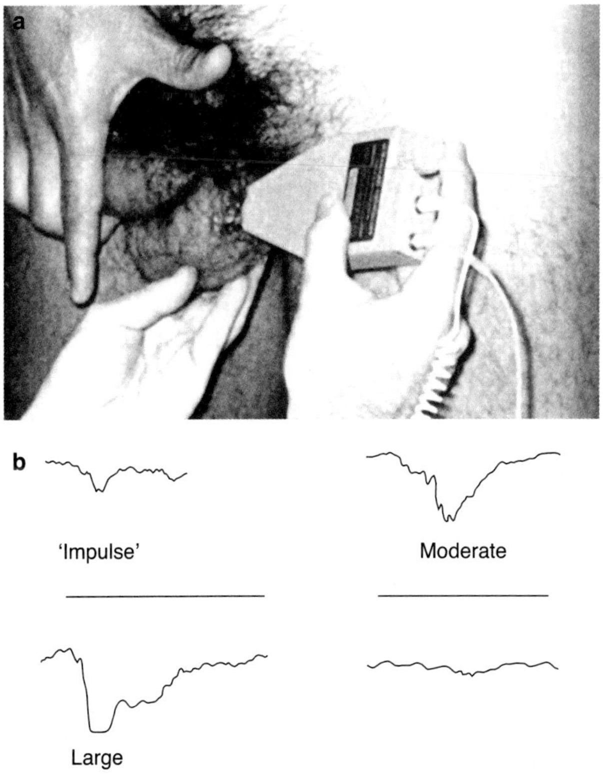

Figure 5.4 (**a**) Patient being examined with Doppler ultrasonic stethoscopy. (**b**) Recordings of varicoceles using the Doppler stethoscope. Courtesy Professor L. Lipschultz

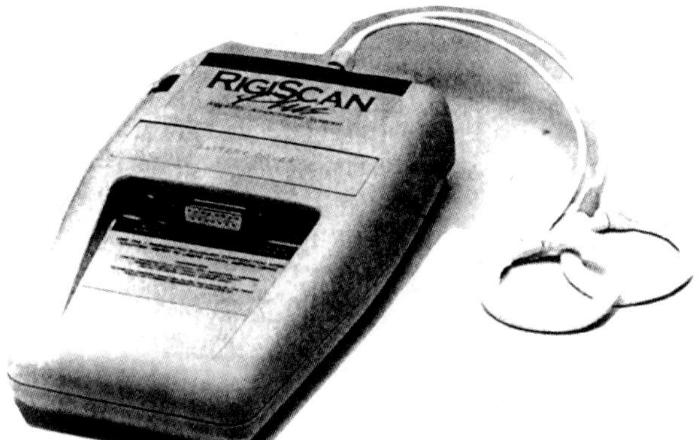

Figure 5.5 RigiScan™ portable monitoring device for at-home or in-office assessment of penile tumescence/rigidity changes. It comprises a microcomputer, loops placed around base/tip of shaft of penis and a logging unit (courtesy *Archives of Andrology*)

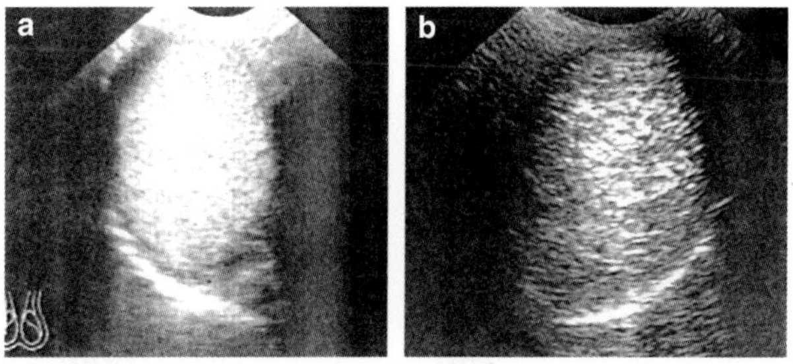

Figure 5.6 Scrotal sonography performed with a 7.5-MHz sector scanner of (**a**) normal and inhomogeneous parenchyma with numerous small hyperechogenic areas, and (**b**) inhomogeneous parenchyma carcinoma *in situ*. From Kamischke and Nieschlag (2002), with permission

late-phase disease, which consist of penile deviation when the penis is erect and erectile dysfunction.

Peyronie's disease affects 1–3% of the male population. Some 10% of men with erectile dysfunction have Peyronie's disease. The disease most commonly affects men older than 40 years and more than 75% of patients are between 45 and 65 years. The disease was first described in correspondence between Fallopius and Vesalius, but was later named after Francois de la Peyronie, who reported it in the medical literature in 1743. Although Peyronie's disease was described several centuries ago, the pathophysiology of the disease remains elusive.

While surgery is the main therapy for Peyronie's disease requiring correction of angulation, interest has grown in the application of extracorporeal shockwave therapy (ESWT) as a minimally invasive approach.

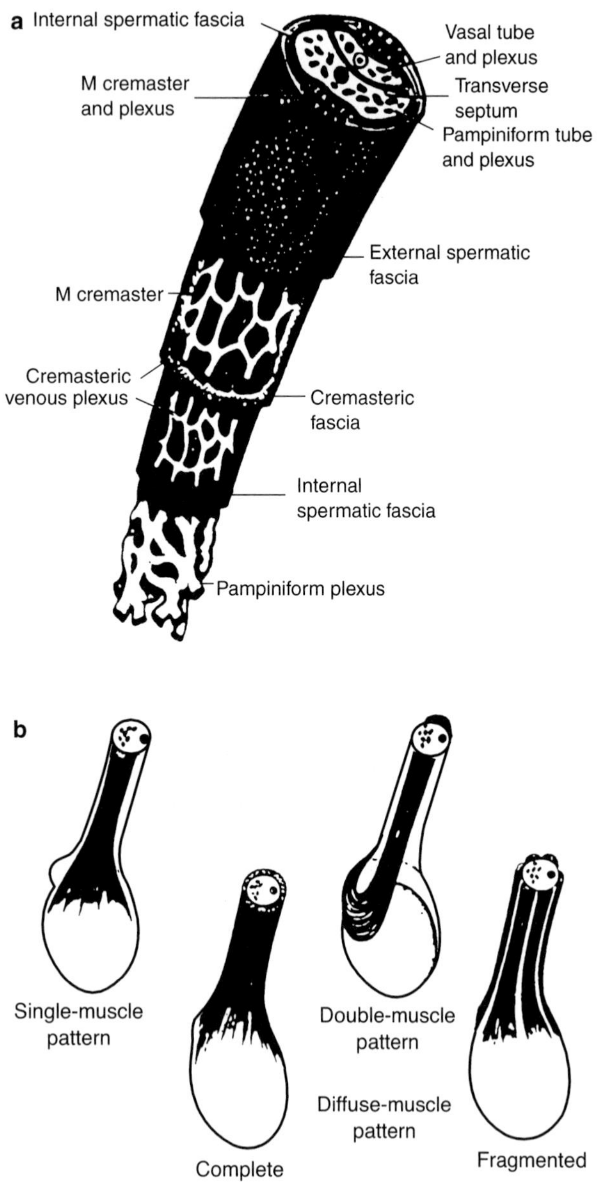

Figure 5.7 (**a**) Fasciomuscular tube (FMT) and the related venous plexuses. The FMT is divided into anterior pampiniform and posterior vasal compartment by a transverse septum. It acts as an 'autoelastic' stocking supporting cord veins and as a 'pump' pushing blood up the spermatic cord. It has 'sphincter' action, which prevents blood regurgitation. (**b**) Cremasteric 'externus' patterns. The muscle has thermoregulatory function. In cold weather its contraction 'internus' helps ductus deferens draining. (**c**) The scrotal ligament binds dartos muscle to lower testicular pole. It serves two functions: first, a thermoregulatory function, harmonizing testicular movement with dartos; and second, a synchronizing effect on the action of both dartos and cremasteric muscles throughout testicle. Absent ligament or aligomentous testicle syndrome leads to infertility. Courtesy Shafik and Olfat

Traditional therapy

Several modalities have been applied including oral, topical, injection and surgery therapy. Oral regimens employed include vitamin E, colchicines and tamoxifen. In addition to oral medication several intralesional injection therapies have been used, including steroids, verapamil and interferons. Unfortunately, the localized side-effects of steroids can be quite severe and have included tissue atrophy and skin thinning. These side-effects can make surgery, if required, technically difficult to perform. Furthermore, interferon and the calcium channel blocker verapamil have only moderate success. Iontophoresis has been used to deliver both verapamil and dexamethasone. Surgical treatment is used primarily in cases refractory to conservative management. There are three categories of surgery for penile curvature. They include tunical shortening and lengthening procedures, as well as placement of prostheses. The Nesbit and modified Nesbit techniques are shortening procedures and have met with positive results. However, complications of both procedures have included erectile dysfunction, penile hematoma, penile narrowing, urethral injury, herniation, glans numbness and phimosis.

Extracorporeal shockwave therapy

ESWT has been the gold standard in treating urolithiasis, and has also been used as an efficient method to treat calcification of connective tissue in orthopedics; furthermore, ESWT of salivary stones may be viable.

Table 5.3 Testicular torsion. Adapted from Dimbro, 2003

Description

Twisting of testis/spermatic cord resulting in acute ischemia

Intravaginal torsion: occurs within tunica vaginalis

Extravaginal torsion: involves twisting of testis, cord/processus vaginalis (especially in newborns)

Symptoms

Scrotum is enlarged, red/edematous

First symptom is pain (sudden or gradual onset, increasing in severity)

Testis may be high in scrotum with a transverse position

Absence of cremasteric reflex

Nausea/vomiting

Fever may occur

Testicle exquisitely tender

Causes

Torsion, spontaneous/idiopathic

History of trauma in 20% of patients

One-third of patients have had prior episodic testicular pain

Contraction of cremasteric or dartos muscle may be stimulated by trauma, exercise, cold, sexual stimulation

Possible alterations in testosterone levels during nocturnal sex response cycle; possible elevated testosterone levels in neonates

Testis must have inadequate, incomplete or absent fixation within scrotum

Risk factors

May be more common in winter

Paraplegia

Diagnosis

Epididymo-orchitis

Incarcerated/strangulated inguinal hernia

Acute hydrocele

Traumatic hematoma

Idiopathic scrotal edema

Torsion appendix testis

Acute varicocele

Testicular tumor

Scrotal abscess

Leukemic filtrate

Imaging

Ultrasound may confirm testicular swelling, Doppler is diagnostic

Surgery

Bilateral testicular fixation

At least 304-point fixation with no absorbable sutures

Excision of window of tunica albuginea with suture to dartos fascia

Any testis that is not clearly viable (and obvious) removed

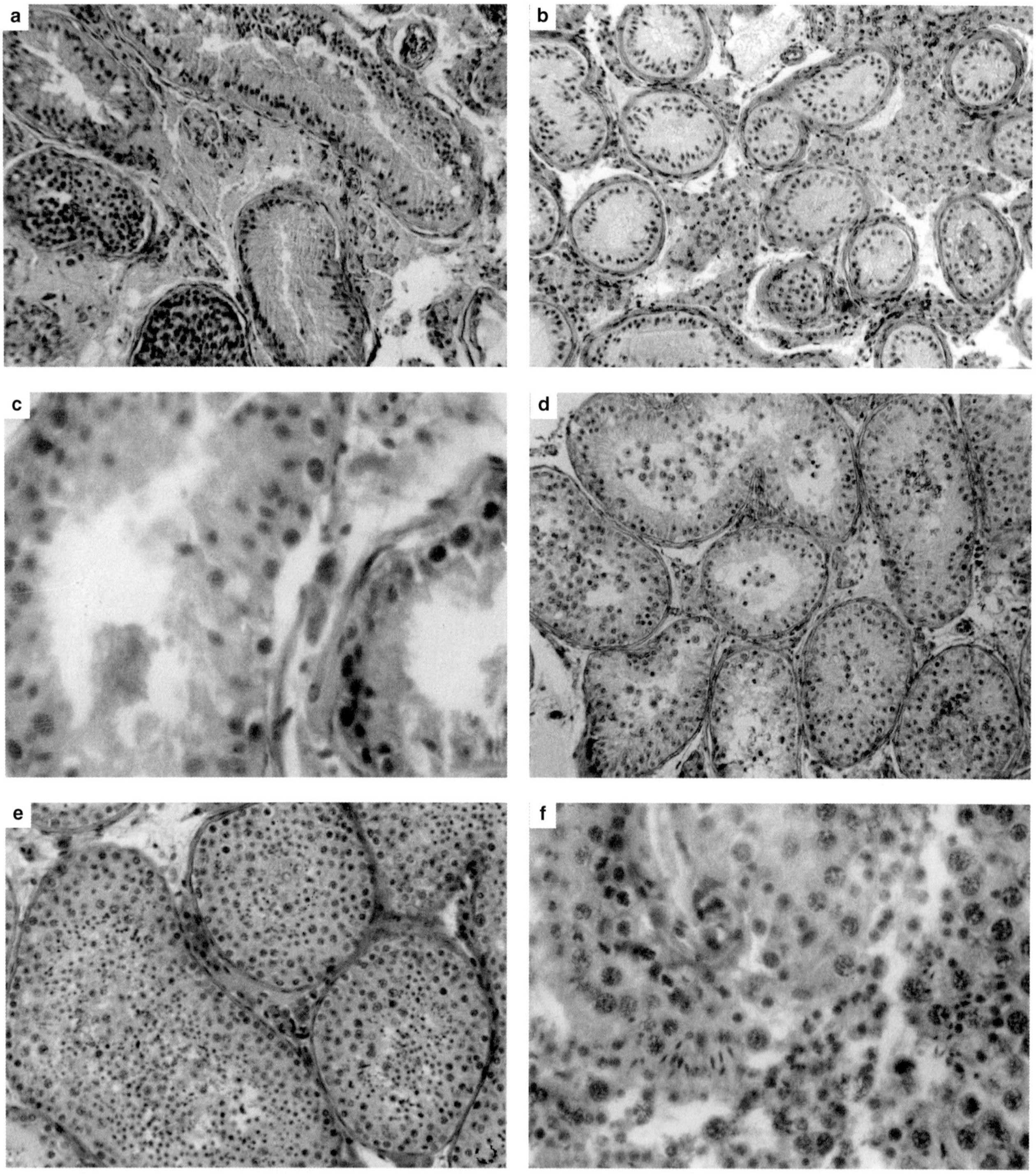

Figure 5.8 (**a**) Severe oligozoospermia 'Sertoli cell only', few tubules with inhibited spermatogenesis (150×). (**b**) Severe oligozoospermia, 'Sertoli cell only' (150×). (**c**) Spermatogenic arrest of spermatocyte stage (450×). (**d**) Spermatogenic arrest at primary spermatocyte stage (150×). (**e**) Spermatogenic arrest at spermatid stage (180×). (**f**) Spermatogenic arrest at late spermatid stage (400×)

Testicular torsion

Testicular torsion is a form of ischemia–reperfusion (I/R) injury, which requires early diagnosis and surgical intervention. Testicular torsion causes testicular injury and subfertility (Table 5.3). The pathophysiology of testicular torsion is associated with two types of cell death: necrosis and apoptosis.

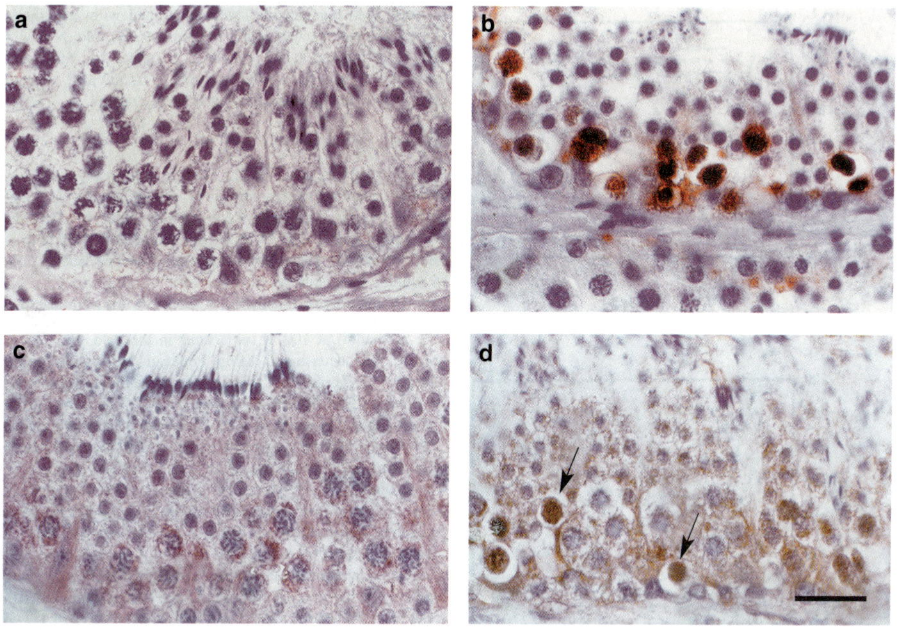

Color Plate 5.11 *In situ* detection of germ cell apoptosis in monkeys before (**a**) and after heat treatment (**b**). Cellular localization of apoptosis was characterized by terminal deoxynucleotidyl transferase mediated dUTP nick end labeling (TUNEL) assay. Methyl green was used as a counterstain. Many apoptotic germ cells (dark brown in color) were noted in testicular biopsies obtained 3 days after the first heat treatment (**b**) but not from control animal (**a**). Bax immunoactivity in the testis before (**c**) and after heat treatment (**d**). A portion of seminiferous tubule from a normal adult monkey showing that Bax is localized in the cytoplasm of germ cells, Sertoli cells and a small amount in Leydig cells (**c**), and from a monkey 3 days after the first heat treatment (**d**) displaying intense immunoactivity of Bax in apoptotic germ cells (arrows). Scale bar 25 μm. From Lue *et al.*, 2002, with permission

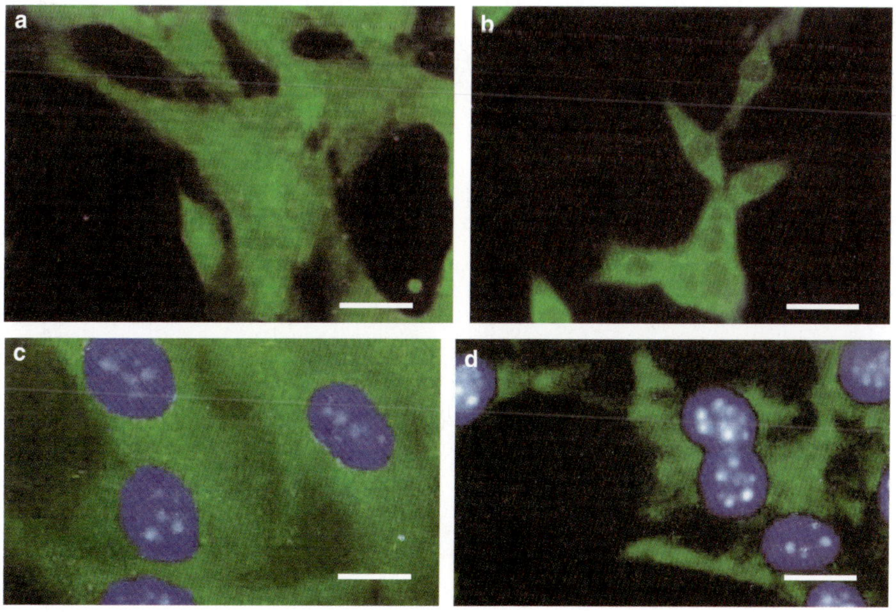

Color Plate 5.12 (**a**) and (**b**) Immunofluorescence of epididymal cell lines cultured for 1 week after approximately 30 passages on a glass slide with supplemented IMDM with 10% fetal calf serum and stained with PEB-like protein antibody (20 μg/ml). (**c**) and (**d**) Immunofluorescence of the cell lines cultured for 1–2 weeks after approximately 30 passages on glass slides with supplemented IMDM with 10% fetal calf serum, stained with a cytokeratin antibody (68 μg/ml). Cytokeratin immunofluorescent staining was green and Hoechst 33342-stained nuclei were blue. (**a**) PCl; (**b**) DC1; (**c**) PCl; (**d**) DC1. Bar 10 μm. From Araki *et al.*, 2002, with permission

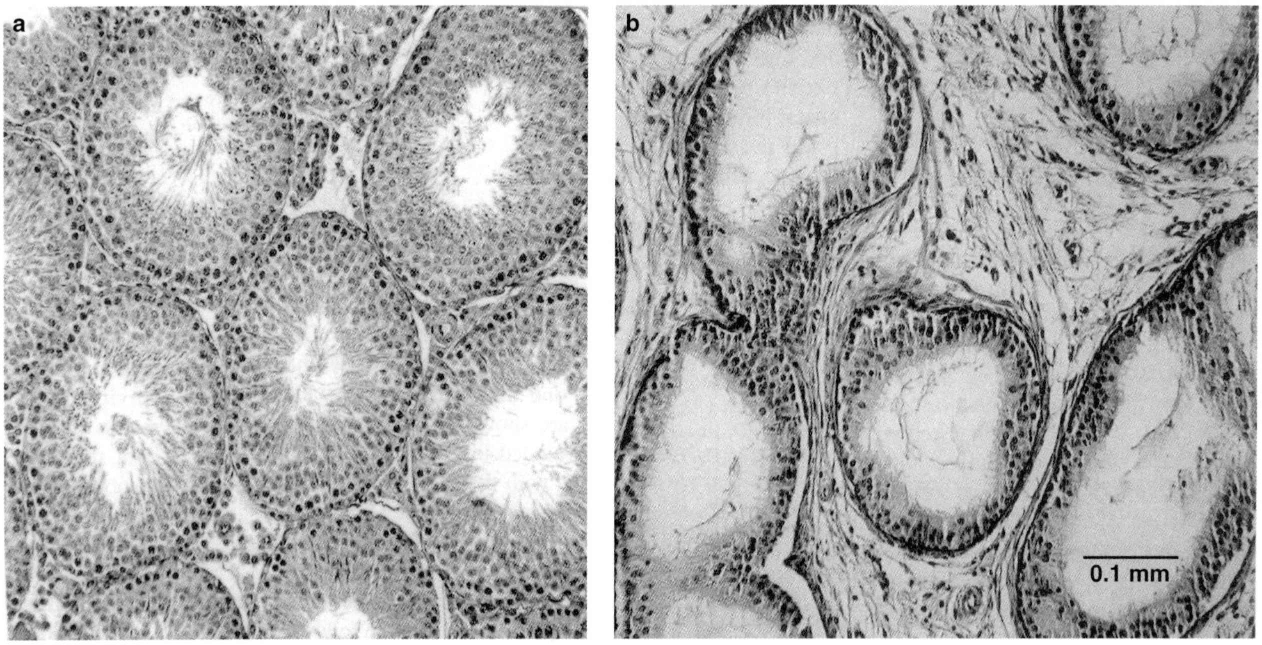

Figure 5.9 Comparison between normal testis (**a**) and altered testis with 'diffuse' abnormalities (**b**) obtained from rat rollowing unilateral vasectomy and stained with hematoxylin and eosin. From Chehval *et al.*, 2002, with permission

Unilaterial testicular torsion (UTT) increases the biochemical changes due to tissue hypoxia and the level of noradrenalin; also, chemical sympathectomy prevents the hypoxic changes after UTT in the contralateral testis. Testicular torsion can provoke contralateral hypoxia due to reduced blood flow through an autonomic nerve reflex. Nitric oxide (NO), derived from vascular endothelium, relaxes vascular smooth muscle. Basal NO release regulates vasodilatation and focal blood flow. NO also plays an important role in the induction of apoptosis, whereas NO protects the heart during I/R through protein kinase C (PKC) activation.

ANOMALIES OF SPERMATOGENESIS

There are different degrees of anomalies of spermatogenesis; spermatogenesis arrest may occur at different stages of spermiation (Figures 5.8–5.12; Table 5.4).

Azoospermia and aspermia

'Azoospermia' is the absence of sperm in a centrifuged semen sample, while 'aspermia' is an absent ejaculate. Azoospermia occurs in 5–20% of infertile men. Azoospermia can be obstructive or non-obstructive. Testicular biopsy of obstructive azoospermia shows sufficient spermatogenesis associated with physical occlusion of the reproductive tract distal to the testis that prevents sperm from entering the semen. The location of obstruction can be at one of several sites: caput epididymis, cauda epididymis, ejaculatory duct or congenital or non-congenital obstruction of the vas deferens. All forms of obstructive azoospermia can be circumvented with sperm retrieval and intracytoplasmic sperm injection (ICSI). Non-obstructive azoospermia (NOA) is caused by severely reduced sperm production. Several drugs affect sperm production and/or function: alcohol, alkylating agents, allopurinol, anabolic steroids, cimetidine, cocaine, colchicine, cyclosporin, erythromycin, gentamicin, marijuana, neomycin, nitrofurantoin, spironolactone, sulfasalazine and tetracyclines.

Further research is needed to evaluate the inheritance of chromosomal and genetic abnormalities in spermatogenesis that are transmitted only by ICSI. Chromosomal analysis of the male partner should be performed before ICSI treatment is initiated. There is an increased rate of chromosomal aberrations in ICSI patients with poor reproductive outcome. Chromosomal analysis is recommended not only for the male partner but

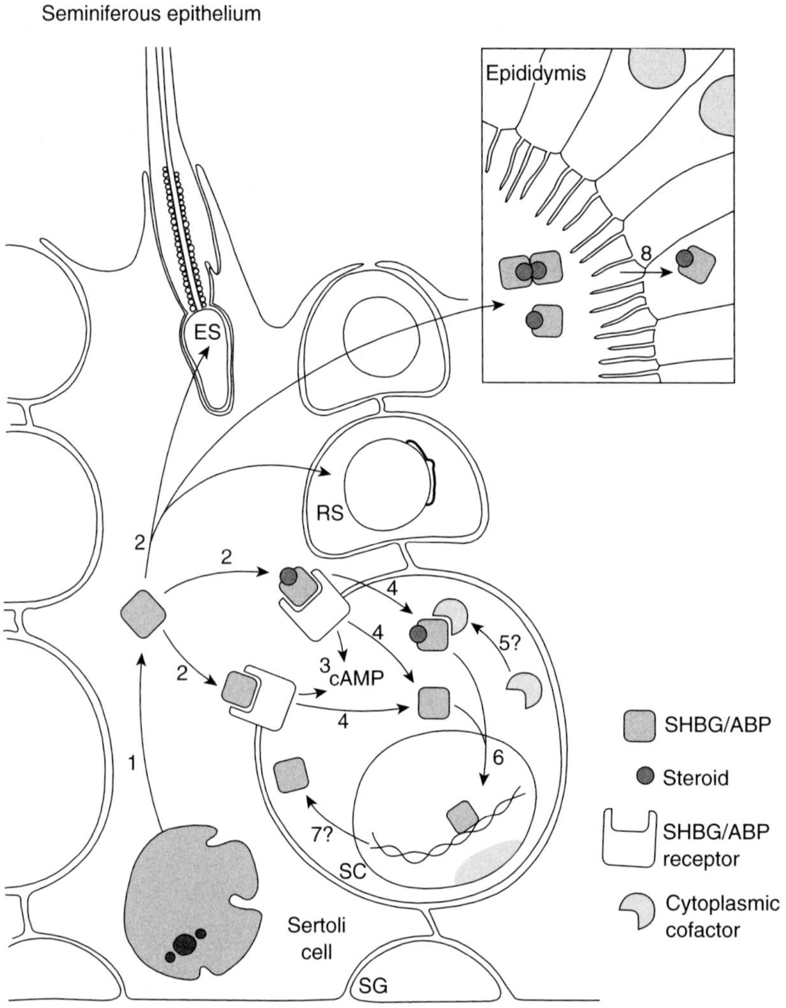

Figure 5.10 Diagrammatic illustration of the metabolic/molecular interactions of sex homone-binding globulin (SHBG) within the Sertoli cell. The following remain to be determined: (1) if human testis expresses both the secreted and the alternative form of SHBG/androgen-binding protein (ABP); (2) the proportional amount of each; (3) the cellular type responsible for the expression of each; (4) the steroid affinity of each; (5) the binding capacity of the alternative form of SHBG/ABP; (6) their mechanism of action (the existence and nature of the SHBG/ABP receptor and/or other interacting proteins); (7) the role of the alternative, cytoplasm form; and (8) the epididymal epithelium. From Munell *et al.*, 2002, with permission. ES, engulfing sperm; RS, spermatocyte; SG, spermatogonium; SC, Sertoli cell

also for the female partner in ICSI. In some cases of chromosomal inversion, recombination of chromosomes can occur during spermatogenesis, and eggs injected with such sperm cannot develop. Sperm chromosomal analysis should also be performed for couples with chromosomal aberrations diagnosed by peripheral cells. Chromosomal analyses of oligozoospermic men have usually been performed using heterologous ICSI of hamster eggs with human sperm, and metaphase chromosomes have been analyzed. However, this technique is not simple and more relevant and straightforward techniques for sperm chromosomal analysis should be developed. Preimplantation genetic diagnosis can be a powerful tool to exclude embryos that cannot develop due to the presence of such recombinant chromosomes.

Testicular hypoplasia

Hypoplasia of the testes is a congenital defect in which the potential for development of the spermatogenic epithelium is lacking. Inherited testicular hypoplasia is best known in Swedish Highland cattle and is caused by a recessive autonomic gene with incomplete (about 50%) penetrance.

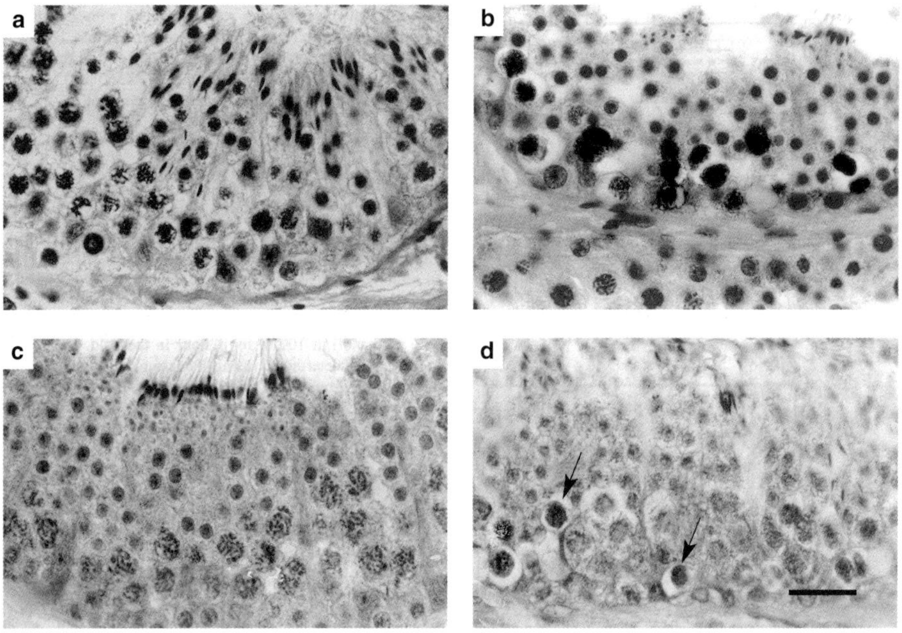

Figure 5.11 *In situ* detection of germ cell apoptosis in monkeys before (**a**) and after heat treatment (**b**). Cellular localization of apoptosis was characterized by terminal deoxynucleotidyl transferase mediated dUTP nick end labeling (TUNEL) assay. Methyl green was used as a counterstain. Many apoptotic germ cells (dark brown in color) were noted in testicular biopsies obtained 3 days after the first heat treatment (**b**) but not from control animal (**a**). Bax immunoactivity in the testis before (**c**) and after heat treatment (**d**). A portion of seminiferous tubule from a normal adult monkey showing that Bax is localized in the cytoplasm of germ cells, Sertoli cells and a small amount in Leydig cells (**c**), and from a monkey 3 days after the first heat treatment (**d**) displaying intense immunoactivity of Bax in apoptotic germ cells (arrows). Scale bar 25 μm. From Lue *et al.*, 2002, with permission. See also color plate

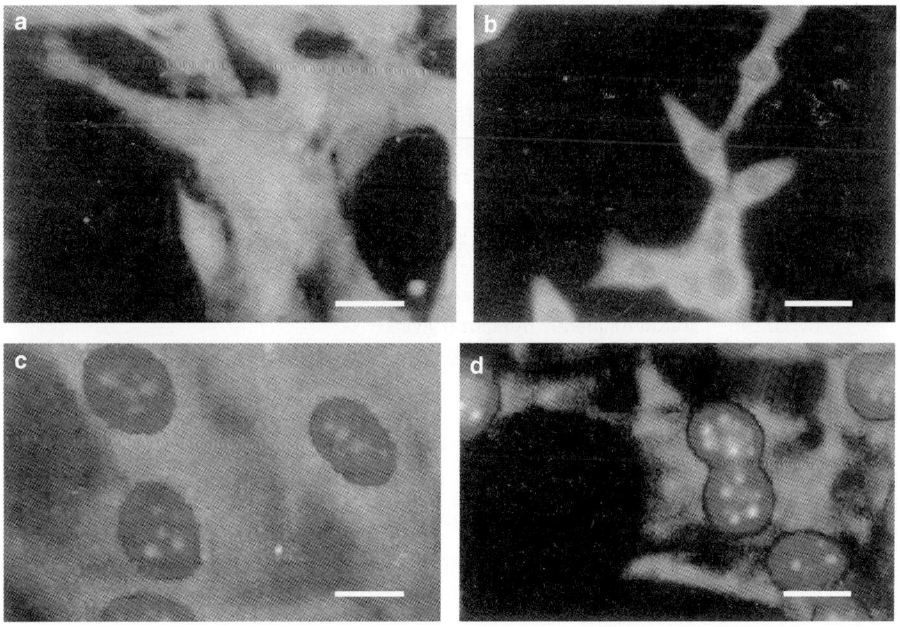

Figure 5.12 (**a**) and (**b**) Immunofluorescence of epididymal cell lines cultured for 1 week after approximately 30 passages on a glass slide with supplemented IMDM with 10% fetal calf serum and stained with PEB-like protein antibody (20 μg/ml). (**c**) and (**d**) Immunofluorescence of the cell lines cultured for 1–2 weeks after approximately 30 passages on glass slides with supplemented IMDM with 10% fetal calf serum, stained with a cytokeratin antibody (68 μg/ml). Cytokeratin immunofluorescent staining was green and Hoechst 33342-stained nuclei were blue. (**a**) PCl; (**b**) DC1; (**c**) PCl; (**d**) DC1. Bar 10 μm. From Araki *et al.*, 2002, with permission. See also color plate

Table 5.4 Testicular biopsy findings related to semen analysis and secondary sexual characteristics

Testicular biopsy interpretation		*Nature*	*Semen analysis*
Normal	Adult tubular size, thin wall and basement membrane	Obstructive	
		Complete	Azoospermia no sperma-togenic cells, pus cells may be present
	Regular and full spermatogenesis up to sperm formation	Incomplete	Severe oligospermia with spermatogenic cells
	Lumen present, interstitium narrow, with adult Leydig cells	Intermittent	Varying between azoo- and oligospermia
Spermatogenic arrest	Adult tubular size, wall thin or may show early thickening	Functional	
Spermatogonium	Only basal cell is intact with spermatogonia and Sertoli cells, wide lumen		Azoospermia
Primary spermatocyte	Spermatogenesis up to primary spermatocyte, few or no spermatids, hypo- or hypercellularity		Azoospermia few or no spermatogenic cells
Spermatid complete or partial arrest	Spermatogenesis up to early to late spermatid, often associated with hypercellularity; no or few spermatozoa		Spermatogenic cells few or no sperm
Sertoli cell only	Tubular size small or normal, wall thin or shows early thickening, complete absence of spermato-genic cells, only Sertoli cells, and their cytoplasms	Congenital	Azoospermia no spermatozoa or spermatogenic cells
	Leydig cells normal or show hyperplasia		
Mixed Sertoli cell only	Sertoli cell-only tubules mixed with normal tubules or tubules with disturbed spermatogenesis	Functional	Azoospermia or oligospermia
Prepubertal	Tubules of small diameter, thin wall, no basement membrane, lumen absent or small, only two types of cells: primary spermatogenic cells and undifferentiated cells	Hypogonado-tropic hypopituitarism	Azoospermia, very small volume with no spermatozoa
	Leydig cells are absent		
Multiple lesions	Appearance is not uniform, with mixed areas of Sertoli cell-only tubules	Functional	Azoospermia or severe oligospermia
	Partially and completely hyalinized tubules		
	Leydig cells often show hyperplasia, which is more pronounced in areas completely hyalinized giving an appearance similar to Klinefelter's syndrome		
Azoospermatogenesis	Tubules are of normal adult size	Functional	Severe oligospermia or azoospermia
	Thinning of spermatogenic cells, tubular hyalinization		
Early diffuse (TH)	Diffuse early to moderate peritubular thickening	Functional	Oligospermia
	Various grades of inhibited spermatogenesis		
Focal TH	Areas of TH mixed with tubules showing disturbed spermatogenesis	Functional	Severe oligospermia
Progressive	Generalized, moderate to severe peritubular thickening	Functional	Azoospermia
	Residual Sertoli cells and few spermatogenic cells		
	Leydig cells commonly show diffuse hyperplasia		

Table 5.4 (Continued)

Testicular biopsy interpretation		*Nature*	*Semen analysis*
Klinefelter's syndrome	Tubules of small diameter, completely hyalinized or show Sertoli cells, hyperplasia of Leydig cells in clumps so that tubules appear relatively empty with few cells and wide lumen	Chromosomal aberration	Azoospermia
Sloughing	Tubules are of normal adult size tubular wall is thin Basal cells layers are intact, the more mature cells are sloughed in lumen so that only few spermatozoa are formed and their passage is blocked by the sloughed cells Leydig cells are normal	Functional	Oligospermia or severe oligospermia many spermatogenic cells
Sloughing and disorganization	As above in addition to disordering arrangement of cells commonly associated with mild to moderate diffuse peritubular thickening Leydig cells are normal or show mild degree of diffuse hyperplasia	Functional	Severe oligospermia or azoospermia with spermatogenic cells, both normal and abnormal

Disease of testes and/or accessory glands

Pathological conditions of the testes, epididymis and seminal vesicles may interfere with fertilization by disturbing spermatogenesis of sperm maturation, causing abnormal semen characteristics, or preventing the passage of sperm from the testes to the urethra.

CHROMOSOMAL AND GENETIC ANOMALIES (TABLE 5.5)

Chromosomal arrangements occur during mitosis and meiosis. Normally the ovum (X) is fertilized by sperm bearing an X or a Y chromosome. In abnormal cases of non-disjunction of oogenesis or spermatogenesis, fertilization may occur between an abnormal sperm and/or an abnormal egg, resulting in various chromosomal anomalies. Structural anomalies of the chromosomes include translocations, deletions, rings and inversions of chromosomes during either mitosis or meiosis. Such anomalies affect individual autosomes or sex chromosomes. The human cell comprises a nucleus, protein-manufacturing units and energy-production points. The sequence or layout of the DNA contains all the instructions the cell needs to function. Recent advances in genetic engineering have

Table 5.5 Chromosomes and genetic inheritance phenomena

Dominant inheritance
New mutations
Incomplete penetrance
Variable expressivity
Gonadal mosaicism
Mechanisms of dominance
Autosomal recessive inheritance
X-chromosome inactivation
X-linked dominant inheritance
X-linked recessive disorders
Genomic imprinting
Unstable DNA
Fragile X syndrome (MIM 309550)
Other disorders
Myotonic dystrophy (MIM 160900)
Huntington's disease (HD; MIM 143100)
Spinocerebellar ataxia type I (olivopontocerebellar degeneration; SCA1; MIM 164400)
Dentatorubropallidoluysian atrophy (DRPLA; MIM 125370)
Machado–Joseph disease (MIM 109150)
Kennedy's disease (spinal and bulbar muscular atrophy, partial androgen resistance)
Genetic diagnosis by linkage (gene tracking)

enabled scientists to uncover, rearrange and make copies, or clones, of genes. For example, each cell contains some 100 000 genes. At least 22 000 of these genes have been isolated, and some of their specific functions have been identified.

Chromosomal defects (Table 5.6)

Male infertility may be caused by a variety of chromosomal abnormalities:

(1) Abnormalities in sex chromosomes or autosomes;

(2) Gain or loss of an entire single chromosome resulting in aneuploidy, whereas a polyploid state occurs when the entire chromosomal content is multiplied (polyploid cells are most commonly associated with malignancies);

(3) Structural abnormalities which include the rearrangement or translocation of fragments of chromosomes, as in Robertsonian translocations, or deletions of single genes or portions of a chromosome (Maduro *et al.*, 2003).

DNA fragmentation in testicular sperm

There is a negative correlation between sperm DNA fragmentation and embryo cleavage and pregnancy rates obtained with ICSI, underlining the importance of sperm DNA quality. Aging affects chromosomal structural abnormalities and generation of reactive oxygen species. Because the sulfhydryl (SH) bonds are not oxidized until transit through the epididymis, testicular sperm DNA packaging is not complete, and their DNA may be more susceptible to assault. DNA integrity is determined by modified alkaline single-cell gel electrophoresis.

Of the structural anomalies of chromosomal aberrations in ICSI fetuses, ten have been reported to be of paternal origin. It is suggested that chromosomal anomalies after ICSI are the result of not only the incidence of cytogenetic anomalies of the male infertility patient but also the ICSI technique itself. There are some differences in the 'choreography' of the cell cycle of fertilization between *in vitro* fertilization (IVF) and ICSI using non-human primates as a model.

Decondensation of sperm nuclei occurs initially in the basal region and the apical region remains condensed, surrounded by the perinuclear theca, a structure typically removed during sperm incorporation into the egg. This unusual nuclear remodeling in the first cell cycle of ICSI may not allow the

Table 5.6 Genetic etiologies of human male infertility. Developmental disorders causing human male infertility result from a failure of gonadal development or testis determination, endocrinopathies, well-known genetic syndromes, and numerical and structural chromosomal abnormalities (translocations, deletions and inversions). From Maduro and Lamb, 2002

Sex determination/development
Pseudohermaphroiditism (NRSAI)
Sex reversal (SOX9, SRY, NROBI)
Denys–Drash (WT1)
Pseudovaginal perineoscrotal
Hypostasis (SRD5A, SRD5A2)
Cryptorchidism (HOXA10, INSL3, GREAT)
CBAVD (CFTR)
PMDS (AMH, AMHR)
Endocrinopathies
Hypogonadotropic hypogonadism (GNRH, KAL, PCI, GNRHR, LEP, PCSK1)
Pituitary/gonadotropin defects (LHB, CGLHR, HESXI, LHX3, PROP1)
Steroid biosynthesis (SIAR, CYP21, TDD, CYP17)
Steroid metabolism (SRD5, SRD5A)
Steroid action (AAR, ESA1)
Sperm production/function
Mytonoic dystrophy (DMPK)
Noonan syndrome (PTPN1)
Sickle cell anemia (HRB)
Kartagener syndrome (DNAI1, DNAH5)
β-Thalassemia (HBB)
Primary ciliary duskiness (DNAI1, DNAH5)
Fancon anemia (FANCA)
Ataxia telangiectasia (ATM)
Chromosomal (numerical/structural)
Klinefelter's syndrome (XXY; XXXY)
Mixed gonadal dygenesis (45X; 46XXY)
Translocations (including Robertsonian)
Inversions
Deletions
Y chromosome microdeletions
XX male
XY female

CBAVD, congential bilateral absence of the vas deferens; PMDS, persistent Müllerian duct syndrome synchronized decongestion of chromosomes and may introduce a delay of the S-phase entry of the male pronucleus, leading to mitotic errors during the first cleavage. Karyoanalysis is used to elucidate the relationships between various types of congenital disorders and the abnormalities in chromosomes. Although, to date, only light microscopy has been used for this type of study, scanning electron microscopy can be applied to this field and serves to elucidate the changes of chromosomes at the submicroscopic level.

Klinefelter's syndrome

The most common chromosomal anomaly in infertile men is Klinefelter's syndrome (KS). In men with non-obstructive azoospermia, such as men with non-mosaic KS, there is no clinical marker to predict the success of sperm recovery with testicular sperm extraction (TESE). Serum inhibin B is a useful predictor of spermatogenesis in men with oligozoospermia and azoospermia. Diagnostic TESE has been successfully applied to identify the presence of sperm in men with KS. The application of TESE with subsequent ICSI results in pregnancy. Inhibin B is not predictive of successful surgical sperm recovery in men with non-mosaic Klinefelter's syndrome. Even a concentration of serum inhibin B below the level of detection does not exclude foci of spermatogenesis. We recommend that all our azoospermic men with Klinefelter's syndrome have a diagnostic TESE before treatment unless donor sperm backup is available and fully accepted by the couple (Westlander *et al.*, 2003).

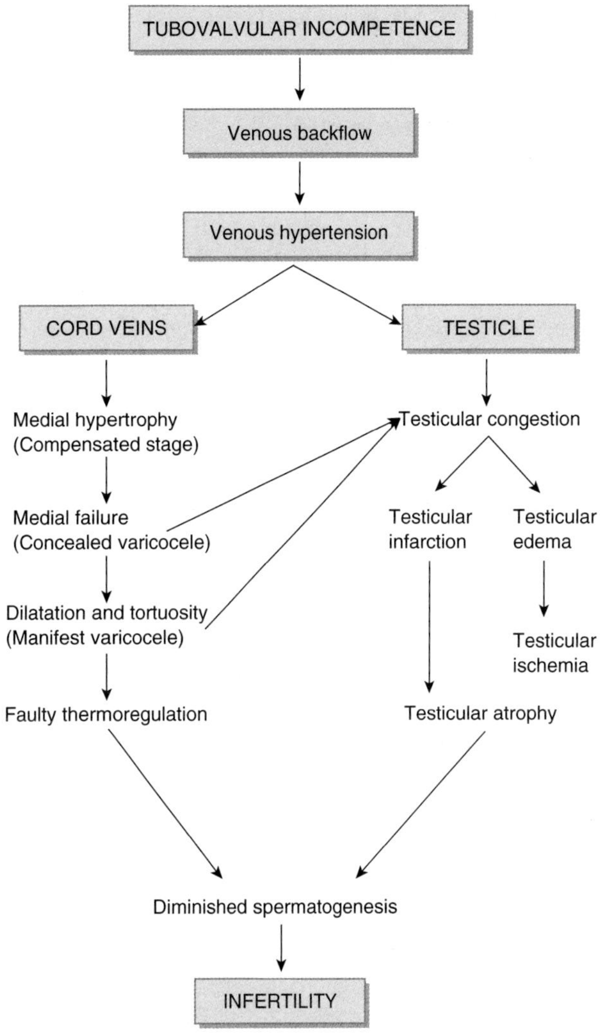

Figure 5.13 Mechanism of varicocele formation. Upon venous backflow and hypertension, three pathological stages occur in varicocele: medial hypertrophy – no blood stasis, symptomless (compensated); medial failure – leading to venous stasis but no clinical varicocele (concealed varicocele) leading to infertility; dilatation – prolonged stasis leading to varicosity (manifest varicocele) leading to infertility

BIOCHEMICAL PARAMETERS

Varicocele and antioxidant capacity

The damage inflicted to sperm by reactive oxygen species (ROS) plays a major role in male infertility. Sperm have a high content of polyunsaturated fatty acids within the plasma membrane and a low concentration of scavenging enzymes in the cytoplasm, and they are susceptible to peroxidation in the presence of elevated seminal ROS levels. Seminal plasma and sperm possess a variety of antioxidant systems to counteract the effects of ROS. The seminal plasma is endowed with antioxidant buffer capacity, and the protective system includes chain-breaking antioxidants capable of reducing oxidant radical levels and blunting the propagation of free radical chain reactions. However, sperm possess a small amount of cellular ROS defense system that consists of catalase, superoxide dismutase, glutathione peroxides and vitamin E.

Meucci *et al.* (2003) evaluated a possible molecular defect linked to infertility, studying total antioxidant capacity (TAC) of seminal plasma in varicocele (VAR) (Figure 5.13). The latency phase, proportional to antioxidant concentration, showed significantly greater values in all VAR patients. VAR patients undergoing surgery may suffer from ejaculatory dysfunction after treatment.

Proacrosin, acrosin and idiopathic infertility

Acrosin (EC 3.4.21.10) is a trypsin-like endprotease localized on the sperm acrosome, that aids in sperm penetration by limited proteolysis of zona pellucida (ZP) lipoproteins. Acrosin protease activity is involved in dissolution of the acrosomal matrix, and in a regulated release of acrosomal contents at the time of the acrosome reaction. Independent of its proteolytic activity, acrosin binds lipoproteins from the extracellular egg coat, supporting its participation in secondary sperm binding to the ZP. Acrosin is synthesized and stored as its inactive zymogen, proacrosin. During the acrosome reaction, proacrosin is converted to the mature enzyme B-acrosin and released. Proacrosin activation involves processing the 53–55-kDa proenzyme to 50–40-kDa activation intermediates, the 34-kDa mature enzyme and lower molecular weight forms. The presence of human proacrosin/acrosin in whole sperm can be detected by immunocytochemistry with specific antibodies.

Biochemical and molecular evaluation of the proacrosin–acrosin system in patients undergoing treatment with standard IVF–embryo transfer (ET) has been performed. Male patients diagnosed with unexplained infertility were only included in the study group to avoid other factors that could contribute to abnormal fertilization. The studies involved evaluation of acrosin activity in ejaculated sperm, the proacrosin–acrosin system in whole sperm by immunocytochemistry, proacrosin activation patterns in sperm protein extracts, and nucleotide sequence around the amino acids of the catalytic triad by single-strand conformation polymorphism (SSCP) analysis. In the study group, the mean value of acrosin activity was 53 μIU/million spermatozoa (range 5.8–135). Five of the 27 cases (19%) showed abnormal activity (Hafez, unpublished data).

SYNDROMES OF MALE INFERTILITY

Idiopathic male infertility

Routine semen analysis using light microscopy is used for the initial evaluation of the male of an infertile couple. However, the diagnosis of defective sperm function by standard semen analysis is difficult because sperm are highly specialized cells that express a diverse array of biological properties to achieve fertilization. Sperm DNA damage is significantly increased in men with idiopathic and male factor infertility, and in men who fail to initiate a pregnancy after assisted reproductive techniques. Such an increase in sperm damage may be related to high levels of seminal oxidative stress (Saleh *et al.*, 2003).

Psychosocial parameters of the infertile couple

Infertile couples are characterized by various psychosocial parameters: anger, grief, guilt, frustration, depression, feelings of isolation and powerlessness, marital problems, separation and divorce. However, sporadic conception is noted in infertile couples after or during romantic holidays, after adoption or after abandoning treatment in an infertility clinic. Spontaneous pregnancy occurs in some 10% of untreated infertile couples with oligozoospermic men, in patients placed for 1–2 years on a waiting list for IVF or ICSI. 'Psychogenic infertility' is associated with chronic and acute stress, with transitory azoospermia or oligospermia. De Gennaro *et al.* (2003) studied normozoospermic and oligozoospermic men for differences in alexithymia (difficulty identifying feelings, difficulty describing feelings, externally oriented thinking), personality traits (extroversion, neuroticism, psychoticism) and coping style toward stressors (task-oriented coping, emotion-oriented coping, avoidance-oriented coping). Significant relationships were noted between these variables and semen characteristics.

Testicular germ cell tumor

Germ cell tumor of the testis (TGCT) is the most common malignancy in 15–35-year-old men. The combination of surgery, radiotherapy and chemotherapy has made TGCT curable in 90% of patients with newly diagnosed disease (Figure 5.14; Tables 5.7– 5.9). Most of the patients have decreased baseline spermatogenesis at the time of diagnosis, a pre-existing defect in spermatogenesis, a history of cryptorchidism, hormone production by the tumor, antisperm antibodies, possible contralateral or intraepithelial germ cell neoplasia, and/or generalized stress associated with illness. Cryptorchidism is

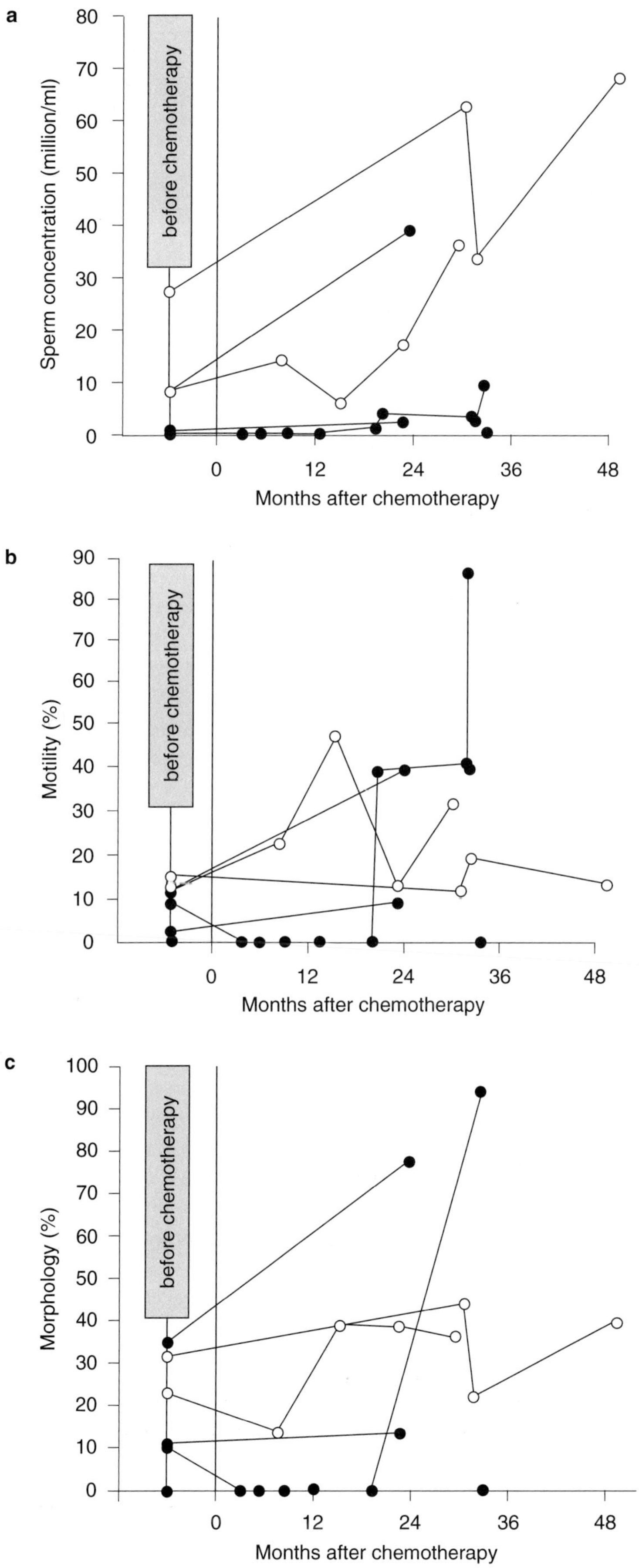

Figure 5.14 Seminal parameters after chemotherapy in patients with testicular germ cell tumor: (**a**) sperm concentration, (**b**) motility and (**c**) morphology. Open circles, patients with normal β-human chorionic gonadotropin (βhCG); closed circles, patients with high βhCG. Courtesy Professor Tomomasa

Table 5.7 Testicular malignancies

Description

Primary testicular neoplasms may arise from any testicular or adnexal cell component. They are divided into germinal (90–95%) and non-germinal tumors. The germinal tumors are further divided into seminomatous/non-seminomatous types (embryonic, teratoma, choriocarcinomas, yolk sac)

Clinical staging

A: tumor limited to testis cord
B: tumor of testis and retroperitoneal nodes
B1: <6 nodes >2 cm in diameter
B2: >6 nodes >2 cm in diameter
B3: positive retroperitoneal nodes >5 cm in diameter (bulky)
C: metastases above diaphragm or involving abdominal solid organs

Symptoms

In adults

testicular nodule or swelling most common
sensation of fullness or heaviness of scrotum
previously 'small' testicle enlarging to size of 'normal' contralateral one
firm, non-tender mass within confines of tunica albuginea usually palpable distinct from cord structures
acute or chronic epididymitis/epididymo-orchitis resulting in delay of diagnosis (10%)
manifestations due to metastasis, e.g. neck mass (supra-clavicular node), respiratory symptoms (lung metastasis), low back pain, uni- or bilateral lower extremity swelling, palpable abdominal mass
hydrocele (10–20%)
gynecomastia (may or may not be due to elevated hormones (5%))
rapid tumor growth resulting in hemorrhage/necrosis

In children

non-tender, non-painful scrotal mass
non-transilluminable, large, non-tender testicle
hydrocele (15–20%)
with hormonally active tumors, the scrotal examination may be unrevealing

Causes

No real clear cause and effect relationships identified

Diagnosis

Hernia
Hydrocele
Hematoma
Spermatocele
Syphilitic gumma
Varicocele
In children – epidermis/dermoid cyst, paratesticular rhabdomyosarcoma, macroorchidism, torsion epididymitis

Imaging

Scrotal ultrasound – with mass clearly originating within testis with echo-texture pattern (hypoechoic) distinct from surrounding normal testicular tissue.
Echo-texture may be mixed

Treatment

Commonly used chemotherapeutic agents include cisplatin + etoposide ± blood, palliate (taxol)
Salvage chemotherapy includes cyclophosphamide (Cytoxan), ifosfamide (with mesna to protect against hemorrhagic cystitis), carbolated, chemotherapy intensification with granulocyte colony stimulating factor (G-CSF) or autologous bone marrow transplant (BMT)
In children – incrusting, dactinomycin (actinomycin D, cyclophosphamide, doxorubicin)

Table 5.8 Clinical staging of testicular germ-cell tumors according to the Lugano classification

Clinical stage	*Description*
I	No evidence of metastases
IA	Tumor limited to testis and epididymis
IB	Infiltration of spermatic cord or tumor in cryptorchid testicle
IC	Infiltration of the scrotum, trans-scrotal surgery, tumor developing after trans-scrotal or inguinal surgery
IX	Extent of primary tumor cannot be evaluated
II	Retroperitoneal lymph-node metastases
IIA	All lymph nodes ≤2 cm
IIB	More than one lymph node 2–5 cm
IIC	Lymph nodes >5 cm
IID	Abdominal tumor palpable, fixed inguinal tumor
III	Mediastinal and supraclavicular lymph-node metastases, visceral metastases
IIIA	Mediastinal and supraclavicular lymph-node metastases only
IIIB	Pulmonary metastases only
IIIC	Hematogenous metastases outside the lung
IIID	Persistent elevated markers without evidence of metastases

Table 5.9 A prognostic factor-based staging system for metastatic germ cell cancers. From International Germ Cell Consensus Classification Group, 1997

Good prognosis
Non-seminoma
primary testicular cancer or extragonadal retroperitoneal cancer, AFP < 1000 ng/ml, hCG < 5000 IU/ml, LDH < 1.5 × normal
Seminoma
no extrapulmonary visceral metastases
all primary locations
all elevated serum markers
Intermediate prognosis
Non-seminoma
primary testicular cancer or extragonadal retroperitoneal cancer, AFP 1000-10 000 ng/ml, hCG < 5000–50 000 IU/ml, LDH 1.5–10 × normal
no extrapulmonary visceral metastases
all primary locations
all elevated serum markers
extrapulmonary visceral metastases (liver, bones, CNS)
Poor prognosis
Non-seminoma
extragonadal mediastinal germ cell tumor
primary testicular/retroperitoneal germ cell tumor with extrapulmonary metastases

AFP, α-fetoprotein; hCG, human chorionic gonadotropin, LDH, lactate dehydrogenase; CNS, central nervous system

associated with both testicular cancer and infertility. Although the majority of patients with testicular cancer have fulfilled their wishes with regard to children, it seems to be more difficult to father a child after treatment compared with the general population. Because it is not possible to predict which patient will have fertility problems after treatment, cryopreservation of sperm should be offered to every testicular cancer patient (Spermon *et al.*, 2003). Deterioration of spermatogenesis occurs after adjuvant radio- or chemotherapeutic treatment in a dose-dependent fashion. Some patients remain azoospermic after treatment while others undergoing surgery may suffer from ejaculatory dysfunction after treatment.

6

Semen, sperm anomalies and infertility

Sperm are antigenic when injected subcutaneously into females. Thus, there are several physiological mechanisms to remove sperm from the female reproductive tract after intercourse. This removal takes the form of phagocytosis; deposition of sperm induces an influx of phagocytic cells (neutrophils, macrophages and dendritic-like cells) into the reproductive tract. Seminal plasma contains various molecules that can inhibit lymphocyte activation. Lymphocytes in the lymph nodes draining the uterus can become activated by seminal plasma, perhaps because immunosuppresants are inactivated as sperm antigens reach the lymph nodes. Despite the presence of mechanisms to prevent immune responses to sperm, females can develop anti-sperm immunity, and antibodies directed towards sperm can occasionally be recovered from the reproductive tract (Hansen, 2000).

In oligozoospermic men there is a higher rate of apoptotic DNA in sperm. In fertile men, the simple selection of motile sperm can eliminate most of the apoptotic sperm. However, the higher percentage of apoptotic sperm from severe oligoasthenozoospermic men could lead to the risk of injection of sperm with fragmented DNA.

SEMINAL PLASMA

Male accessory sex organs, made of epithelial/mesenchymal components, require androgens for proliferation and maintenance of their function. There are three types of epithelial cells: secretory glandular cells, non-secretory basal cells and neuroendocrine cells:

(1) Basal cells, which are stem cells for secretory epithelial cells, are androgen-independent because they do not express androgen receptors.

Table 6.1 Some biochemical markers to identify the source of secretions within the ejaculate by the presence of different ejaculate components

Source of secretion	*Biochemical markers*
Testes	Androgen-binding protein Inhibin Testosterone Transferrin
Epididymal ducts	Carnitine Glycerophosphorylcholine Inositol
Seminal vesicles	Fructose Prostaglandins
Prostate	Acid phosphatase Citrate Calcium, zinc Spermine Vesiculase
Bulbourethral/urethral glands	IgA Mucoproteins

(2) Neuroendocrine cells play a role in regulating the growth and function of secretory cells.

(3) Mesenchyme comprises smooth muscle cells, fibroblasts, lymphocytes and neuromuscular tissue embedded in an extracellular matrix.

Several biochemical markers are used to identify the source of secretions within the ejaculate by the presence of different components (Table 6.1).

SPERM ANOMALIES

The World Health Organization (1999) has developed 'strict criteria' for sperm normality. Several classifications

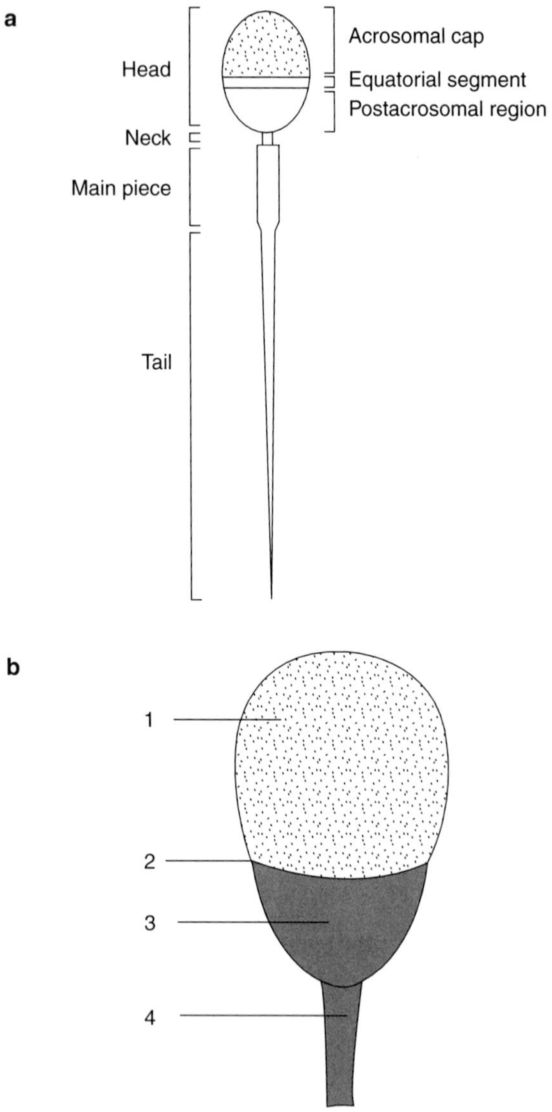

Figure 6.1 (**a**) Sperm membrane regions. Reproduced with permission of Hemisphere Publishing. (**b**) Plasma membrane surface domains: (1) the acrosomal segment with some particles; (2) the equatorial segment showing a striated morphology; (3) the post-acrosomal segment with abundant particles; and (4) the tail segment (middle piece and main piece) with dispersed particles. (From Calamera (1998), with permission)

have been designed to describe sperm abnormalities (Figures 6.1–6.5; Tables 6.2 and 6.3). The following groups are of special physiological significance:

(1) Head abnormalities (Figures 6.6–6.9):
  (a) large heads;
  (b) small heads;
  (c) elongated/tapering heads;
  (d) duplicated heads;
  (e) amorphous heads;
  (f) loose heads;
(2) Tail abnormalities;
(3) Neck/middle piece abnormalities;
(4) Cytoplasmic droplets.

Every man has a certain percentage of sperm that are defective in one or more attributes. Such sperm are unlikely to be able to fertilize an oocyte. Many sperm are defective in more than one attribute. Also, many sperm that are not detected as defective may have a problem that prevents them from fertilizing an oocyte. There are several laboratory assays which can predict if an individual male is likely to be subfertile or sterile. Subfertile men may be able to fertilize an oocyte by the application of *in vitro* fertilization (IVF) or intrauterine insemination (IUI). Cleavage is probably the best measure for fertility in IVF, but passage through two to three cleavage divisions is not predictive that an embryo will complete embryogenesis and fetal development. The number of sperm in an IVF droplet or IUI dose is substantially in excess of the minimum number needed to maximize 'success', although it is balanced with the requirement to minimize polyspermy.

Table 6.4 summarizes the andrological terminology used to describe semen deviations. Since it is often the practice to describe all deviations from normal semen variables with words, the international nomenclature was introduced, because these terms may have different values in different laboratories.

Sperm surface in HIV patients

In the initial stages of HIV infection, the patient may ejaculate motile (and fertile) sperm. Some patients undergoing highly active antiretroviral therapy (HAART) produce active sperm with normal motility (Figure 6.10). Antiviral regimens affect lymphocytes and sperm chromosomes, morphology and semen quality in HIV patients. HIV particles are present on the sperm membrane as determined by labeling with monoclonal or polyclonal anti-HIV antibodies.

Atomic force microscopy (AFM) is a powerful technique to evaluate any alterations in the sperm of HIV patients, and the effects of HAART including minute details, e.g. viral particles on sperm membrane. AFM, unlike electron microscopy, permits virions to be imaged in almost their natural environment and identification of possible membrane penetration or any budding (Joshi *et al.*, 2000, 2001a, 2001b). An AFM unit

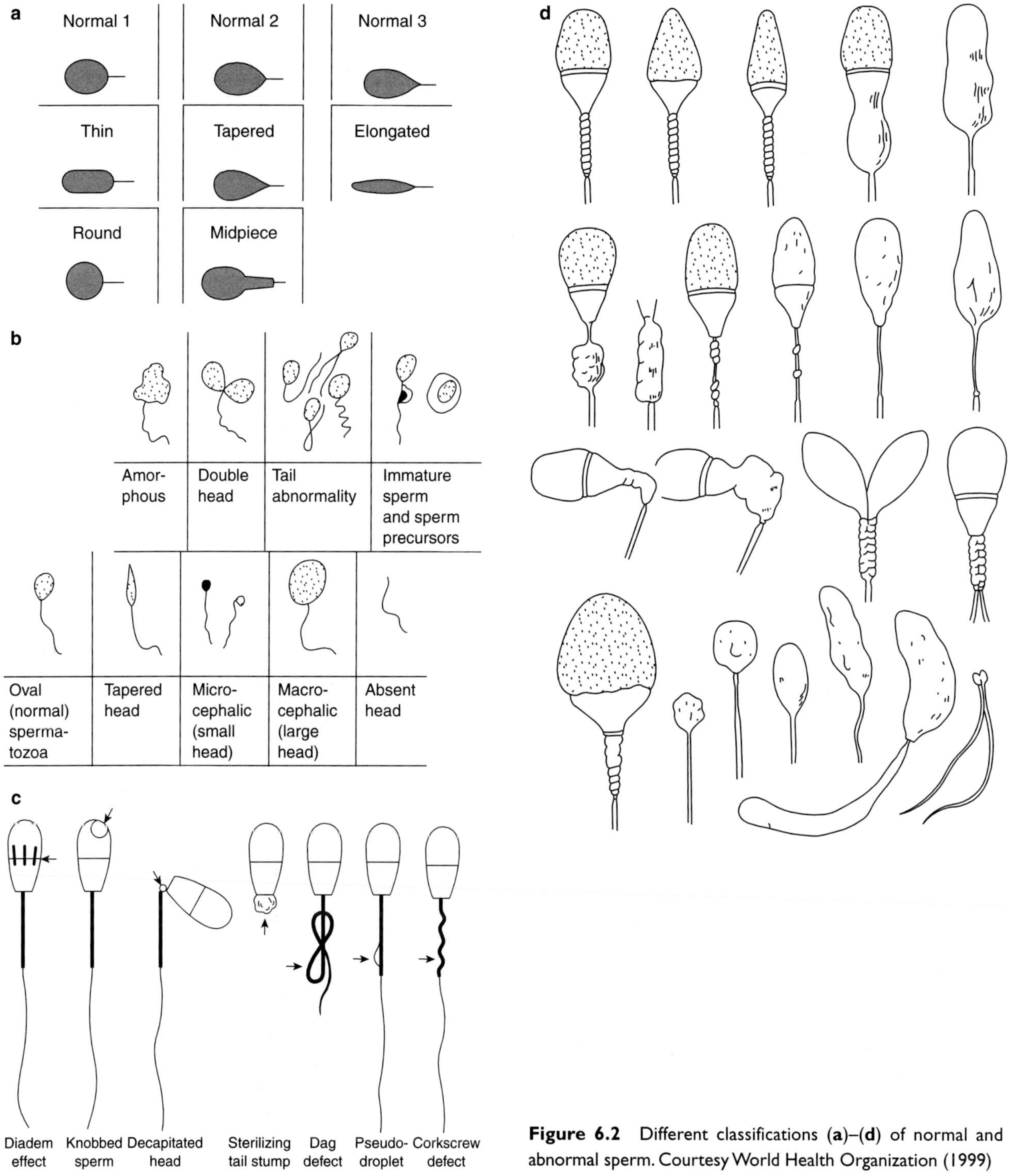

Figure 6.2 Different classifications (**a**)–(**d**) of normal and abnormal sperm. Courtesy World Health Organization (1999)

(Surface Imaging System ultraobjective; Surface Imaging System, Germany) attached to a conventional Olympus microscope (BX60, Japan) is employed for investigation. Cantilevers of silicon of length 450 µm, width 50 µm and thickness 2 µm are attached to the objective. The spring constant of the cantilever is 15 N/m, operated at frequency 159 266 kHz.

PATHOLOGY OF INFERTILITY

Infertile patients can be classified as having the following conditions: subfertile semen (Figure 6.11), periodic oligozoospermia, permanent oligozoospermia, oligozoospermia, azoospermia (Figure 6.12), hypogonadotropism (pre- and postpuberty) and

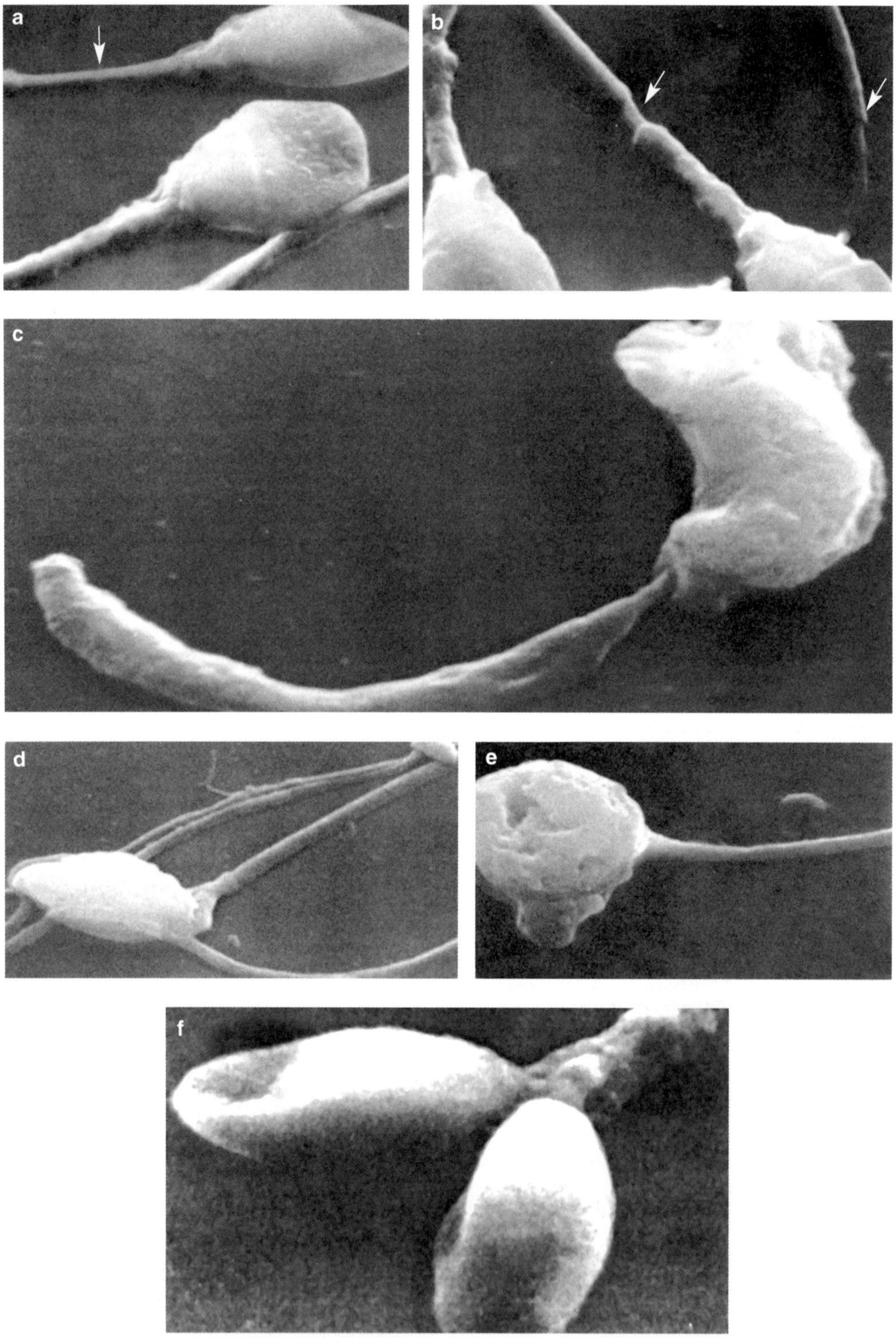

Figure 6.3 Morphological anomalies of spermatozoa (all are of immotile type, being devoid of mitochondrial thickening in the middle piece). (**a**) Mitochondria thickening is lacking (arrow). This deformed spermatozoa, being deprived of its 'motor', would have been immotile in the ejaculate (12 000×). (**b**) The constricted boundary of the middle and main pieces of the tail probably represents a mechanically weak point as shown by a spermatozoon broken at this site. The main piece abruptly joins the short end-piece (arrow) (12 000×). (**c**)–(**e**) Abnormal spermatozoa from patients with suspected male infertility. (**c**) Spermatozoon with a monstrous head and a short and irregularly thick tail (10 000×). (**d**) Spermatozoon with a rudimentary and bipartite head and two tails (8700×). (**e**) Sperm with unusually small, oval and rough-surfaced head. without an acrosome (20 000×). (**f**) Spermatozoon with two heads found in the same normal semen. The acrosome is probably failing in these heads. Although deformities are found in no more than 15% of the total spermatozoa in normal semen, they occur more or less in excess or even exclusively in the ejaculates of sterile males (10 000)

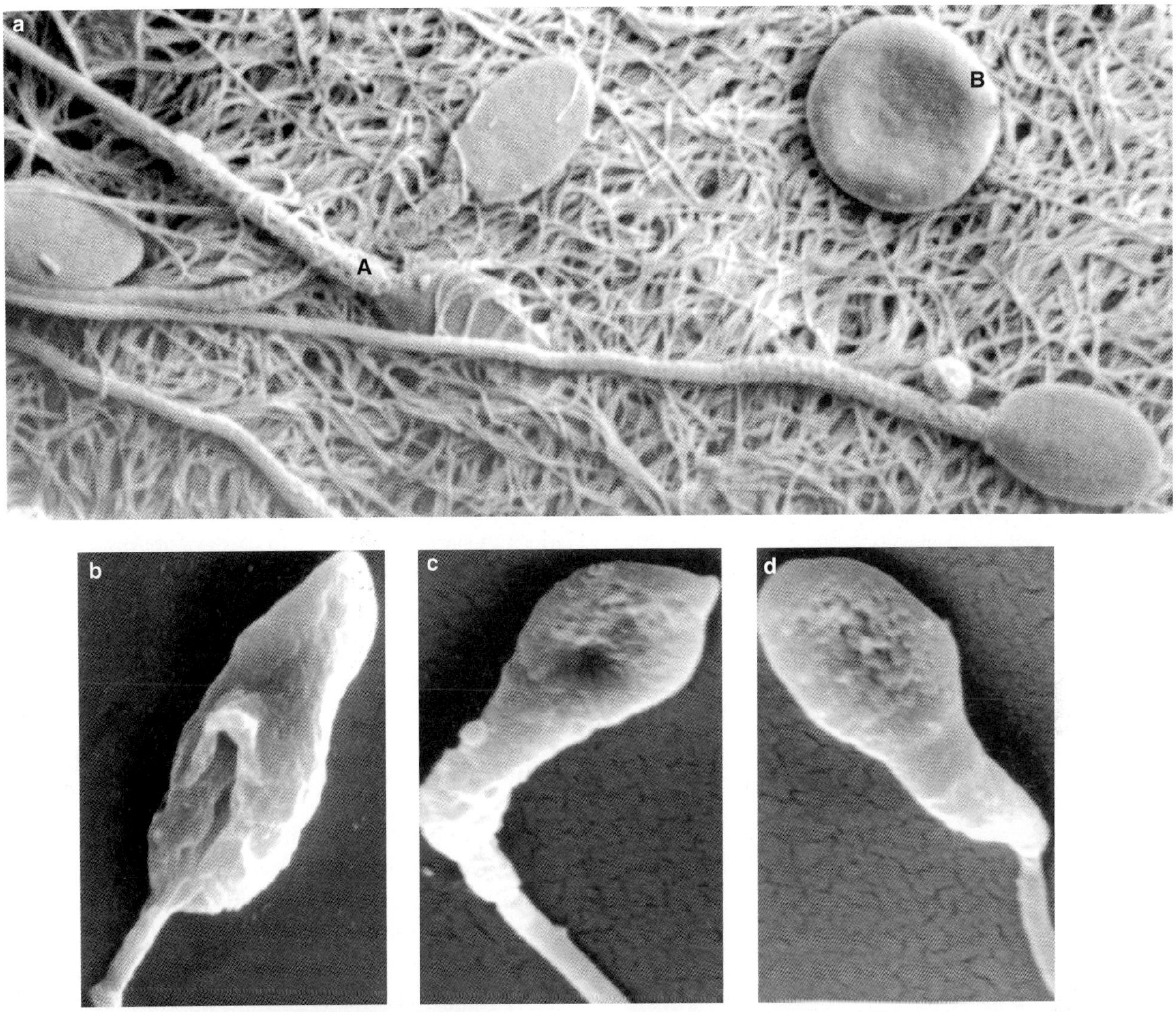

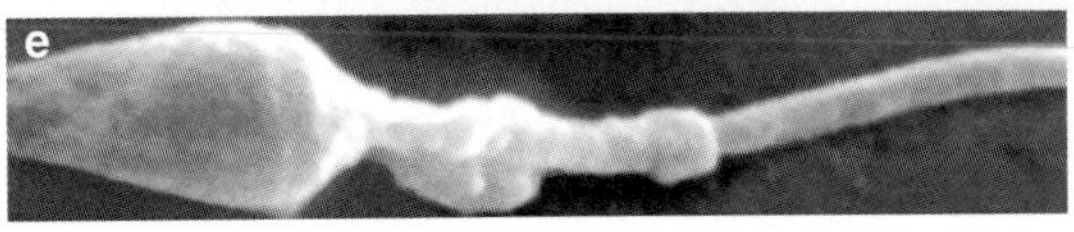

Figure 6.4 (**a**) Scanning electron microscopy (SEM) of normal sperm (A) and red blood cell (B). (**b**)–(**e**) SEM of common sperm anomalies. Courtesy of Professor T. Fujita

immunological infertility. The step-by-step scheme for the evaluation of cervical mucus in infertility patients is shown in Figure 6.13.

Non-obstructive azoospermia (NOA)

Once a single viable sperm is injected into a normal metaphase II oocyte it has the potential to achieve successful fertilization, and normal embryo development can proceed. The task of extracting a single viable sperm from an azoospermic man is a specialty in itself. This task is even more complicated in a man with non-obstructive azoospermia (NOA). The diagnosis of azoospermia should include: complete semen analysis, careful inspection of semen sediment obtained by ultracentrifugation of seminal plasma, and clinical examination for the presence of vasa deferentia. The differentiation between obstructive azoospermia and NOA is achieved by testicular biopsy and endocrine profile. The degree of spermatogenesis impairment should then be evaluated. Tesarik *et al.* (2000) incubated testicular tissues in hormone- and growth factor-supplemented media *in vitro* in order to stimulate maturation of spermatogenic cells. Hypospermatogenesis provides good chances for isolating viable, intact spermatozoa with fertilizing capacity. Tiny focal spermatogenesis may take place in the testis without sperm appearing in the selected biopsy specimen or released in the ejaculate (Tournaye *et al.*, 1996). In such cases it is possible to isolate sperm

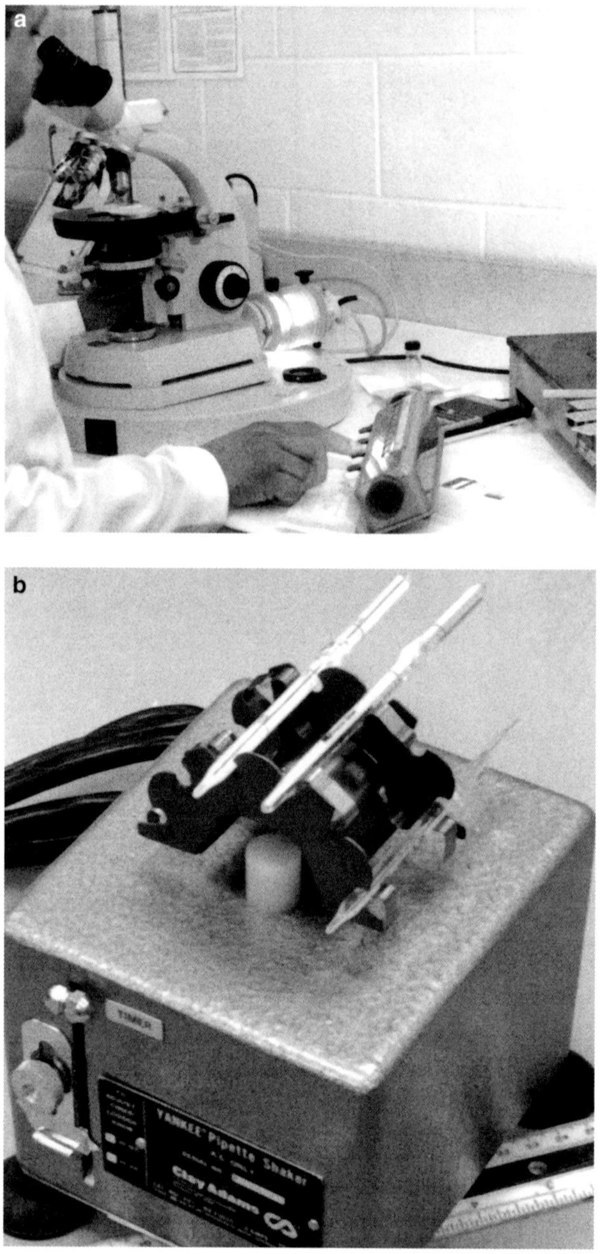

Figure 6.5 (**a**) Semen evaluation using stained semen smear under phase-contrast microscopy. (**b**) Automatic shaker for proper mixing of semen in calibrated pipettes

from additional testicular specimens and to use them in IVF–intracytoplasmic sperm injection (ICSI) (Ben-Yousef *et al.*, 1999). Careful evaluation of the histology (cytology of the specimen) is crucial to determine the number, location and size of biopsies to be obtained (Ezeh *et al.*, 1998).

Modern diagnostic tools have been used in the management of NOA. Biopsy techniques utilize isolated testicular tissue or spermatogenic cells obtained by testicular sperm extraction (TESE), (open biopsy under local anesthesia) or testicular sperm aspiration (TESA) (fine-needle biopsy) (Craft *et al.*, 1997).

A multiple TESE is superior in cases of NOA because it may enhance diagnostic accuracy and increase the chance of sperm cell retrieval. The sperm isolated from the testis may occasionally have morphology as good as that of ejaculated sperm. The rate of bivalent formation of homologous chromosomes in spermatocytes increases the prospect of focal spermatogenesis in the testes of men with NOA. Bivalent formation can be analyzed with fluorescence *in situ* hybridization (FISH) using alpha-satellite centromere probes for the evaluation of autosomes (Hauser *et al.*, 1998; Paz *et al.*, 2003). Men with NOA have the highest risk for Y-chromosome microdeletions, which are associated with impairment of spermatogenesis. In cases of spermatogenesis or meiotic arrest in men with NOA, techniques are attempted to advance the maturation of spermatogenic cells *in vitro*. Tesarik *et al.* (2000) incubated testicular tissues in hormone-supplemented medium *in vitro* to stimulate maturation of spermatogenic cells.

Leukospermia

Routine application of antibiotics for leukospermia may have a negative impact on semen parameters as well as increasing the possibility of inoculating the reproductive tract of the female partner with antibiotic-resistant bacteria.

The presence or absence of bacteriospermia or leukospermia do not correlate with each other. Leukospermia does not correlate with semen parameters. In a study by Rodin *et al.* (2003) staphylococcus species were the most common isolates and did not correlate with semen parameters or leukospermia. *Streptococcus viridians* and *Enterococcus faecalis* were the next most common isolates and were associated with statistically significantly poorer semen quality (Rodin *et al.*, 2003). Leukospermia is a poor marker for either bacteriospermia or impaired semen quality. Staphylococcus species are commonly isolated but appear to be innocuous. *Streptococcus viridians* and *Enterococcus faecalis* are associated with poorer semen quality and may warrant treatment.

Azoospermia and oligozoospermia

Azoospermia and oligozoospermia are associated with a wide variety of genetic anomalies. Chromosomal anomalies are more frequent in infertile men compared with fertile men, with a frequency of 2% in all

Table 6.2 Evaluation of sperm morphology. From Acosta and Kruger, 1996

Sperm head anomalies

Large heads
Small heads
Elongated/tapering heads
Duplicated heads
Amorphous heads
Normal sperm heads with neck/middle piece and/or tail and/or cytoplasmic droplet defects

Abnormalities or no sperm cells counted

Precursors
Tail abnormalities
Neck/middle piece abnormalities
Cytoplasmic droplets
Loose heads

Acrosome disorders

Type A: slight disorders where small or missing acrosomes are present. The outline (form) of the sperm is normal or slightly narrowed
Type B: sperm shows the same acrosome defects, but the sperm heads are round with a compact condensation of the chromatin
Combination of type A and type B

Sperm tail defects

Type A: broken tails
Type B: broken tails at neck or middle piece area with coiling of the tails
Type C: short rudimentary (tadpole-like) tails

Structural shaft disturbance of tail based on Shorr staining technique (Dusseldorf classification)

Size defects, too small or too large
Different degrees of hyperelongation
Hyperelongation with acrosome defects
Different degrees of acrosome disorders
Duplicated forms
Middle piece and/or tail defects
Combination of head and tail defects

Table 6.3 Strict criteria for sperm normality according to the World Health Organization (1999)

Domain	*Criteria for normality*
Sperm head	
Shape	Oval, acrosome occupying 40–70% of head area
Length	4.0–5.0 μm
Width	2.5–3.5 μm
Aspect ratio	1.5–1.75
Middle piece	
Shape	Slender, attached axially to the head
Length	One and a half times the length of the head
Width	< 1 μm
Cytoplasmic droplet	Less than half the size of the head
Tail	

men attending infertility clinics. In azoospermia, the frequency rises to 15%, including about 13% with a 47,XXY chromosome constitution. The remaining azoospermic cases are characterized by specific anomalies, which include other numerical structural anomalies, such as reciprocal and Robertsonian translocations, inversions, ring chromosomes, aneuploidies and supernumerary chromosomes. Congential bilateral absence of the vas deferens (CBAVD) leading to obstructive azoospermia in healthy males is a relatively frequent cause of male infertility, occurring at the rate of 1–2% of cases with sterility and ≥6% of cases with obstructive azoospermia. Most men with CBAVD have mutations in the cystic fibrosis transmembrane conductance regulator (CFTR) gene, with an increased risk of carrying the 5T variant.

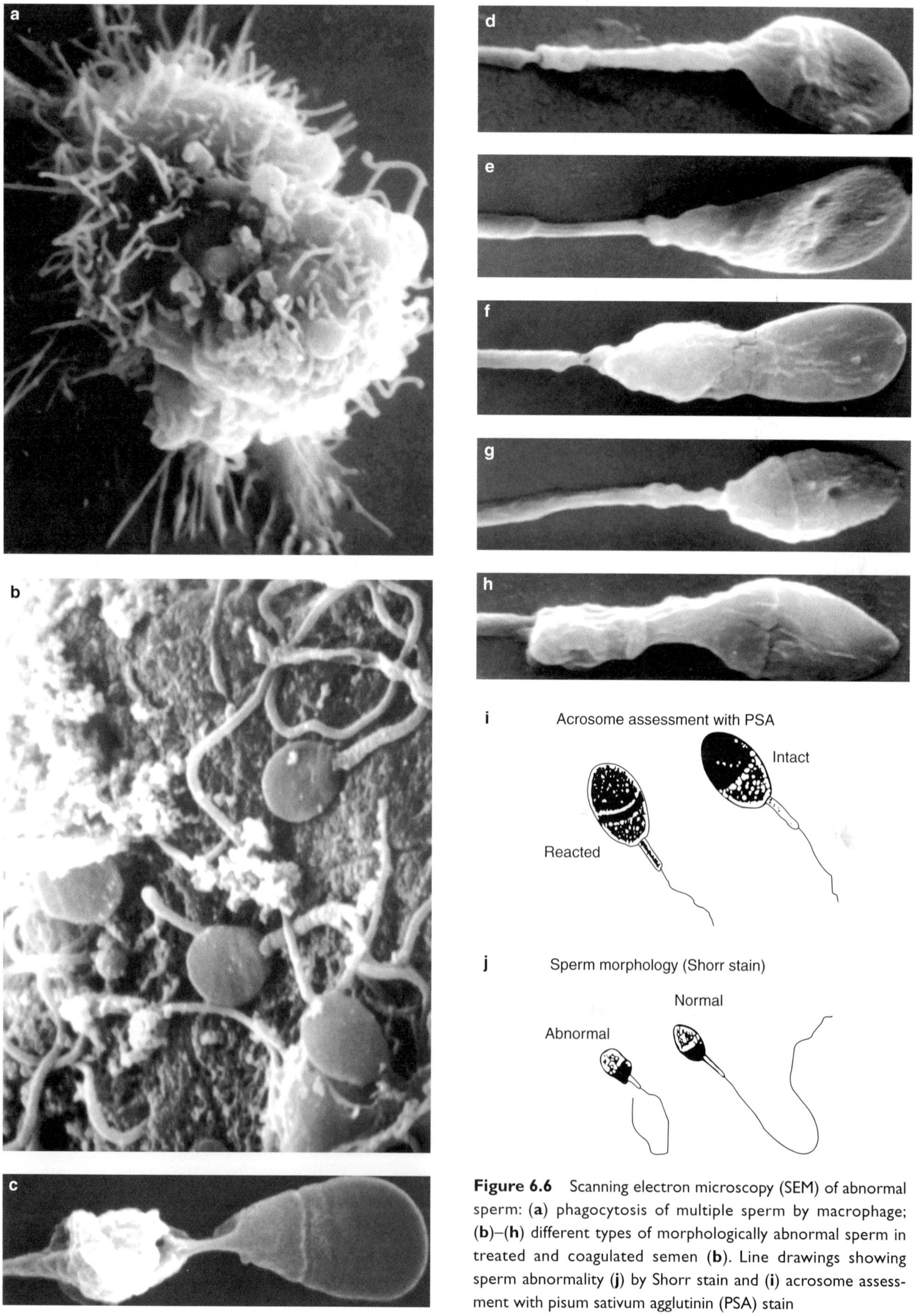

Figure 6.6 Scanning electron microscopy (SEM) of abnormal sperm: (**a**) phagocytosis of multiple sperm by macrophage; (**b**)–(**h**) different types of morphologically abnormal sperm in treated and coagulated semen (**b**). Line drawings showing sperm abnormality (**j**) by Shorr stain and (**i**) acrosome assessment with pisum sativum agglutinin (PSA) stain

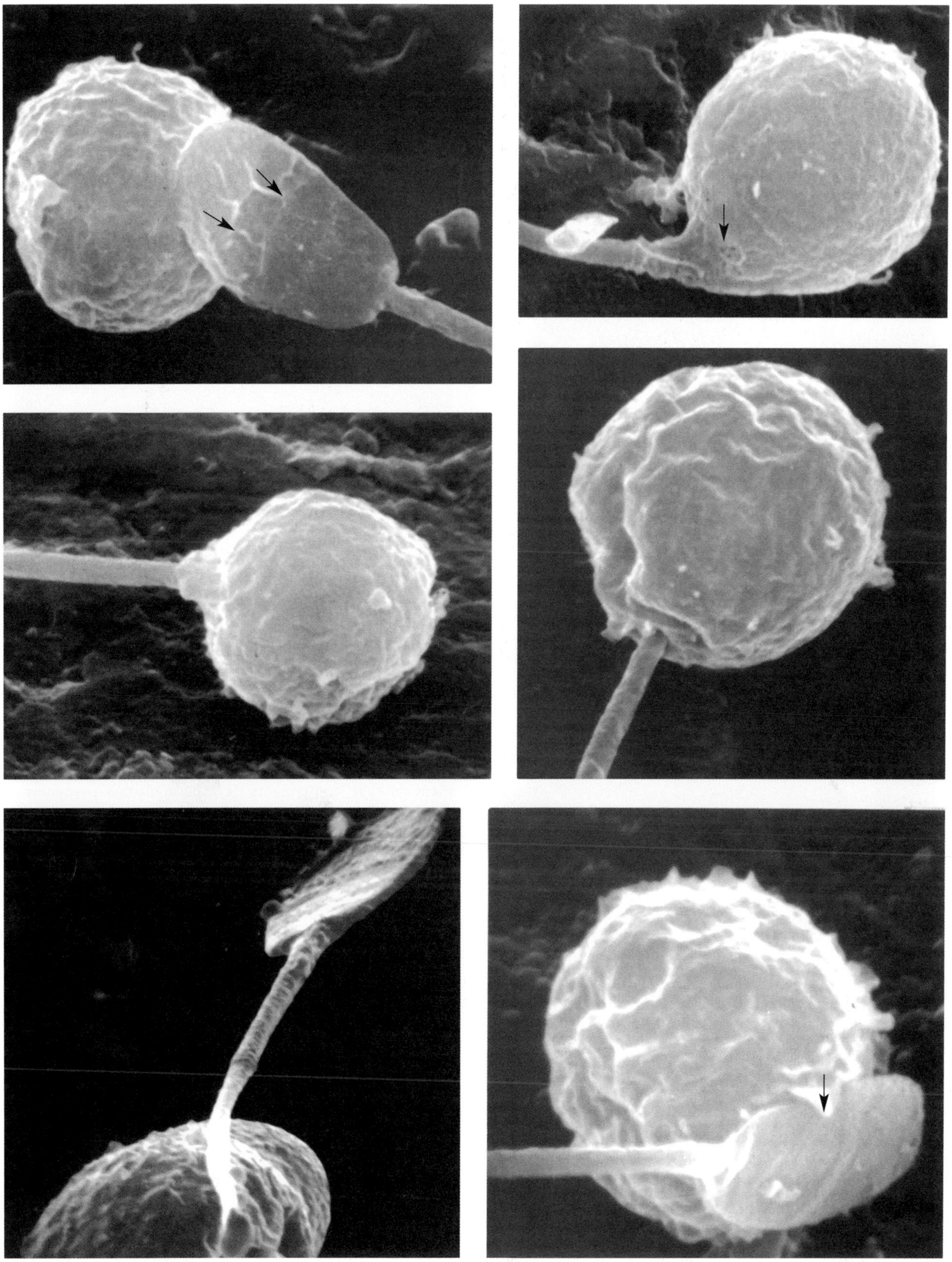

Figure 6.7 Different types of ultrastructural sperm abnormalities as shown by scanning electron microscopy (SEM). Arrows indicate early stage of phagocytosis. Courtesy of Professors Zaneveld and Polakaski, Chicago, IL, USA

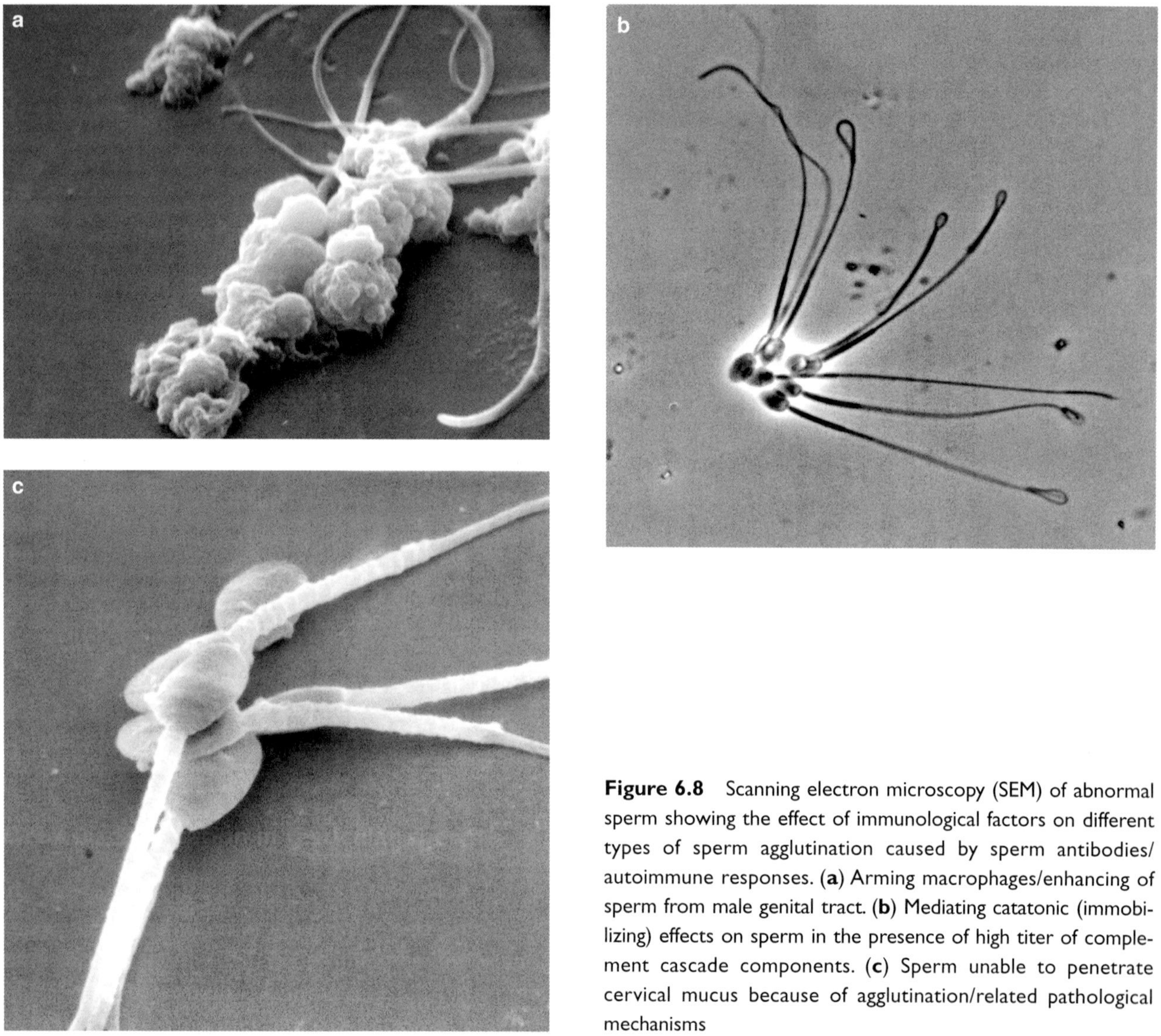

Figure 6.8 Scanning electron microscopy (SEM) of abnormal sperm showing the effect of immunological factors on different types of sperm agglutination caused by sperm antibodies/autoimmune responses. (**a**) Arming macrophages/enhancing of sperm from male genital tract. (**b**) Mediating catatonic (immobilizing) effects on sperm in the presence of high titer of complement cascade components. (**c**) Sperm unable to penetrate cervical mucus because of agglutination/related pathological mechanisms

Idiopathic oligozoospermia

Several drugs have been used in the treatment of male infertility to improve spermatogenesis or epididymal maturation. However, there is no 'standard' therapy for idiopathic oligozoospermia. Various substances, such as kallikrein, vitamins and Kampo (Japanese herbal medicine), have been administered orally as an empiric therapy for male infertility, but the exact mechanism of efficacy has not been established. A novel treatment of male infertility focuses on the role of mast cell blockers, which inhibit the release of histamine and other vasoactive substances from mast cells. The rationale of this approach is based on mastocytosis of the testis in infertile men.

Several factors could potentially be involved in male unexplained infertility including cytokine-mediated immune response and sperm-membrane lipid peroxidation. Reactive oxygen species (ROS) produced by sperm and white blood cells can attack the sperm membrane, thereby increasing the level of lipid peroxidation. Human sperm are particularly susceptible to oxidative attack, not only because of the high concentration of unsaturated fatty acids within their plasma membrane, but also because of the low concentration of scavenging enzymes in their cytoplasm. The occurrence of any imbalance between ROS production and total antioxidant capacity correlates with male infertility. An increased production of cytokines can increase ROS production in the male genital tract. Male infertility is correlated with increased levels of cytokines in human semen. Urogenital infections increase the concentration of semen cytokines as well as affecting sperm parameters. Studies

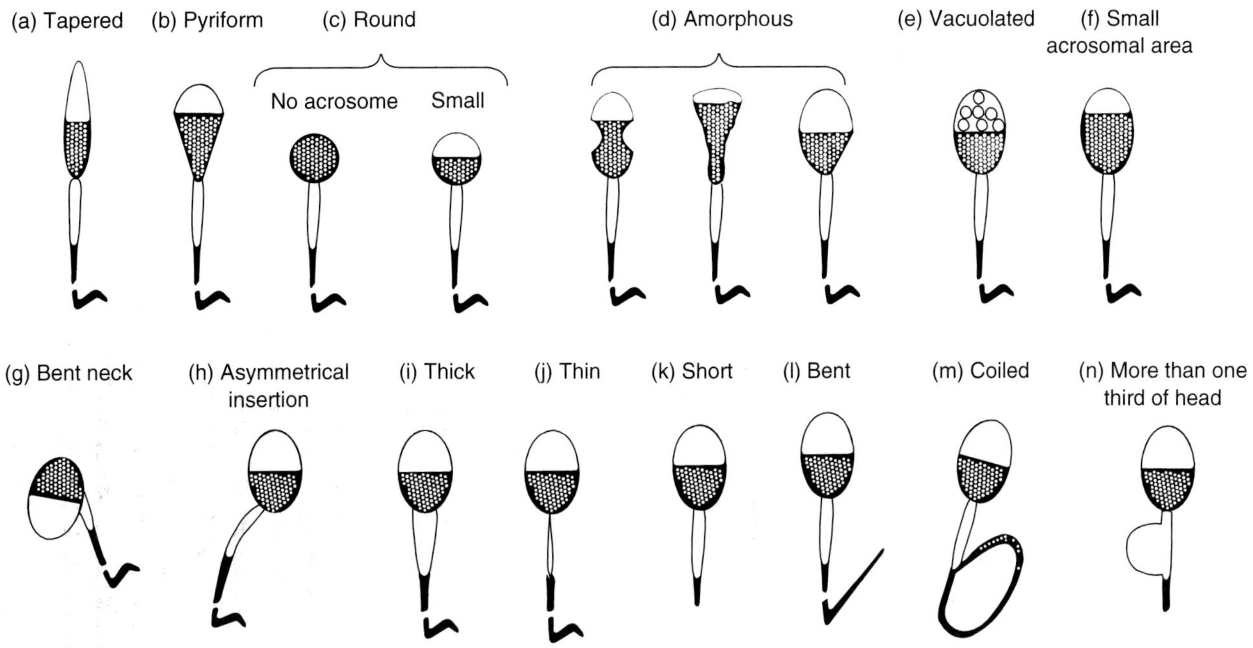

Figure 6.9 Classification of abnormal sperm according to head defects (a)–(f), neck/middle piece defects (g)–(j), tail defects (k)–(m) and cytoplasmic droplet defects (n) as used to evaluate the functional three-dimensional ultrastructure of affected sperm

Table 6.4 Descriptive terminology for semen variables according to WHO guidelines (WHO, 1999)

Term	*Definition*
Normozoospermia	Normal ejaculate as defined in Table 6.3
Globozoospermia	Round-headed acrosomeless spermatozoa
Oligozoospermia	<20 million spermatozoa/ml
Asthenozoospermia	<50% sperm with forward progression
Teratozoospermia	<30% spermatozoa with normal morphology
Oligoasthenoteratozoospermia (OAT)	Signifies disturbance of all three variables (combinations of only two prefixes may also be used)
Azoospermia	No spermatozoa in the ejaculate
Necrozoospermia	All spermatozoa are dead as judged by supravital staining
Hemospermia (hematospermia)	Presence of fresh or altered blood in ejaculate derived from pathology in accessory sexual glands, urethra or bladder. Related to emission and ejaculation; associated with infertility, hematuria, lower urinary tract infection, vascular abnormalities, ductal obstruction or cysts, neoplasms and systemic or iatrogenic factors
Parvisemia	Ejaculate volume <2 ml
Leukocytospermia	Leukocytes present in ejaculate
-zoospermia	Refers to sperm in ejaculate
-spermia	Refers to the ejaculate
-aspermia	No ejaculate

with pancreatic islet beta-cells have demonstrated a toxic effect of cytokines, mediated by generation of ROS and lipid peroxidation. *In vitro* studies have demonstrated stimulation of sperm-membrane peroxidation in the sperm of fertile donors, by interleukin-α (ILα) and tumor necrosis factor-α (TNF-α).

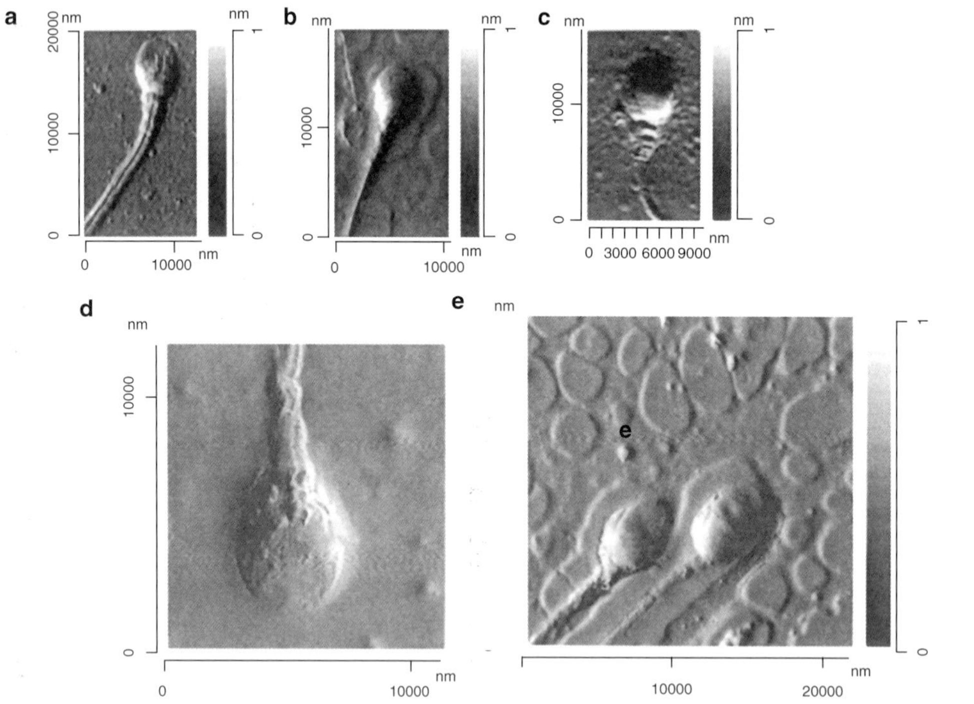

	Normal (nm)	HIV without treatment (nm)	HIV with HAART (nm)
Longitude of the head	4200–6700	5000–7200	4600–6500
Width of the head	3800–5800	4000–4700	4200–5400
Length of the head	700–1200	600–900	700–1000
Width connecting pieces	1500–2100	1300–2500	1400–2900
Length of neck	200–500	100–301	100–400

Figure 6.10 Scanning electron microscopy (SEM) of sperm of normal (**a**), HIV-infected without treatment (**b**) and HIV-infected patients treated with highly active antiretroviral therapy (HAART) (**c**). Higher magnification shows HIV-infected sperm (**d**) and normal sperm (**e**). The infected sperm (**d**) shows complete absence of the central canal, the neck piece is not well marked or is obscured by the sudden increase in width near the neck. From Barboza *et al.*, 2004, with permission

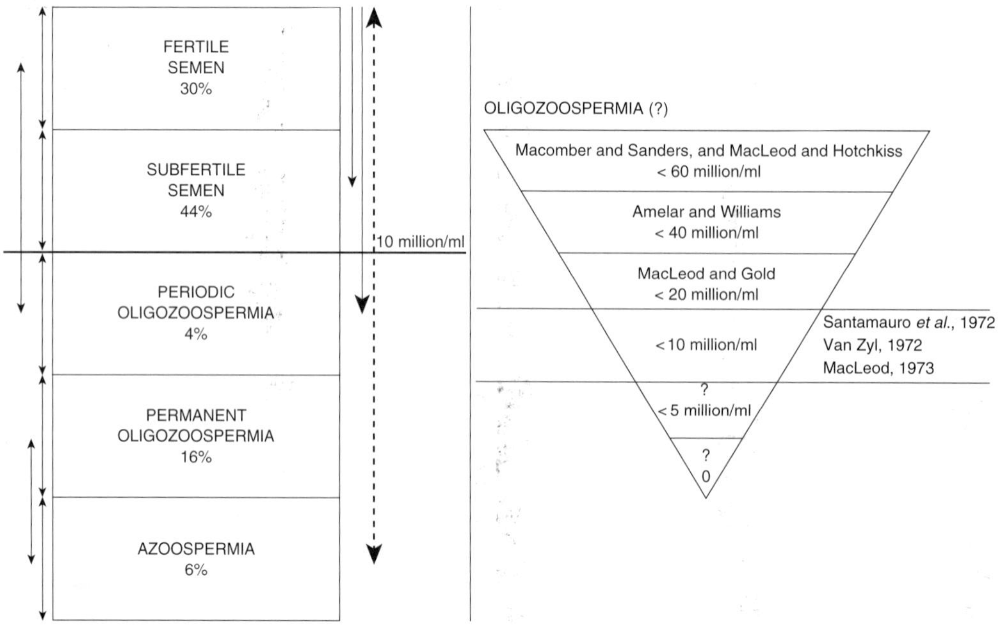

Figure 6.11 Classification of subfertility, periodic and permanent oligozoospermia and azoospermia

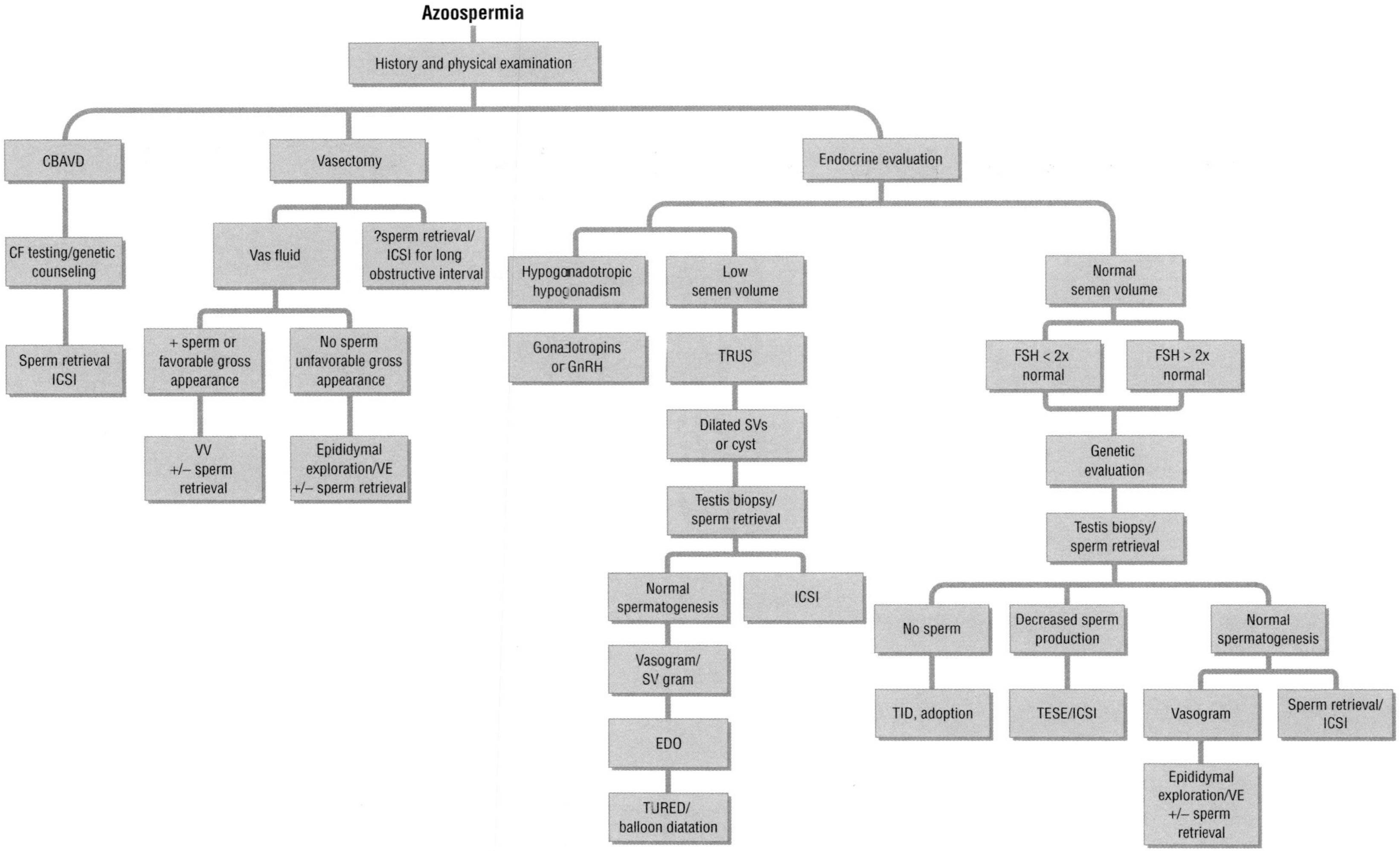

Figure 6.12 Flowchart of treatment for azoospermia. CBAVD, congenital bilateral absence of vas deferens; CF, cystic fibrosis; ICSI, intracytoplasmic sperm injection; VV, vasovasostomy; GnRH, gonadotropin releasing hormone; VE, vasoepididymostomy; SV, seminal vesicle; EDO, ejaculatory duct obstruction; TRUS, transrectal ultrasound; TURED, transurethral resection of ejaculatory ducts; TID, therapeutic insemination with donor sperm; TESE, testicular sperm extraction. From Kolettis, 2002, with permission

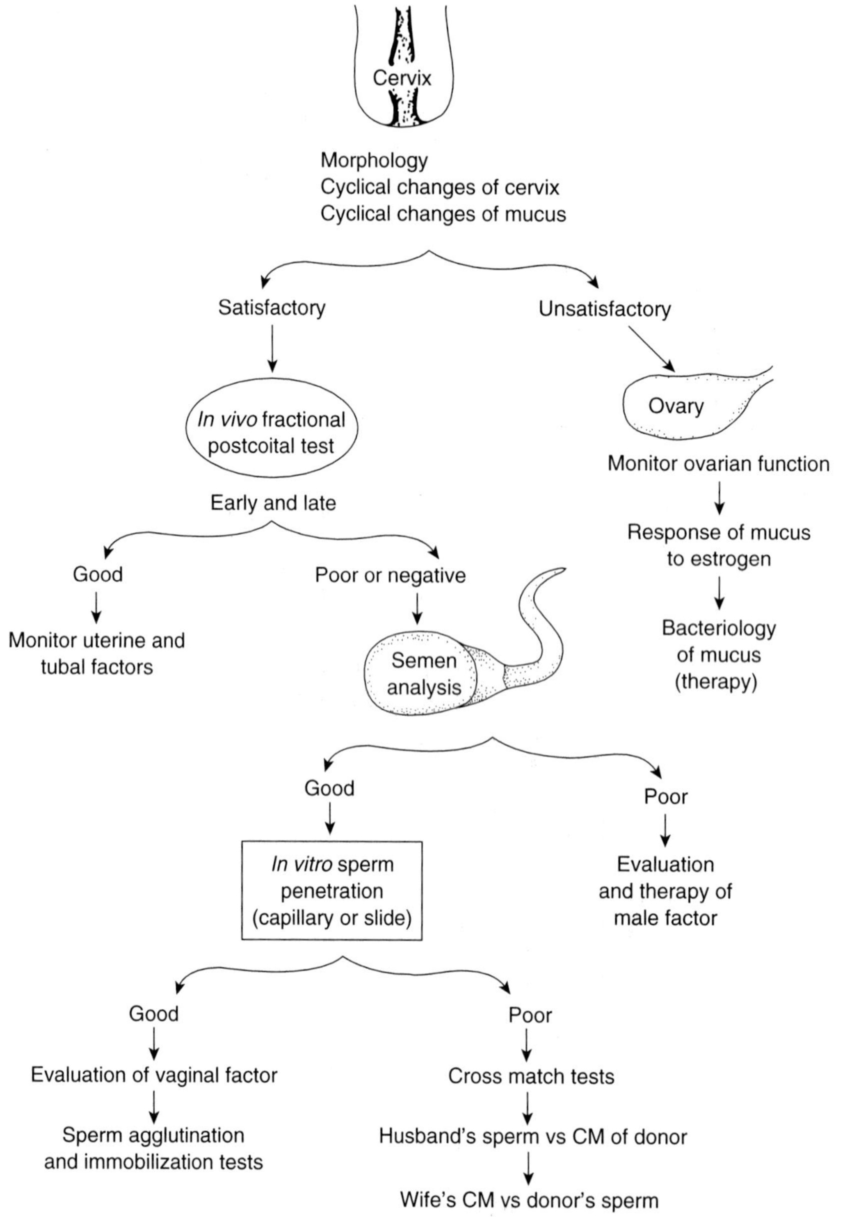

Figure 6.13 Step-by-step scheme for the evaluation of cervical factor in infertility patients. CM, cervical mucus

Hypogonadotropism

Hypogonadotropism may be acquired either before or after puberty (Table 6.5).

THERAPEUTIC APPROACHES TO MALE INFERTILITY

Several hormonal and surgical procedures have been used to treat the following major causes of infertility: azoospermia, transurethral resection of ejaculatory ducts (TURED), antegrade ejaculatory duct canalization/balloon dilatation and vasovasostomy microsurgery (Table 6.6).

Azoospermia due to defects in the hypothalamic–pituitary–gonadal axis associated with low hormone levels is treatable. Defects may also be associated with hyposmia or anosmia in patients with Kallmann's syndrome, hyperprolactinemia hypogonadism with erectile dysfunction/infertility. Non-obstructive azoospermia is treated exclusively by hypogonadal hormones to reinitiate spermatogenesis.

Vasal occlusion can be due to a variety of factors, including previous vasectomy, inflammation and damage as a result of surgery (such as hernia

Table 6.5 Manifestion of hypogonadotropism acquired before or after puberty

Hypogonadotropism acquired prepubertally
Scant body hair and facial terminal hair
High-pitched voice
Female escutcheon
Small testes: volume < 6 ml; length < 2.5 cm
Small penis: length < 5 cm
Little or no scrotal rugae or hyperpigmentation
Small prostate
Eunuchoidal proportions
Hypogonadotropism acquired postpubertally
Loss of libido
Facial terminal hair present but slow growth
Body hair present but decreased
Normal male voice pitch
Testes > 10 ml; sometimes soft
Normal penile length
Scrotal rugae and hyperpigmentation present
Adult prostate size
Decreased bone and muscle mass
Normal skeletal proportions

repair) or accident (trauma). Both vasectomy and non-vasectomy patients should undergo a full medical examination and evaluation prior to undergoing vasovasostomy. As with infertility patients, routine assessment should include semen analysis, serum hormone levels and radiographic examination.

Various micromanipulation techniques are used to treat infertility (Table 6.7).

Chromosomal abnormalities/ polymorphisms

Abnormalities in either sex or autosomal chromosomes are frequent in infertile men; therefore, disorders in spermatogenic processes could be directly related to changes in the number or structure of chromosomes. Aneuploidy has been shown in the sex chromosomes of some sterile men. There is an association between alterations in gamete production and genetic disorders, such as Klinefelter's syndrome or 45,X/46,XY gonadal dysgenesia. This may be due to the presence of the AZF gene

Table 6.6 Hormonal and surgical procedures for major infertility cases (data from Acosta and Kruger, 1996; Hafez *et al.*, 2003; Hafez and Hafez, 2000; Jeyandran, 2003)

	Treatment
Azoospermia	1500–3000 IU of hCG intramuscularly 3 times a week; recombinant FSH in conjunction with hCG for 6–9 months to initiate spermatogenesis and stimulate Sertoli cells
Transurethral resection of ejaculatory ducts (TURED)	Spinal or general anesthesia plus prophylactic antibiotics; patient prepared in sterile fashion in dorsal lithotomic position; O'Conor sheath used to facilitate digital transrectal prostate massage/manipulation during procedure; standard cystoscopy to inspect urethra/bladder; cystoscope removed to insert electroscope with a resection loop into urethra; same instruments used as for transurethral resection of prostate (TURP); electrical current at 100 W (set for pure cutting); guide wire passed into seminal vesicle with advancement into ejaculatory duct
Antegrade ejaculation duct canalization/balloon dilatation	Cystoscopy used to gain control of distal end of guide wire; Seldinger technique to place 4-mm wide, 2-cm long balloon dilating catheter over guide wire; dilating catheter advanced over guide wire to ejaculatory level duct; proper position confirmed fluoroscopically/visually with cystoscope; dilating balloon inflated/left in place for 2–3 min/balloon inflated; instruments withdrawn to address other side similarly as required; the following complications could be minimized or avoided by careful identification of pertinent anatomical landmark before resection: bleeding, rectal injury, prostate capsule perforation, external sphincter injury with urinary incontinence, bladder neck resection (leading to retrograde ejaculation or a bladder neck contracture)
Vasovasostomy microsurgery	Local or general anesthesia before bilateral, two-layered anastomosis; slight patient movement may cause injury to vas deferens and anastomosis site; pressure points of elbows, hands, ankles, and heels of feet are padded; TED Hose compression boots may diminish risk of deep vein thrombosis; patient offered concurrent sperm retrieval; epididymovasostomy performed if vasovasostomy does not cause patency

hCG, human chorionic gonadotropin; FSH, follicle stimulating hormone

Table 6.7 Micromanipulation techniques used to treat infertility

Insemination
Donor insemination (DI)
Artificial insemination (husband) (AIH)
Intrauterine insemination (IUI)
IVF-related
Gamete intrafallopian transfer (GIFT)
Pronuclear stage tubal transfer (PROST)
In vitro fertilization and embryo transfer (IVF–ET)
Tubal embryo stage transfer (TEST)
Others
Direct intraperitoneal insemination (DIPI)
Peritoneal ovum and sperm transfer (POST)
Fallopian replacement of eggs and delayed insemination (FREDI)
Intracytoplasmic sperm injection (ICSI)

(azoospermia factor) on the long arm of the Y chromosome, since deletion of the distal portion of that chromosomal region occurs in azoospermic patients. Other structural abnormalities in sex chromosomes, e.g. microdeletions, isochromosomes, translocations and ring chromosomes, have been found. Also, autosomal alterations, mainly Robertsonian translocations, have been shown in infertile males. Cytogenetic analysis of sterile males is needed not only for the diagnosis of sterility, but also as selection criteria for assisted reproduction techniques, e.g. ICSI.

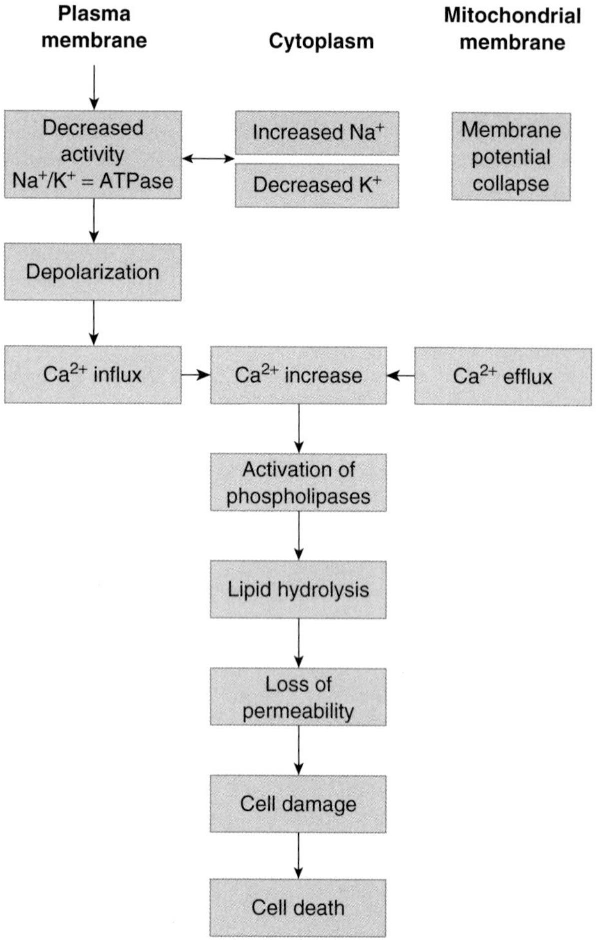

Figure 6.14 Progression of events associated with imbalanced ATP synthesis/degradation and subsequent death of spermatozoa

Molecular parameters of infertility

Severe defects in sperm production cause infertility in 2% of infertile men. Genetic infertility is due to chromosomal abnormalities and microdeletions of the Y chromosome. In azoospermic and oligozoospermic men there are three non-overlapping AZF regions, designated AZFs a, b and c, residing in intervals 5 and 6 of the human Y chromosome. Each of the AZF regions contains many genes that have not been fully characterized. These genes may be potential candidates for AZF. The VCY2 (variable charge, Y chromosome, 2; alias BPY2) gene is located in the most frequently deleted AZFc region in infertile men. Tse *et al.* (2003) performed testicular biopsy in infertile men with different testicular histologies, then carried out immunohistochemical analysis to determine the possible relationship of VCY2 and the pathogenesis of male infertility. VCY2 was weakly expressed at the spermatogonia and immunonegative in spermatocytes and round spermatids in testicular biopsy specimens, with maturation arrest or hypospermatogenesis. The impaired expression of VCY2 in infertile men suggests its involvement in the pathogenesis of male infertility.

The death of spermatozoa occurs as a consequence of molecular changes in the plasma membrane, cytoplasm and mitochondrial membrane (Figure 6.14).

Immunological infertility

Antisperm antibodies, especially sperm-immobilizing antibodies found in the sera of immunologically infertile women, cause infertility by interfering with fertilization and by blocking penetration through the cervical mucus. There is an immunoglobulin-binding protein capable of binding antisperm antibodies which trap any penetrating sperm. One of the mechanisms

Table 6.8 Endocrine profile of the blood of infertile men

Syndrome	*FSH*	*LH*	*Testosterone*	*Total estrogen*
Primary hypogonadism	Very little	Very high	Normal or low	Low
Hypogonadotropic hypogonadism	Undetected	Undetected	Low	Very low
Idiopathic oligospermia (maturation arrest at spermatocyte stage)	Normal	Normal	Low	High
Varicocele (left)	Normal	Normal	Normal	Normal
Oligozoospermia (with non-bacterial chronic functional prostatitis)	Very low	Very high	Very low	Very high
Sertoli cell-only syndrome	High	Normal	Normal	Normal

Table 6.9 Endocrine profile and diagnosis of azoospermia

Category	*LH*	*FSH*	*Testosterone*	*Diagnosis*
Hypergonadotropic azoospermia	—	—	—	Testicular dysfunction
Hypogonadotropic azoospermia	Nil	Nil	Nil	Abnormal hormonal stimulation/endocrine evaluation Normal testicular function, unexplained obstruction
Eugonadotropic azoospermia	Normal	Normal	Testosterone	Obstruction Maturation arrest Sertoli cell-only syndrome Ejaculatory dysfunction Sexual dysfunction

LH, luteinizing hormone; FSH, follicle-stimulating hormone

by which sperm-immobilizing antibodies exert their anti-fertility effect is by inhibition of the acrosome reaction (AR). Spontaneous AR is almost completely inhibited by sperm-immobilizing antibodies; this inhibitory effect on AR can be abolished by incubation of antisperm antibody-treated sperm in antibody-free medium, as demonstrated in an *in vitro* human fertilization test, in which the blocking effect of the antibody on the sperm–zona pellucida interaction is reversed by incubation of the antibody-bound spermatozoa in antibody-free medium. Only capacitated sperm undergo AR.

Diagnosis of male infertility

Evaluation of the endocrine profile of the blood of infertile men is used for the diagnosis of primary hypogonadism, hypogonadotropic hypogonadism, idiopathic oligozoospermia (maturation arrest at spermatocyte stage), varicocele (left), oligozoospermia (with non-bacterial chronic functional prostatitis) and Sertoli cell-only syndrome (Tables 6.8 and 6.9). Azoospermia may be due to the congenital bilateral absence of the vas deferens (CBAVD), cystic fibrosis (CS) and ejaculatory duct obstruction (EDO).

7

Erectile dysfunction

Erectile dysfunction (ED) is the persistent inability to achieve and maintain an erection sufficient for satisfactory sexual intercourse, and has a reported prevalence of about 50% in men aged 40–70 years. The penis might be erect, but the erection may not last long enough before it fades away. Extensive investigations have been conducted into the etiology of ED, its endocrine profile, the effects of testosterone and prostate cancer, and the application of animal models (reviewed by Hafez and Hafez, 2004). ED may lead to depressive symptoms, low self-esteem, other signs of psychological distress and decreased quality of life. ED can be due to organic and psychological mechanisms associated with psychological, neurological, endocrinological, vascular (venous or arterial), traumatic or iatrogenic factors (drugs and surgery).

PREVALENCE OF ERECTILE DYSFUNCTION

ED is a common problem in general medical practice affecting especially the elderly and those with hypertension, ischemic heart disease, peripheral vascular disease and diabetes mellitus (Jaffe *et al.*, 1996; Panser *et al.*, 1995). ED is manifested in 10–60% of men depending on the demography of the population (Table 7.1).

Some 40% of diabetic men > 60 years of age have ED all the time (complete ED). Men with ischemic heart disease are 1.9 times more likely to have complete ED than those who do not have ischemic heart disease.

PATHOPHYSIOLOGY AND PSYCHOPATHOLOGY OF ERECTILE DYSFUNCTION

Two major psychopathological/emotional factors play a significant role in the etiology of ED: performance anxiety and relationship discord. Changes associated with ED are shown in Tables 7.2 and 7.3.

Table 7.1 Demographic distribution of erectile dysfunction

Country	*Age (years)*	*ED (%)*
USA	40–80	10–12
France	18–70	39
Spain	25–70	73
Nigeria	21–84	34
Korea	>50	59

Pathophysiology of erectile dysfunction

Vascular dysfunction results from arterial insufficiency and/or incompetence of the veno-occlusive mechanism (venous leak) (Brow *et al.*, 2000). Differentiating between the two has prognostic and therapeutic implications (Table 7.4). Corporal fibrosis, which causes venogenic (venous leak) impotence, develops secondary to abnormalities in the regulation of collagen synthesis and degradation, probably related to chronic ischemia (Nehra *et al.*, 1996). Erectile and sexual functions are regulated by dopamine and oxytocin release by the neurons of the hypothalamus. However, hypogonadism does not seem to contribute to the impaired penile reflex, as testosterone replacement does not cause the centrally mediated penile reflexes to recover (Sarapura and Schlaff, 1993; Sobrinho, 1993). Potassium (K) channels are key regulators of membrane potential and, therefore, of transmembrane Ca^{2+} flux, and, subsequently, the degree of contraction of many types of smooth muscle, including human corporal smooth muscle (Christ *et al.*, 1995). Corporal smooth muscle tone, in turn, modulates penile blood flow and intracavernous pressure and, as such, affects both penile rigidity and erectile capacity. At least four subtypes of K channels are present in human corporal myocytes, with the high conductance calcium-sensitive potassium channel (maxi-K or K_{Ca} channel) and the metabolically regulated potassium channel (K_{ATP}) being the most physiologically relevant. The low po_2 in patients with arteriogenic impotence, and the subset of men with severe venous leak impotence, support a concept of low cavernosal po_2 as a mechanism for both arteriogenic and venogenic impotence (Brow *et al.*, 2000).

Reproductive function is suppressed by hyperprolactinemia, but little is known about its effect on penile erection. Hyperprolactinemic men exhibit decreased libido and an inability to either obtain or maintain a rigid erection. Monga *et al.* (2001) evaluated the long-term efficacy of testosterone supplementation for ED, using parenteral Depo-testosterone, Testoderm scrotal patches as compared to Testoderm-transdermal therapeutic system (TTS) non-scrotal patches. They reported a better response with Depo-testosterone and Testoderm-TTS non-scrotal patches as compared to Testoderm scrotal patches. Testoderm-TTS non-scrotal patches were significantly better than Depo-testosterone with regard to satisfaction with sexual intercourse.

Table 7.2 Changes associated with erectile dysfunction (ED)

Hormonal, metabolic and pathophysiological
Loss of serum testosterone circadian rhythmicity
Psychosexual behavior of hypopituitary
Long-term consequences of castration in men
Testosterone effects on spatial cognition
Androgen–brain–behavior interactions
Hormonal therapy of male hypogonadism
Lack of sexual activity from ED associated with reversible reduction in serum testosterone
Endocrine profile
Depressive symptoms
Testosterone replacement and sleep-related erection
Androgen deficiency or aging
Effect of human growth hormone in men aged over 60
Geriatric psychiatry/psychopharmacology
Sexual health in later life
Love–sex–aging interactions
Sexuality and aging

Table 7.3 Sexuality and aging responses (Bhasin, 2000; Carani *et al.*, 1990; Cohan and Korenman, 2001; Heim, 1981; Korenman *et al.*, 1990; Schiavi and Rehman, 1995)

General effects
Anxiety, chronic fatigue and sleep disturbances, decreased lean body mass and muscular strength, and increased visceral fat distribution, decreased bone mineral density. Regression of secondary sexual characteristics
Sexual responses
Prolonged arousal response and decreased penile sensitivity. Erection is less rigid and delayed, and orgasm less intense. Rapid detumescence and a prolonged refractory period. Decrease in sexual desire, fantasy, spontaneous erections and masturbation
Histomorphology
Reduction in number of Leydig and Sertoli cells, thickening of the basal membrane of the seminiferous tubules, and arteriosclerotic lesions
Effects of androgen therapy
Chronic testosterone administration in physiological dosages sperm production by suppressing gonadotropin secretion.
After 6 months of weekly intramuscularly testosterone enanthate injections, 65% of subjects became azoospermic. In these individuals, the effectiveness of testosterone injections after 1 year was comparable to the effectiveness of oral contraceptives
These effects are reversible after treatment discontinuation
Specific sexual responses
Low–normal range concentrations of testosterone are sufficient to maintain sexual activity; there is a threshold level of testosterone above which no further improvement ensues in response to therapy
Administration of testosterone to normal eugonadal men enhances penile rigidity, but does not change the circumference or frequency of erections during nocturnal penile tumescence. In hypogonadal men, it improves libido and sexual performance
In all, 50% of castrated sex offenders could achieve and sustain an erection. Although nocturnal penile tumescence is inhibited by androgen deficiency, erections in response to visual erotic stimuli may be partly androgen independent
ED and secondary hypogonadism are two common independent disorders

Table 7.4 Pathophysiology of organic erectile dysfunction (ED)

Endocrine
Low testosterone levels associated with decreased libido, due to central effect of androgens on sexual function
Bioavailable testosterone levels related to nocturnal penile tumescence
Decline in nitric oxide synthase (NOS) activity in castrated animals reversed by androgen supplementation
NOS mRNA increases with androgen supplementation
Hypogonadism may be due to primary testicular failure, decreased gonadotropin releasing hormone (GnRH) secretion (e.g. in hyperprolactinemia), or alterations in steroid hormone protein binding (e.g. in alcoholism, liver failure)
Pharmacology
Centrally acting pharmacological agents, such as phenothiazines, opiates, tricyclic antidepressants and H_2-antagonists cause erectile dysfunction by increasing prolactin levels or decreasing dopaminergic stimulation
Vascular etiology of ED expected in 60% of patients. Small vessel vascular disease (e.g. diabetic) and large vessel arteriosclerosis (e.g. in hypertension) cause arterial insufficiency/ED; ED occurs in 25% of men treated for hypertension in diabetics
Hemodynamics
Tobacco alters penile arterial hemodynamics, causing ED in 81% of elderly smokers; pelvic radiation leads to fibrosis/stenosis of pelvic arteries/accelerates existing arteriosclerosis; veno-occlusive dysfunction may be due to decreased ability of corpora cavernosa or inherent abnormalities in tunica albuginea; elastic concentration in tunica albuginea/trabeculae decreased in ED; collagen type I increased in tunica albuginea of patients with arterial ED while collagen type IV increased in patients with venous ED
Molecular parameters
Vascular endothelial growth factor (VEGF) may play a role in modulation of normal vascularity of penile architecture; presence of four splice variants of VEGF mRNA (VEGF 120, 144, 164, 188) and two of its receptors (flt-l, KDR) in human cavernosal smooth muscle cells; VEGF 164 is most abundant form of mRNA, whereas flt-1 is the most prominent receptor type in these cells
Clinical disease
Diabetes, alcoholism and vitamin deficiencies contribute to somatic/autonomic neuropathy
Demyelinating diseases (e.g. multiple sclerosis) decrease penile sensation
Effects of aging
Aging elevates sensory thresholds to vibratory/electrical stimulation, pelvic/retroperitoneal surgery (e.g. radical prostatectomy) may damage autonomic nervous system controlling physiology of penile erection/ejaculation
Cellular senescence alters collagen content in corpora cavernosa and tunica albuginea, leading to veno-occlusive dysfunction and/or decreased neuronal transmission to cavernosal smooth muscle
Aging alters endothelial function/decreases basal NO release/up-regulation of basal endothelial-1 (ET1)
Reproductive aging in animals impairs erectile response: increase in latency period to attain an erection/decrease in maximal intracavernosal pressure; loss of functional integrity of endoluminal structures; imbalance in expression of vasoconstricting/vasorelaxing modulators of penile erection/decrease in e-NOS/increase in ET1 levels

Devices used to treat ED include those which are malleable, mechanical, inflatable (self-contained) and inflatable (multicomponent). These devices are inserted in the corpora cavernosa through an incision between the penis and scrotum. The inside of each chamber in the penis is stretched open to allow placement of the device. The chambers are then closed and the skin is stitched closed (Figure 7.1).

Biochemical parameters

ED can be due to organic and psychological mechanisms associated with psychological, neurological, endocrinological, vascular (venous or arterial), traumatic or iatrogenic factors (drugs and surgery). Selective inhibition of the enzyme phosphodiesterase (PDE) type 5, the enzyme responsible for the breakdown of cyclic guanosine monophosphate (cGMP) in the corpora cavernosa, has been used to treat ED. Persistence of cGMP leads to smooth muscle relaxation, resulting in erection. Extensive studies have been conducted on the etiology, pathophysiology, pharmacokinetics and therapy of ED (Chew *et al.*, 2000; Christ, 1995; Christ *et al.*, 1995; Fabbri and Aversa, 1997; Govier *et al.*, 1997; Jaffe *et al.*, 1996; Lee *et al.*, 2000; Sarteschi *et al.*, 1998).

Nitric oxide (NO)-mediated smooth muscle relaxation is a critical event during sexually stimulated penile erection. Subsequent to activation of neuronal and endothelial NO synthases, NO diffuses into penile

Table 7.5 Clinical manifestation/psychophysiological mechanism and management of different types of erectile dysfunction (ED) and related phenomena

	Management
Honeymoon impotence common in Middle East, especially in the first sexual relationship in Islamic man's life	Oral sildenafil (Viagra) and intracorporeal injection of papaverine-phentolamine are both effective
Hypercholesterolemia, occlusive atherosclerosis of aorta/common iliac arteries	Chronic oral arginine
Congential penile curvature causing penile deformity, that precludes sexual intercourse	Nesbit corporoplasty with plication sutures or incisional corporoplasty (longitudinal incision/transverse closure) Heineke–Mikuletz principle; convex side of curvature exposed by a degloving subcoronal incision
	Both techniques are effective; modified Nesbit procedure achieves higher rate of correction of curvature, yet incisional corporoplasty is easier, simpler and safer. Urethral stricture may develop following any type of phalloplasty
Esthetic appearance of abnormal/ normal penis	Buccal mucosa is ideal, urethral substitute can be used in any type of phalloplasty. Graft takes reliability within 7 days and can be grafted onto fat, dermis, granulation and scar tissue
Invasive therapy in selected cases where (semi-)conservative treatment is ineffective, precarious or not accepted	Yohimbine first administered in clinic under supervision, then patients allowed to increase dose at home (titration) under more conducive circumstances, nocturnal emission main side-effect
Over 100 different variations of surgeries entitled 'penile revascularization'	In successful arteriovenous fistulae to deep dorsal penile vein dilatation, stenosis or occlusion can occur. Color duplex sonography recommended for early detection of postoperative change
	Operation for young patients with pure arteriogenic impotence with no vascular risk factors, prognosis for success of surgery is the presence of a branch from the dorsal artery to the cavernous tissue

vascular smooth muscle cells and binds the heme moiety of soluble guanylyl cyclase to stimulate the synthesis of cGMP, an important intracellular messenger that transduces extracellular signals in cavernosal smooth muscle cells. These events result in smooth muscle relaxation within the resistance arteries and cavernosal trabeculae, enabling exposure to systemic arterial blood pressure and corporal volume expansion.

Little is known about the effect of stress-related hormone changes on the neurobiological correlates of psychogenic impotence. future research is needed to evaluate parameters of blood biochemistry, hormone profile and the corpora cavernosa associated with ED. Patterns of ED have been examined using frequency distributions and contingency tables generated with Microsoft Graph software. Statistical associations were assessed using the χ^2 test. The relationships between various grades of ED and self-reported comorbidity were examined using logistic regression and EGRET software, with the final multivariate model being derived using backwards stepwise elimination (Chew *et al.*, 2000). Color power Doppler sonography is a valuable technique in the initial evaluation of penile circulation in ED (Aversa *et al.*, 2000). This procedure is employed to achieve a full penile erection and complete smooth muscle relaxation by an intracavernous injection (ICI) of several vasoactive drugs to evaluate fully both the morphodynamic features of the cavernous arteries and to obtain information about the corpora cavernosa (Table 7.5).

Neurological mechanisms

Penile erection (PE), a psychoneuroendocrine vascular phenomenon, involves three simultaneous steps: arterial dilatation with subsequent increase in flow; lucunar space dilatation with filling of the corpora cavernosa; and, decreased venous outflow (Fabri and

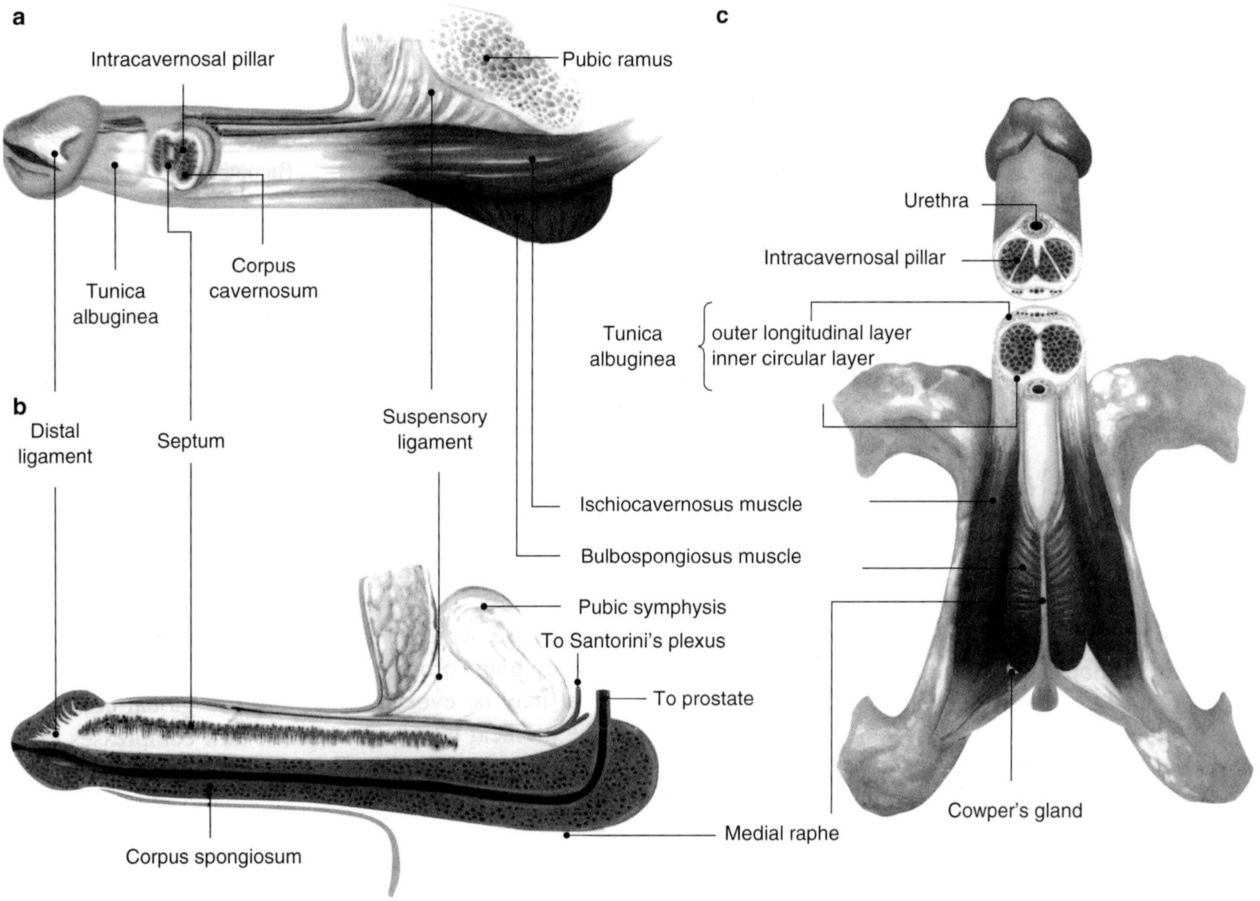

Figure 7.1 Schematic illustration of the human penis. (**a**) Lateral aspect. The penis leans on and is supported by a suspensory ligament, which is an extension of the linea alba. It is capped by the glans penis. Proximally, the corpus spongiosum is held by the bulbospongiosus muscle in which the fibers are mostly transverse. The corpora cavernosa are surrounded by the tunica albuginea, which is a bilayered structure (an inner circular and an outer longitudinal layer with multiple sublayers). The intracavernosal pillars, which may be considerably larger distally, are a continuation of the inner circular layer. Each corpus cavernosum is entrapped in the ischiocavernosus muscle with the muscle fibers aligned in the longitudinal direction. (**b**) Medial aspect. The distal ligament is aggregated from the collagen bundles of the outer longitudinal layer of the tunica albuginea. It is a non-elastic fibrous structure that forms the trunk of the glans penis. The incomplete septum is dorsally fenestrated. The corpus spongiosum contains the urethra. (**c**) Ventral aspect. The three-dimensional structure of the human penis is evident. The ischiocavernosus muscle is paired with and situated at the lateral boundary of the perineum. Each segment covers its ipsilateral penile crus. Meanwhile, the anterior fibers of the bulbospongiosus muscle partly radiate to encircle the corpus cavernosum and insert mainly into the ventral thickening of the tunica. From Hsu *et al.* (2004), with permission

Aversa, 1997). PE is associated with increased arterial flow, smooth muscle relaxation and increased venous outflow resistance. Psychological distress can have a grave detrimental effect on sexual function. However, psychiatric disease does not predispose or protect against the development of cardiac, diabetic or endocrine conditions (Blazer *et al.*, 1994; Feldman *et al.*, 1994; Helmchen *et al.*, 1996). There is concern about the possible negative effects of psychiatric medications on erectile function and libido. The increased size of the cavernosal bodies creates stretching and compression of the subtunical venules, leading to functionally rigid penile erections.

CLINICAL PARAMETERS

Clinical testing

A simple, inexpensive test is to provide the patient with test strips to determine nocturnal erections and the rigidity of the erection. This can be accomplished with commercially prepared strips or even with postage stamps placed on the penis at bedtime. Dorsal nerve conduction studies may be obtained if neural origin is suspected and the patient wishes to pursue nerve grafting. Doppler color flow studies can help to assess the arterial flow to the cavernosa. This may be of benefit to those who are seeking surgical revisualization (Basson, 2001; Baum and Spiefer, 2001; Colpo, 1988; Lue, 1992; Rendell *et al.*, 1999).

Priapism (Table 7.6)

Priapism, prolonged erection unaccompanied by sexual desire or stimulation, is manifested in two categories: high flow (non-ischemic) and low flow (ischemic) depending upon the veins involved, severity of the disease and duration of venous occlusion (Ramos *et al.*, 1995; Seftel *et al.*, 1998). High-flow priapism is characterized by adequate (or increased) arterial inflow with normal venous outflow, but helicine arteriolar bypass, or a defect in regulation, prevents detumescence (Sartenshi *et al.*, 1998). Causes of low-flow priapism include sickle cell anemia, leukemia, secondary penile cancer, prostatitis, urethritis, prolonged sexual intercourse/erection, pelvic thromboses, congenital neonatal priapism, spinal stenosis, spinal cord injury, antipsychotic drugs, clozapine, chlorpromazine, antihypertensives, hydralazine, guanethidine, antidepressants, marijuana, alcohol, cocaine, heparin and testosterone (Hoffman *et al.*, 2000).

THERAPY (TABLES 7.7–7.9)

Factors that affect erections can be of five different etiologies or any combination of these causes. Psychogenic and organic are the major classifications of etiology for erectile dysfunction. Organic origin is further designated as neurological, hormonal, vascular, cavernosal and mixed etiologies. Treatment could include:

(1) Oral medication – Viagra®, Vasomax, apomorphine, pentoxifylline, yohimbine and other oral agents, including testosterone replacement;

(2) Mechanical devices – vacuum erection devices (VED);

(3) Injection therapy – including Caverject®, Edex, alprostadil, papaverine and Regitine®;

(4) Surgical treatment – penile implants, vascular surgery to improve blood flow, treatment for Peyronie's disease, plication or plaque removal.

Intracavernous vasoactive injections

Several intracavernous vasoactive injections have been used alone or in combination for the evaluation and diagnosis of ED: papaverine, phentolamine,

Table 7.6 Priapism

Symptoms
Penile erection persistent, prolonged, painful/tender
Urination difficult during erection
Loss of sexual function if treatment is not prompt
Low flow or ischemic priapism – glans penis flaccid
High flow or arterial priapism – glans penis rigid
Causes
Intracavernosal injections of vocative drugs for erectile dysfunction; most common causes
pelvic vascular thrombosis
sickle cell anemia/leukemia
cerebrospinal tumors
bladder calculus
prolonged sexual activity
pelvic hematoma or neoplasia
tertiary syphilis
injury to penis
Urinary tract infections, prostatitis, arthritis, cystitis
Several drugs: chlorpromazine, prazosin, trazodone, and certain corticosteroids, anticoagulants, antihypertensives
Diagnosis
Full blood count
Coagulation profile
Platelet count
Urinalysis
Imaging
Penile Doppler testing may be necessary to differentiate high- from low-flow priapism
Treatment
Continuous caudal or spinal anesthesia if etiology is neurogenic
Treat any underlying cause
In sickle cell anemia: intravenous hydration; partial exchange or repeated transfusions to reduce sickle cells below 50%
Surgery
Introduction of 12- or 16-gauge needle into corpora cavernosa
first: aspiration of 20–30 ml of blood from corpora cavernosa with 12–16-gauge needle
then: if caused by injected vasodilator, use intracavernous injection of 10–25 mg ephedrine sulfate or 510 μg epinephrine or 125–250 μg phenylephrine
may repeat once after 20–30 min if no response
Create fistula between glans and corpus cavernosa
Semipermanent division by saphenous shunt from one or both corpora
Cavernosa–spongiosum shunt to permit re-establishment of pelvic circulation
Medication
Narcotics for pain if needed
Vasoconstrictors may be injected after dilution
Metaraminol 1 mg into penis

Table 7.7 Erectile dysfunction (ED) treatment options (Aversa *et al.*, 2000; Chew *et al.*, 2000; Costa *et al.*, 1996; Fabbri and Aversa, 1997; Fujisawa and Sawada, 2002; Jarrow *et al.*, 1999; Linet and Ogrinc, 1996; McMahon *et al.*, 2000; Tissot and Johnson, 2002; Wilke *et al.*, 1997)

Behavioral modification/counseling
Stress reduction, rest and exercise may improve sexual function
Patients instructed on techniques of sensate focusing/increased sexual foreplay to enhance arousal, patient and partner encouraged to broaden their sexual dialog and share wants, needs and preferences
Brief psychoeducational counseling improves patient and partner satisfaction with oral pharmacological therapy for erectile dysfunction.
Intraurethral medication
MUSE® (Vivus) is the intraurethral administration of alprostadil (prostaglandin E_1 (PGE_1) suppository), absorption of PGE_1 across the tunica albuginea to reach corporal bodies is limited, with systemic absorption through well vascularized corpus spongiosum, high concentrations of PGE_1 used to maintain efficacy: significant burning in up to 30% of patients
Success rates of 65%, as determined by one successful sexual intercourse
Highly successful for selected patients with adequate tumescene/rigidity whose primary problem is early detumescence due to anxiety or mild–moderate veno-occlusive dysfunction
Vacuum erection device
Cylinder placed over penis and vacuum pressure > 100 mmHg generated using a hand-pump or battery-operated pump to cause passive engorgement of the penis, improved rigidity by 'double-pump': applying a vacuum for 2 min, then releasing and reapplying. Once a good erection is obtained, a constrictive band is placed at base of penis and the vacuum released
Rare side-effects: penile ecchymosed or hematoma and use of vacuum erection device cautioned in anticoagulated patient; penile cyanosis/diminished sensation; rigidity extends proximally only to level of constrictive device; more proximally corpora is flaccid, therefore, crura of corpora cavernosa is not 'fixed' at pubic bone
Penile prostheses
Risks: infection and device malfunction; patient/partner satisfaction rates 77%; inflatable penile prostheses better than malleable penile prostheses
Penile drug delivery implants
A cannula which is inserted into the corpus cavernosum and a combined scrotal reservior and a pump containing a vasoactive drug. Compression of the reservoir pump distributes a bolus of vasoactive agent to the penis and stimulates erectile response. When active, the device works extremely well giving excellent quality erection. Failure may be due to leaking reservoir, blocked tubes, mechanical failure or infection
Remote intracorporeal injection
Self-intracavernous injection (SICI) is the most convenient way to deliver drugs, however, it is difficult to perform and carries the risk of corporeal multipuncture; to overcome these difficulties/risks, a specific device is successfully implanted
Self-injection devices
The use of intracorporeal papaverine, papaverine/phentolamine mixtures is widely used for diagnosis and therapy of ED. Chlorpromazine is a useful substitute for phentolamine when used in combination with papaverine. Advantage of alpha-blocker chlorpromazine over phentolamine is reduced cost of drug with similar or the same effectiveness
Low dose PGE_1
4 μg is effective/safe, intracavernous injection (ICI)

PGE_1, prostaglandin E_1

prostaglandin E_1 (PGE_1), vasointestinal peptide and moxysilite (Costa *et al.*, 1996; Govier *et al.*, 1997). High levels of state-anxiety, measured by psychological tests, are often present in newly diagnosed impotent patients and may lead to an incomplete pharmaco-induced erection with vasoactive agents (Aversa *et al.*, 2000). Since the veno-occlusive mechanism is highly susceptible to psychological factors and to the type and dosage of the vasoactive agent, some authors used to combine intracavernous injection with audiovisual sexual stimulation (AVSS) (Costa *et al.*, 1996). Treatment of 'phallodynamically' challenged individuals without adequately addressing the possible presence of psychopathology accounts for treatment failures and has the potential for leaving untreated serious emotional problems.

Table 7.8 Some medication side-effects

Brand name	*Generic name or generic ingredients*	*Side-effects/comments*
Caverject®	Prostaglandin E_1	Penile injection of drug may result in adequate erection. For use only under urologist's supervision. Improper use may cause priapism or penile scarring
Cerebid®	Papaverine	Penile injection of drug may result in adequate erection. For use only under urologist's supervision. Improper use may cause priapism or penile scarring. Available under other brand names
Regitine®	Phentolamine	Penile injection of drug may result in adequate erection. For use only under urologist's supervision. Improper use may cause priapism or penile scarring
Desyrel®	Trazadone	Oral drug for treating impotence by improving function of the smooth muscles of the penis. Used in higher dosages as an antidepressant. Impotence patients should never take more than the prescribed dosage
Viagra®	Sildenafil	Oral drug for treating erectile dysfunction by increasing blood flow and erectile stimulation. May cause headaches, indigestion and color/brightness visionary disturbances. Should not be taken by patients with severe kidney or liver failure, rare disease retinitis pigmentosa of the eye, or using nitroglycerin or nitrates
Yocon®	Yohimbine	Drug with apparent aphrodisiac properties. May cause elevated blood pressure, rapid heart rate, irritability, tremor, dizziness, headache and nausea. Available in other brand names

Table 7.9 Penile implants used for erectile dysfunction (ED)

Malleable
Slight increase in penis diameter
Least likely to malfunction
Bendable
Always rigid (can be bent)
Mechanical
Slight increase in penis diameter
Easier to bend
Rare malfunction
Always rigid
Inflatable (self-contained)
Sight increase in penis diameter
More risk of malfunction
Pump at end of penis
Increase/decrease rigidity
Inflatable (multi-component)
Slight increase in length and diameter
Increase/decrease rigidity
Most like normal
Most likely to malfunction

Sildenafil (Viagra®)

Sildenafil (Viagra) helps 70% of those treated to achieve sexual function. It was originally developed for heart disease, but was found to have a unique mechanism of action that blocks the enzyme phosphodiestgerase-5, thus maintaining persistent levels of cGMP, which is produced in the penis during sexual arousal and relaxes smooth muscle and increases blood flow. Viagra is effective within 20–40 min without risk of priapism (Tissot and Johnson, 2001).

Alprostadil

Medicated urethral system for erection (MUSE®) (Vivus; Merck) is the intraurethral administration of alprostadil (prostaglandin E_1 (PGE_1) suppository). Absorption of PGE_1 across the tunica albuginea to reach corporal bodies is limited, with systemic absorption through well vascularized corpus spongiosum. High concentrations of PGE_1 are used to maintain efficacy: a significant burning sensation can occur in up to 30% of patients. Sixty-five per cent (65%) success rates are reported, as determined by one successful sexual intercourse; in significant organic disease only 7% sustained rigid erections and 63% erections inadequate for sexual intercourse are reported.

MUSE is most effective in conjunction with use of an Actus Ring to restrict the venous flow. The most commonly used dose for patients at the Charleston V.A. Hospital is 500 μg, with a range of 125–1000 μg. MUSE should be inserted, after urinating, by pushing the button to completely insert the alprostadil into the urethra. Gently massaging or rolling the penis in the hand helps absorb the medication into the tissues. The effect is enhanced with standing for approximately 10 min and sexual stimulation. Sexual positions can affect the erect penis. Standing or being on top help keep the penis erect.

Testosterone supplement

Monga *et al.* (2003) evaluated the effect of various testosterone supplements on improved libido, improved energy and improved erection (Table 7.10).

Devices used to treat ED (Figure 7.2)

Devices and techniques used to treat ED include:

(1) Penile implants:

(a) malleable implant in normal or
(b) erect position;
(c) inflatable implant (Bostwick *et al.*, 1999).

Table 7.10 Comparative effects of various testosterone supplements on patients with erectile dysfunction (Monga *et al.*, 2002)

	DPT	*TSD*	*TTS*
Follow-up (months)	92	38	28
Serum testosterone (ng/dl) post-therapy	662	443	488
Improved libido (%)	73	38	86
Improved energy (%)	53	38	86
Improved erections (%)	40	31	57
Discontinuation rate (%)	13	73	0

DPT, Depo-testosterone; TSD, Testoderm scrotal patches; TTS, transdermal testosterone system non-scrotal patches

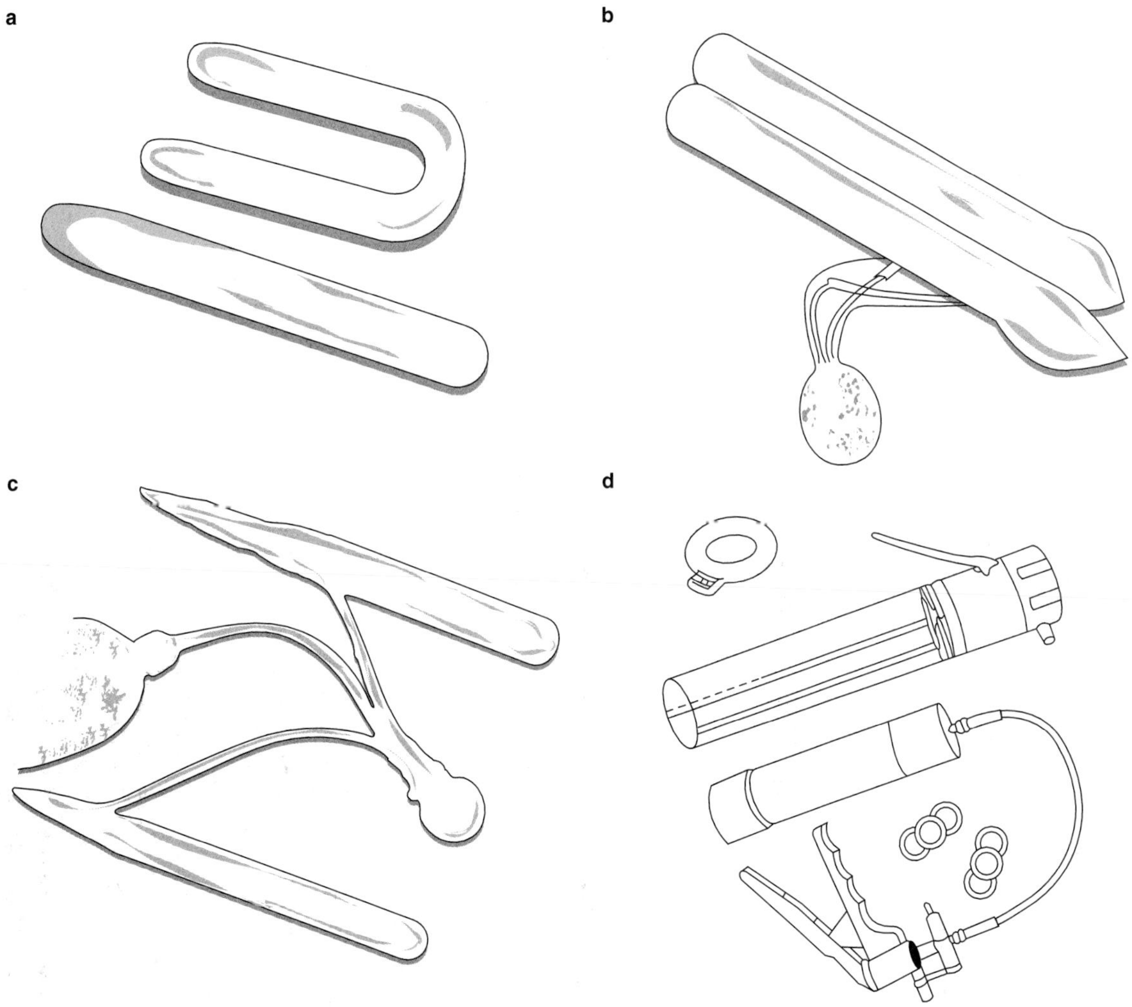

Figure 7.2 Penile implants used for erectile dysfunction. (**a**) Malleable penile implant: a bendable prosthesis placed into both of the corpora can be bent in any direction. There are no moving parts, so problems with malfunction and breakage are rare. Courtesy of Mentor Urology, Inc. (**b**) Multicomponent inflatable penile implant uses a separate pump placed in the scrotum to inflate and deflate separate cylinders in the corpora. A separate reservoir may be used to hold fluid. This device allows for the most natural results. Courtesy of American Medical Systems, Inc. (**c**) Inflatable penile implant with scrotal pump, which is also the reservoir. This is squeezed to pump fluid into the device and results in increased rigidity. From Marks (1999), with permission. (**d**) One-handed unit, including cylinder and pump combined with thick ring and two-handed unit, including clear cylinder, vacuum pump and thin rings

(2) Penile anatomy and self-injection: normal erection develops when blood flows into both corpora cavernosa within the penis. Penile self-injection is an effective technique to produce an erection by stimulating blood flow with medication injected directly into one of the corpora. After the medication is injected through a tiny needle, blood flow increases and an erection develops.

(3) Mechanical penile implant: this movable device, placed into the corpora, is easier to bend and stays in position better than the malleable penile implant.

(4) Malleable penile implant: a bendable prosthesis placed into both of the corpora bent in any direction. There are no moving parts, so problems with malfunction and breakage are rare.

(5) Multicomponent inflatable penile implant: inflatable penile implant uses a separate pump placed in the scrotum to inflate and deflate separate cylinders in the corpora. A separate reservoir may be used to hold fluid. This device allows for the most natural results.

(6) Inflatable penile implant: inflatable penile implant with scrotal pump, which is also the reservoir. This is squeezed to pump fluid into the device and results in increased rigidity.

(7) Penile clamp: penile clamp squeezes urethra shut to prevent urine from leaking.

(8) Artificial sphincter: placed surgically, the artificial sphincter provides relief from severe urinary incontinence. Cuff surrounds bladder neck and urethra and squeezes shut, blocking any urine leakage. Device is activated and deactivated by a pump placed in the scrotum.

(9) Vacuum erection device: uses a pump attached to a plastic cylinder. The cylinder is placed over the lubricated penis, and a vacuum is created by the pump. This results in blood flowing into the two chambers in the penis to create an erection. An elastic ring is then slipped off of the cylinder onto the base of the penis to keep the blood in place and the erection intact.

8

Ejaculatory anomalies

The physiological and psychological disorders of sexual desire, arousal and orgasm are summarized in Table 8.1 and illustrated in Figures 8.1 and 8.2. Sexual dysfunction may be due to drug administration and/or medical–neural–psychogenic interaction (Table 8.2).

There are two main ejaculatory abnormalities: retrograde flow of semen is the complete or incomplete flow of semen into the bladder; and anejaculation is the complete absence of ejaculate due to total failure of seminal emission into the posterior urethra. Anejaculation is differentiated from retrograde flow by conducting a postorgasmic urinalysis test, which in anejaculation reveals a non-viscous, fructose-negative and sperm negative result.

RETROGRADE FLOW OF SEMEN

'Retrograde flow of semen' erroneously referred to as 'retrograde ejaculation' involves the flow of semen into the urinary bladder during orgasm. In normal men the urinary sphincter remains closed during ejaculation to prevent retrograde semen flow into the bladder. However, if the sphincter is not contracted for any reason, the ejaculate may flow backwards into the bladder rather than flow normally through the urethra. Thus, retrograde flow of semen is caused by several physiological anomalies which interfere with sympathetic innervation and anatomical defects of the smooth musculature of the bladder neck. Retrograde flow of semen may be associated with various conditions:

(1) Men with multiple sclerosis, spinal cord injury or extensive pelvic surgery, e.g. prostatectomy;

(2) Retroperitoneal lymph node dissection to treat testicular cancer, probably due to the removal of or damage to sympathetic ganglia/hypogastric plexus;

(3) Transurethral resection of prostate or bladder neck, resulting in interruption in sympathetic innervation to bladder neck;

(4) Diabetic visceral neuropathy, causing erectile dysfunction or retrograde flow of semen;

(5) Pharmacological agents causing psychogenic or idiopathic erectile or ejaculatory dysfunction, including antipsychotic drugs, chlorpromazine, antihypertensive drugs, α-adrenergic blockers, bethanidine, prazosin hydrochloride, phenoxybenzamine hydrochloride (Jeyendran, 2003).

Symptoms and diagnosis

Symptoms of retrograde flow of semen include:

(1) Aspermia (total lack of an ejaculate after orgasm) caused by 'complete' retrograde flow of semen into the bladder;

(2) Absent or intermittent emission of ejaculate;

(3) Presence of sperm within voided urine after orgasm;

(4) Hypospermia (tiny semen volume (<0.5 ml)) caused by 'incomplete' retrograde flow of semen.

Medical treatment

Medical treatment for the correction of retrograde ejaculation is based on either increasing sympathetic tone at the bladder neck or decreasing parasympathetic

Table 8.1 Physiological and psychological disorders of sexual desire, arousal and orgasm

Desire
Deficient sexual fantasies and desire for sexual activity or an extreme aversion to genital sexual contact
Stress-related causes: poor marital adjustment (marital stress), in-built and religious prohibitions, fear of intimacy, fear of loss of control over sexual urges, fear of sexually transmitted diseases and post-traumatic stress disorder as a result of rape or sexual assault
Job/family are not significant causes of such disorders
Aversion disorders are stressful to the individual and to any (potential) partners
Arousal
Inability to attain or maintain a physiological arousal response
Anxiety plays a central role etiologically in interfering with sexual arousal, particularly erectile failure
Sexual arousal/anxiety include both cognitive and physiological components, sexual arousal can be affected through reciprocal inhibition, i.e. incompatible behaviors or other emotions can interfere with arousal
Cognitively, sexual arousal can be affected through cognitive control over arousal, intentional factors including distracting thoughts, and attention focus during performance demand
Physiological/cognitive factors have different effects on sexual arousal when anxiety is induced in individuals with sexual dysfunction compared with those with no sexual dysfunction
In individuals with sexual dysfunction, sympathetic arousal inhibits sexual arousal as indicated by reciprocal inhibition; however, this is not the case in individuals who do not have sexual dysfunction. In fact, in these individuals, sympathetic arousal may even facilitate sexual arousal
Sexually functional men differ from sexually dysfunctional men in that they are aware of this control and they can identify the cognitive strategies they use
When distracted by non-erotic stimuli, penile tumescence decreases in sexually functional men but not in sexually dysfunctional men; instead, a slight increase occurs
Sexually functional men achieve a greater increase in penile tumescence in high-performance demand conditions than in low-performance demand conditions. For sexually dysfunctional men, the opposite is true
When anxiety is induced, physiological and cognitive factors can adversely affect sexual arousal in sexually dysfunctional men, whereas these factors can positively affect sexual arousal in sexually functional individuals. Other etiological factors affecting sexual arousal are psychosocial stress, whereby chronic and acute stress result in erection impairment, and a history of sexual abuse
Orgasm
Premature ejaculation, delay in or absence of orgasm, or ejaculation with minimal sexual stimulation
Stress-related etiological factors include performance disorders
In couples who report a greater number of stressful life events (particularly marital problems), it is more common for sexual dysfunction disorders to be reported than in those with fewer stressful life events
Induced anxiety can affect sexual arousal. It is difficult to differentiate the effects of stress from the effects of anxiety
Inversely, sexual dysfunction can also be a causal factor in stress onset or exacerbate existing stress for the individual and/or couple

activity, when alpha-agonistic or anticholinergic and antihistaminic drugs are used, respectively. At the administered doses, the side-effects of drugs given for the reversal of retrograde ejaculation include various degrees of dizziness, sleep disturbances, weakness, restlessness, dry mouth, nausea or sweating during the medical treatment.

The effect of amezinium, a new type of antihypotensive agent, on retrograde ejaculation has been studied. The patients received 10 mg amezinium orally once a day. All patients achieved antegrade ejaculation. Semen analyses revealed 650×10^6/ml (mean 28.7×10^6/ml) sperm with a motility of 20–50% (mean 36.7%). The wives of two of the patients became pregnant within 6 months of the initial treatment. None of the patients had any side-effects.

Sperm retrieval from urine

Urine, due to its acidity and other factors, is naturally detrimental to sperm quality. In order to obtain viable sperm from urine, the osmolality and acidity of

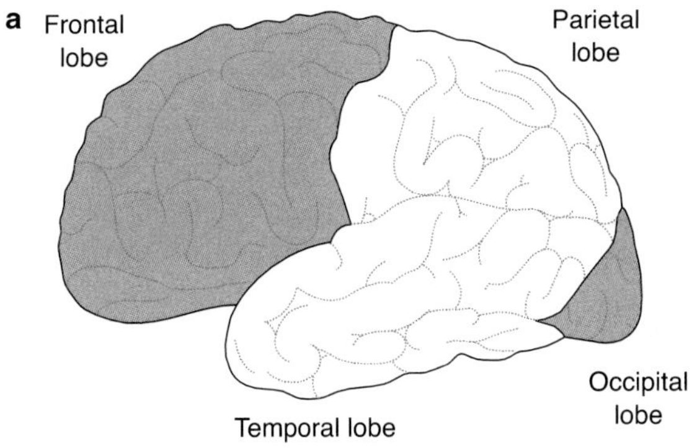

b

Sex steroids support sex behavior

	Desire	Arousal
Male	androgens	androgens
Female	androgens	estrogens

Figure 8.1 (**a**) Areas of the brain that are important for normal sexual desire and responsiveness. (**b**) Types of hormones linked to desire and arousal. From Morrell and Flynn (2003), with permission

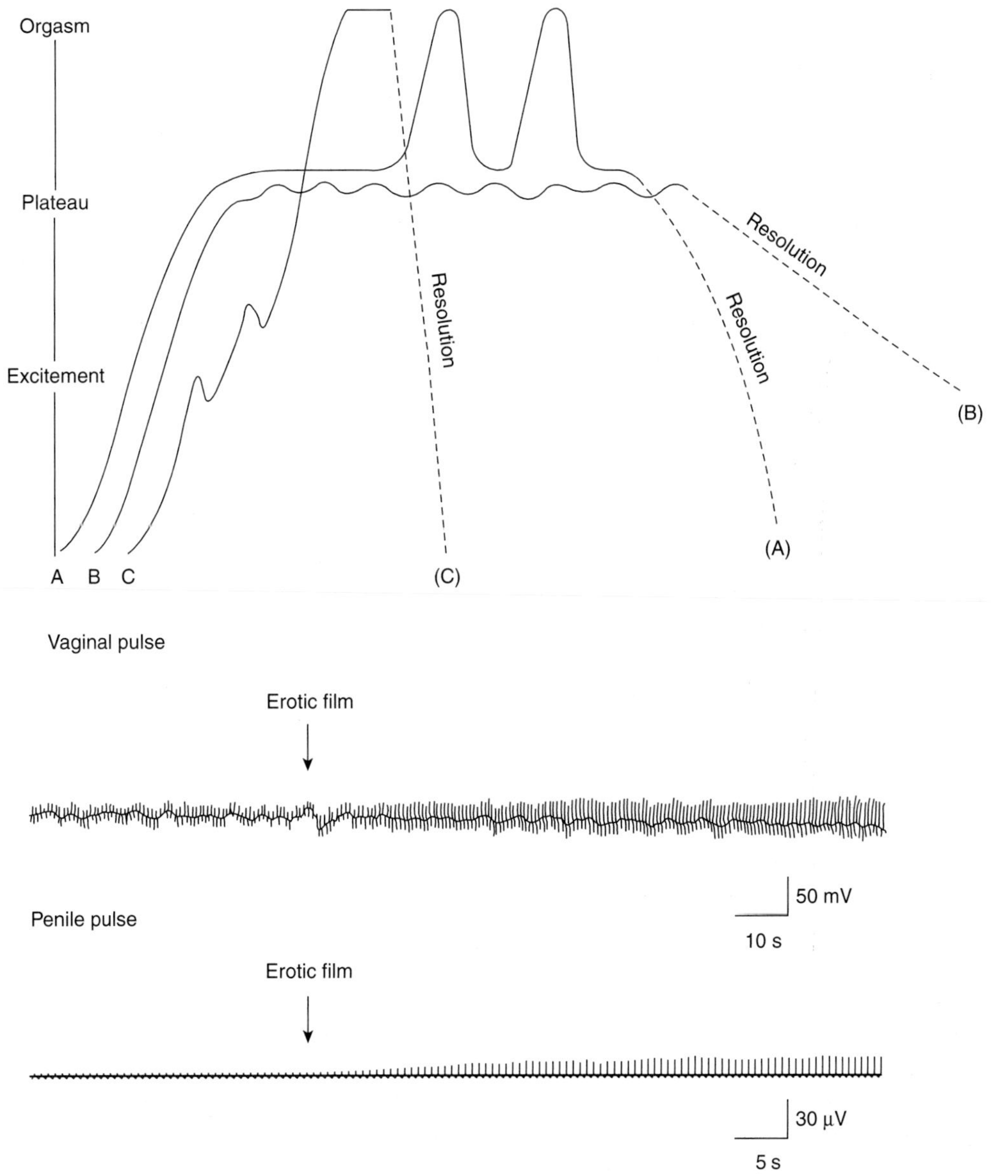

Figure 8.2 Physiological sexual response in men and women (upper panel). Blood flow measurements in male and female genitalia in response to erotic film (lower panel). From Morrell and Flynn (2003), with permission

Table 8.2 Causes of sexual dysfunction (Morrell and Flynn, 2003)

Drugs	
Psychotropic drugs	monoamine oxidase inhibitors, phenothiazines, barbiturates, benzodiazepines, alcohol
Antihypertensive drugs	methyldopa, beta-blockers, α-adrenergic blockers
Other	anticholinergics, stimulants, narcotics
Medical	
Vascular	small-vessel disease secondary to diabetes, hypertension, hyperlipidemia
Endocrine	hyperprolactinemia, hypothyroidism or hyperthyroidism, significantly low testosterone
Systemic illness	renal, hepatic, cardiac or pulmonary; cancer
Urogenital	infections, injury
Neural	
Spinal cord	injury or disease
Neuropathy	peripheral, autonomic
Cortical lesions	frontal lobe, temporal lobe
Psychogenic	
Psychiatric	psychosis, depression, bipolar illness
Intrapsychiatric	result of religious, social, family taboos; early-life sexual experience, low self-esteem
Extrapsychiatric	dysfunctional relationship

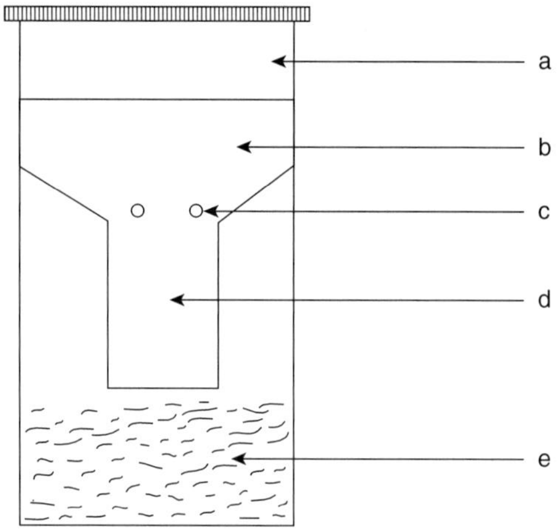

Figure 8.3 Retrograde sperm collection device. Urine collection container (**a**), housing the semen collection device. Reusable semen collection device (**b**), designed to separate initial voided urine flow aliquot. Urine overflow ducts (**c**), facilitating separation of initial voided urine from remaining flow. Initial voided urine flow (high relative semen concentration) aliquot retention receptacle (**d**) and excess voided urine (**e**) (low semen concentration). Jeyendran, 2003

bladder urine are adjusted using chemicals which minimize the detrimental qualities of urine towards semen. Two main methods are used to equalize osmolality and to neutralize the pH effects of urine.

Procedure 1

Aliquots of 5 ml of voided urine are collected, after masturbation, in buffered physiological solution or media.

A reusable device allows for easy and efficient collection of urine containing retrograde semen flow (Figures 8.3 and 8.4). Since such retrograde semen flow typically saturates the urine, the retrograde sperm collection device mechanically isolates only the initial portion of voided urine to facilitate optimal sperm separation.

Procedure 2

The patient drinks large volumes of water to dilute the urine, starting 48 h before and continuing on the morning of urine collection. Urine pH is raised above 7.5 by ingestion of 650 mg sodium bicarbonate tablets 48 h before and on the morning of collection or ingestion of Alka-Seltzer® (two tablets) on the night before and morning of collection. In patients who are unable to void urine, their bladder can be catheterized (30–60 ml media should be instilled into the bladder and sperm should be retrieved rapidly after orgasm to minimize any deleterious effects of urine on sperm quality).

A dose of 10–60 mg nifedipine given orally, singly or in combination with nitroglycerin tablets should be given sublingually 10 min before initiation of the procedure, when blood pressure is normal/stabilized.

Three professionals are needed in the out-patient setting: a nurse to monitor the patient; a clinician to operate the electrostimulator; and an assistant to collect the ejaculate. The patient should be sedated with diazepam, hesperidins or midazolam. Blood pressure should be recorded when the patient is in a wheelchair, then when lying on a table.

The bladder should be emptied, flushed with 10 ml of media and infused with 10 ml media, the catheter then being withdrawn leaving media *in situ*.

If one finger can slip easily into the rectum a 2.5-cm probe should be used; a 3-cm probe should be used if two fingers can slip in easily. The probe should be connected to a stimulator and inserted 10–11 cm inside the anal ring. Ejaculation occurs upon application of 4–10 V with higher cord lesions (T10 and

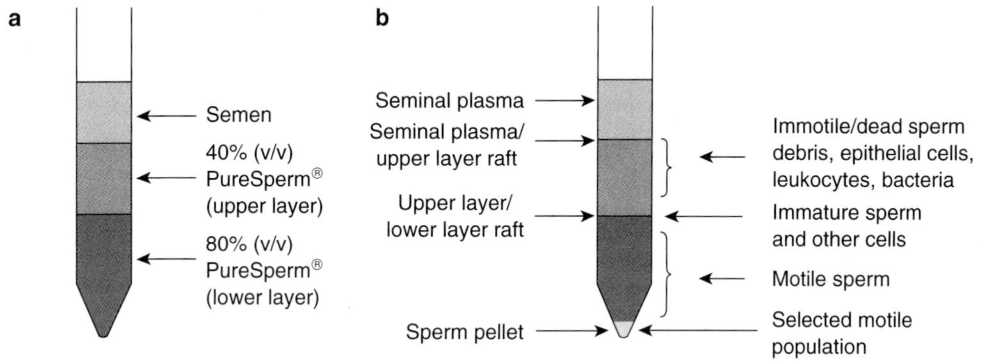

Figure 8.4 Sperm before (**a**) and after centrifugation (**b**)

above. The probe should be withdrawn immediately upon ejaculation, the rectum examined and the bladder catheterized and flushed to obtain any retrograde ejaculate (oral antibiotics may be required for 34 days after the procedure).

Anejaculation

Anejaculation, the physical inability to ejaculate, may result from diabetes, spinal cord injury, neurological disorders and idiopathic or psychogenic factors. In such cases, clinical semen collection can be achieved using mechanical, electrical or pharmacological procedures.

Several instruments have been used for vibratory stimulation of the penis to induce a reflex ejaculation, including 'Swedish massager' and Ling 201 vibrator (Ling Dynamics, Royston, UK).

Unfortunately, these techniques are not effective during the first 6 months after spinal injuries, and patients lose their capacity for reflex hip flexion. The success of such procedures depends on the location of the injury. Central nervous system lesions on T8 and above may tolerate artificially induced ejaculation; however, the procedure is ineffective with injuries to lower vertebrae.

Psychogenic anejaculation

This type of infertility refers to patients who cannot produce a semen specimen for analysis or for use in intrauterine insemination (IUI) and, in some cases, are also unable to ejaculate during intercourse. The patient is unable to ejaculate around the time of his wife's ovulation, although sperm are present in the postcoital test. Vibratory stimulation is recommended because it is simpler and less invasive, and can be performed in the office or at home. Since electroejaculation (EEJ) requires general anesthesia, EEJ can be used in neurologically intact men. In men with a neurological problem, it is more cost-effective to perform *in vitro* fertilization (IVF) rather than IUI. Testicular sperm extraction and IVF/intracytoplasmic sperm injection (ICSI) can be performed for such patients, thus avoiding general anesthesia and EEJ altogether. IUI combined with EEJ or penile vibratory stimulation is cost-effective in patients with spinal cord injury who do not require anesthesia. If the patient cannot ejaculate at ovulation by vibratory stimulation, a semen sample can be cryopreserved. Sex therapy may also help the patient ejaculate intravaginally by gradual desensitization. Open microsurgical vasal aspiration is another option. Sex therapy is considered for patients with initial complaints of erectile dysfunction and retarded ejaculation.

Pharmacology of anejaculation

Pharmacological drugs are not recommended for anejaculation, because of the inherent unpredictability of ejaculatory response, coupled with potentially deleterious side-effects. Tricyclic antidepressant drugs such as imipramine induce episodes of spontaneous ejaculation and orgasm in a dose-dependent manner during yawning and defecation. Such compounds and their metabolites inhibit norepinephrine reuptake by promoting α-adrenergic activity. Intrathecal neostigmine methylsulfate has been applied to obtain semen from physically disabled men.

Therapy

Vibratory stimulation

The patient is placed in the supine position, the vibrator is turned on and adjusted to 100 Hz frequency.

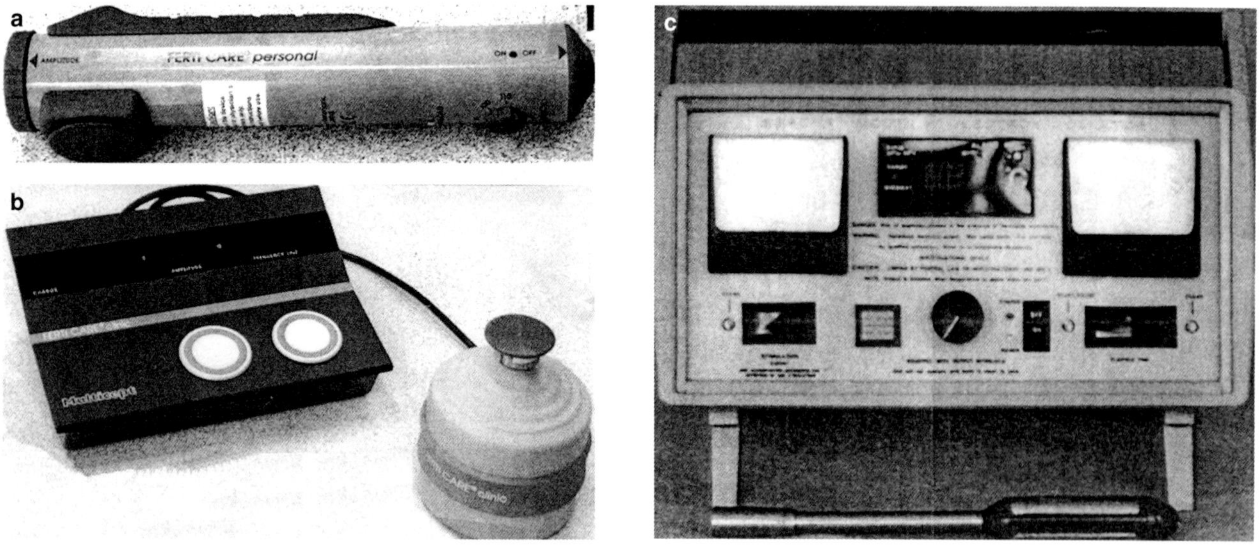

Figure 8.5 Vibratory stimulation for ejaculation in an anejaculatory man. (**a**) Hand-held Multicept A/S Ferti Care® personal vibrator. (**b**) Standard Multicept A/S Ferti Care® clinic vibrator. (**c**) NeuroControl™ Life STM system (NeuroControl Corporation, Valley View, OH). Courtesy of Professor R. S. Jeyendran

Either a large clinic vibrator (Multicept A/S Ferti Care® Clinic Vibrator) (Multicept A/S, Rungsted, Denmark) or a hand-held personal vibrator can be used (Figure 8.5).

Flat applicators of vibrator are used for spinal cord-injury patients, while curved applicators are used for healthy men in a seated position; during the procedure the amplitude is adjusted for a peak-to-peak distance of 4 mm.

The prepuce is retracted and the vibrator is applied to the frenulum of the penis, with the tip of the penis in a sterile cup. The vibrator is applied to the penis and adjusted to a peak-to-peak distance of 2.5 mm. The procedure is repeated for up to 3.5 min if ejaculation does not occur; with an interval of 1.5 min the procedure can be repeated four times. The prepuce is then replaced to normal and the patient observed to ensure no episodes of 'autonomic dysreflexia' or skin discoloration occur. Ejaculation is usually accompanied by a rhythmic reflex contraction of genital/anal abdominal muscles.

Electroejaculation

This procedure is used within 6 months after spinal injury; it requires viability of at least T10–L2 segments (reflex function in the lumbar cord is not necessary). The procedure is used when vibratory stimulation is not effective or if autonomic dysreflexia occurs. A rectal probe is used to affect only the nerve fibers vital to accomplish the procedure; stimulation is limited to the myelinated sympathetic efferent fibers of hypogastric plexus, to avoid any possible thermal or electrolytic damage of rectal mucosa.

Section III Reproductive Anomalies

9

Immunological andrology

CELLS OF THE IMMUNE SYSTEM

B and T lymphocytes

Immunity mediated by B lymphocytes is referred to as humoral immunity because transfer of immunity from one individual to another can be achieved via transfer of blood plasma or serum. T lymphocyte receptors can only recognize antigens if they are expressed on the surface of a cell in association with a protein of the major histocompatability complex (MHC) (Table 9.1).

Cells of the immune system are present in various tissues of the body, especially those in contact with the external environment. Immune system cells prevent establishment of infections and clear up cancerous or damaged cells in the host. These cells, organized in specialized tissues such as the thymus, spleen and lymph nodes, circulate in the blood (Figures 9.1–9.3).

Anatomical sites for immune responses

Activation of immune responses can occur at several levels in the body, including the site of entry of microorganisms (skin, lungs, etc.). Antigens that enter the bloodstream are concentrated in the spleen where T and B cell responses can be initiated. Similarly, another circulatory system, the lymphatic system, drains extracellular fluid from the tissues. Antigen collected in the lymphatic vessels is captured in the lymph nodes, which also contain both T and B cells. Activated effector and memory T cells leave the spleen and lymph nodes, circulate throughout the body, and move specifically to sites of antigen entry. B cells can also be present in peripheral organs, particularly mucosal tissues such as the intestine and reproductive tract. However, many activated cells remain in the spleen and lymph nodes, perhaps because the actions of B cells are dependent upon antibodies, which circulate in the blood (Hansen, 2000).

Table 9.1 Some cellular components of the immune system

Cell type	*Key function*
Phagocytes	
Macrophage	Phagocytosis, antigen presentation
Dendritic cell	Endocytosis and phagocytosis, antigen presentation
Neutrophil	Phagocytosis
Lymphocytes	
B lymphocyte	Secretion of antibody, antigen presentation
T helper lymphocyte type 1 (Th1)	Secretion of cytokines that stimulate macrophages and cytotoxic T cells
T helper lymphocyte type 2 (Th2)	Secretion of cytokines that stimulate B cells and antibody responses
Cytotoxic T lymphocyte	Lysis of target cells
Gamma-delta ($\gamma\delta$) T lymphocyte*	Lysis of target cells, secretion of cytokines and growth factors

*T-cell receptor is of the $\gamma\delta$ type; other T lymphocytes have $\alpha\beta$ type

COMPONENTS OF THE IMMUNE SYSTEM

The reproductive tract contains macrophages, T lymphocytes, B lymphocytes, neutrophils and other cells that participate in maintaining the reproductive tract in a sterile state. Moreover, the reproductive tract is drained by the lymphatic system. Lymph vessels draining the uterus join with similar vessels from

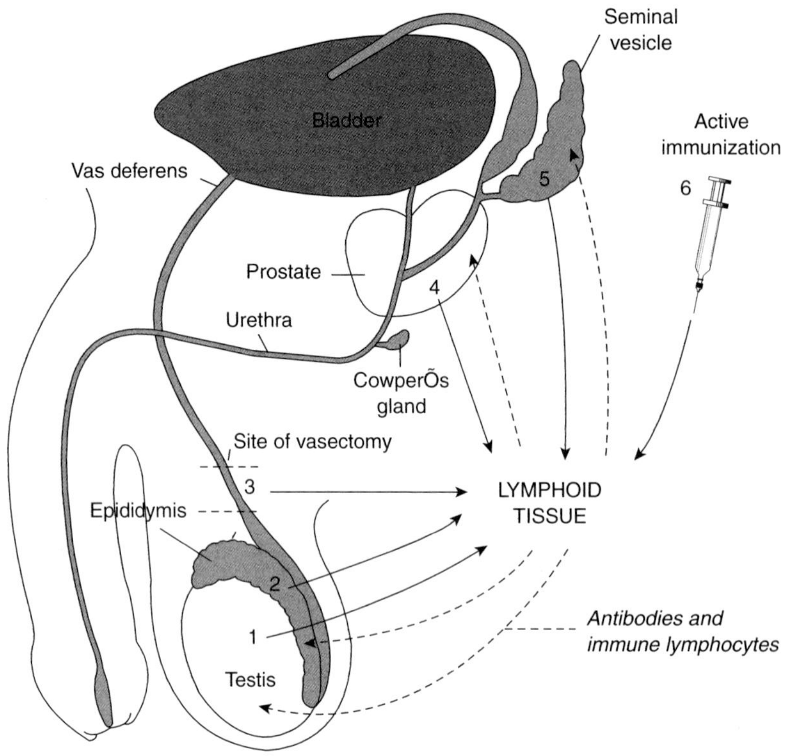

Figure 9.1 Sites of antigen origin and absorption, and lymphocyte and antibody entry into the male reproductive tract. (1) Testis: production of testis- and sperm-specific antigen; absorption of antigens after trauma; seminiferous tubules can be invaded by immune lymphocytes, whereas antibody enters the rete testes and efferent ducts; autoantibodies can cause agglutination and immobilization of spermatozoa. (2) Epididymis: secretion of coating antigens; removal of non-ejaculated sperm by phagocytosis by macrophages; inflammation can occlude duct resulting in sperm extravasation and absorption of antigens; entry site for immune cells and antibodies. (3) Vasectomy: occludes sperm passage resulting in sperm extravasation and granulomas and antigen absorption in epididymis and at site of vas sectioning if not ligated. (4) Prostate: secretion of prostatic antigens; inflammation results in occlusion of ejaculatory duct and absorption of prostatic and sperm antigens; entry of antibodies into ejaculate. (5) Seminal vesicle: major secretion of sperm-coating antigens; inflammation results in occlusion of ejaculatory duct and absorption of seminal and sperm antigens; entry and secretion of antibodies into ejaculate. Autoantibodies against seminal and prostatic secretions cause sperm agglutination. (6) Active immunization: use of sperm or testis antigens can cause autoantibodies and immune lymphocytes, depressed sperm quality and allergic orchitis in man and animals. Use of prostatic and seminal antigens may result in autoagglutinins and possible lesions in respective accessory glands

the ovary so that concentrations of progesterone in utero-ovarian lymph on the side ipsilateral to an ovary with a functional corpus luteum can be 10–1000-fold higher than concentrations in jugular blood.

Innate immune system

The most immediate responses to invasion of foreign organisms are those mediated by phagocytic cells of the innate immune system. Macrophages and neutrophils engulf foreign particles and then kill the organism. This process, called phagocytosis, can be stimulated by other components of the immune system. For example, phagocytes have receptors for antibodies (produced by B lymphocytes) and complement (produced by the liver), and more easily recognize microorganisms coated with these molecules. Also, various regulatory molecules called cytokines produced by T lymphocytes can activate phagocytes and make them more effective. One such cytokine is tumor necrosis factor (TNF).

Natural killer (NK) cells are a type of lymphocyte; however, unlike other cells of this lineage, they do not have receptors that recognize specific antigens. Rather, NK cells kill cells that do not display MHC class I antigens on their cell surfaces or have MHC class I but without the self-peptide usually present in association with the MHC protein (Figure 9.4).

The most common types of cell with either of these conditions are those infected with virus. Like phagocytes, activity of NK cells can be increased by certain cytokines from other lymphocytes. One such molecule is interferon-γ. Also, NK cells contain immunoglobulin receptors and have increased killing

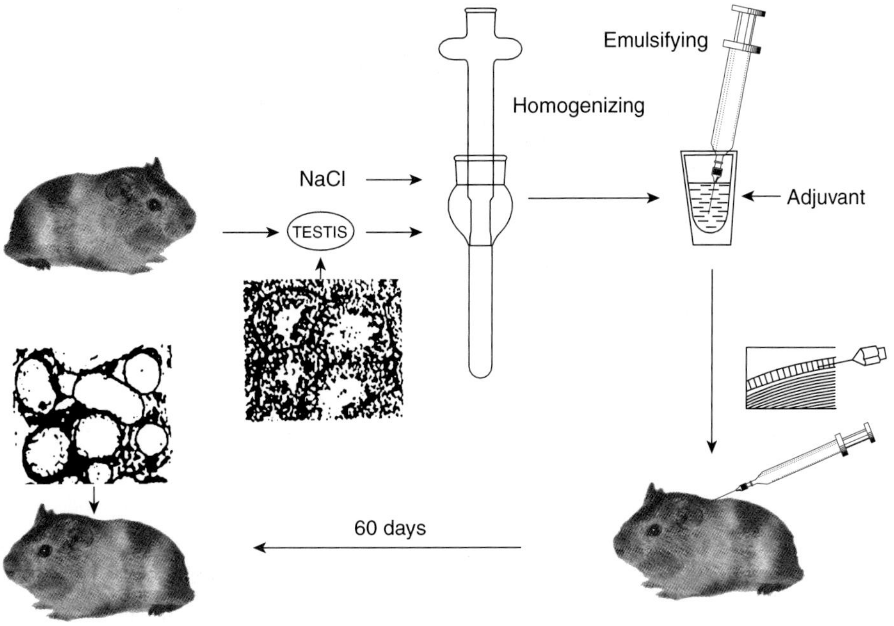

Figure 9.2 Classical example of experimentally induced immunological aspermatogenesis in the guinea pig

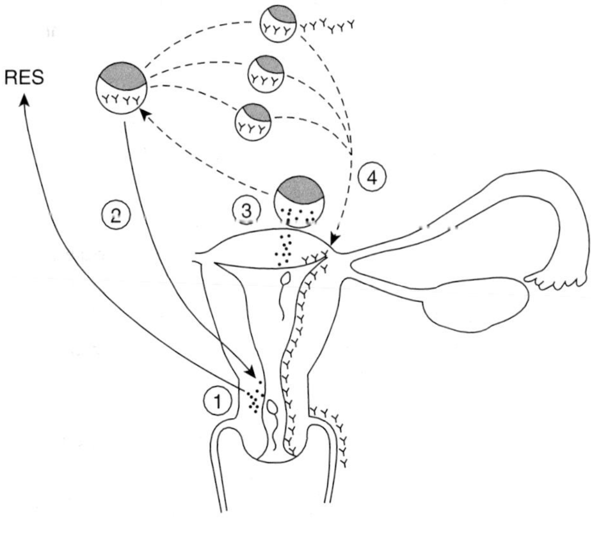

Figure 9.3 Schematic representation of primary and secondary immune response in infertility. (1) Sperm elements are absorbed by macrophages and taken to the reticulo-endothelial system (RES) which produces the large molecular IgM antibody or primary response (2), which then protects the body by attacking the immunogen. (3) On repeated exposure to this antigen the macrophages stimulate this large lymphocyte to produce many circulatory antibodies of IgG type which also attack the antigen (4)

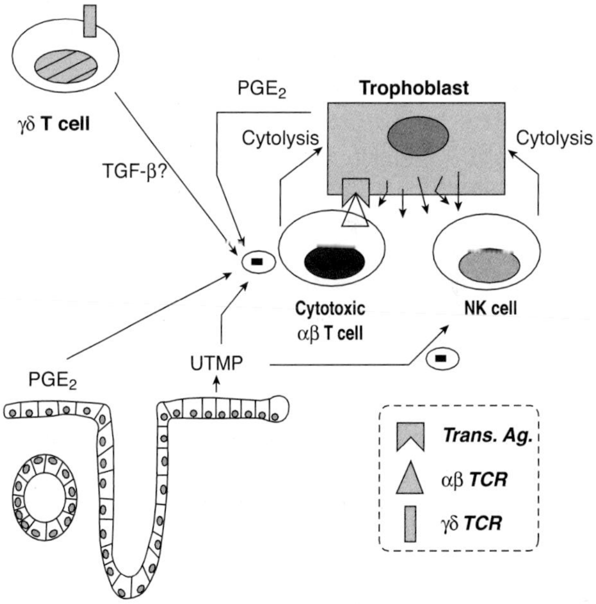

Figure 9.4 Model illustrating how lymphocyte inhibitory molecules from the endometrium and trophoblast inhibit activation and effector functions of maternal lymphocyte. There are at least two cells that could potentially cause cytolysis of trophoblast cells. These are αβ cytotoxic T cells that possess T cell receptors (TCR) specific for trophoblast transplantation antigens (Trans. Ag.), and natural killer (NK) cells which recognize trophoblast without major histocompatibility antigens. These cells are inhibited by molecules secreted from the trophoblast and endometrium. Prostaglandin E_2 (PGE_2), secreted by trophoblast, is among the lymphocyte-inhibitory molecules at the fetal–maternal interface. UTMP, uterine milk protein; TGF, transforming growth factor

activity against cells that have antibody on their cell surfaces. In addition to cellular components, the innate immune system also includes proteins, such as complement which promotes phagocytosis and lysis of microbes, and lactoferrin which can inhibit bacterial growth.

When antigens are placed in the reproductive tract, initial removal is accomplished by phagocytic cells of the innate immune system. Macrophages and dendritic-like cells are located in the reproductive tract. Microbial infection, deposition of semen or other inflammatory stimuli cause the release of chemotactic molecules that stimulate the movement of neutrophils out of the blood and into the lumen of the uterus. Opsonins (from the Greek, opsonein, to prepare food) are molecules that bind to particulate antigens and increase the affinity of phagocytes for that antigen. For example, serum contains complement C3b which can cause opsonization by binding to microorganisms; neutrophils and macrophages have receptors for C3b on their cell surfaces.

Microbial infection is also associated with inflammation accompanied by vasodilatation, increased vascular permeability, movement of serum proteins into the uterine lumen and production of a uterine discharge. These effects may be mediated by mast cells, basophils and eosinophils, which release vasoactive molecules upon activation.

Responses mediated by the innate immune system occur rapidly; however, they do not provide any long-term adjustments for improving the effectiveness of immune responses on subsequent exposure to an antigen.

Cell-mediated immunity (Table 9.2)

T lymphocytes

The actions of T lymphocytes are collectively termed cell-mediated immunity. T cell-dependent immunity from an immunized to a non-immunized animal requires the transfer to T cells themselves. There are two classes of T cells:

(1) Cytotoxic T cells, which are CD8 T lymphocytes, kill cells expressing antigen recognized by the T lymphocyte's receptor. Lysis is caused by secretion of toxic proteins: 'perforin' and 'granzymes'. CD8 lymphocytes are activated by antigen bound to MHC class I antigens, i.e. intracellular antigens such as virus. Thus, cytotoxic T cells kill cells that contain intracellular antigens that are not found by antibody or phagocytosed by macrophages or neutrophils.

(2) T helper (Th) cells regulate the activity of other lymphocytes by providing 'help' in the form of secretion of various cytokines. This activity is exerted primarily by CD4 T cells (that recognize extracellular antigens). In rodents, there are at least two types of T helper cells.

Recognition of antigen by T lymphocytes

One property of T lymphocytes is that the T cell receptor can only recognize antigen if it is expressed on the surface of a cell in association with a protein of the MHC. Thus, most T cells cannot recognize antigen themselves, but require so-called antigen-presenting cells that can process foreign proteins in such a way as to place the processed antigen within an MHC protein. Cells that can function as antigen-presenting cells include macrophages, dendritic cells (phagocytic and endocytic cells located in many tissues) and B lymphocytes (Hansen, 2000).

Role of T helper cells

Th1 cells' function is to promote cell-mediated immunity. Th1 cells produce cytokines, such as interferon-γ, that preferentially stimulate bacterial killing by macrophages; lymphotoxin, which stimulates neutrophils; and interleukin-2, which promotes growth of cytotoxic T cells. The Th2 cells promote primarily antibody-dependent immunity. The characteristic cytokine produced by Th2 cells is interleukin-4, which stimulates B lymphocytes to produce antibody (Hansen, 2000; Pinkert, 2000).

Acquired immune system

Acquired immune responses often take longer to exert their functions but responses are specific for individual foreign molecules (antigen) and result in a process called immunological memory, so that subsequent exposure to the same antigen will lead to a stronger response to that antigen.

The two main types of cells of the acquired immune system are B and T lymphocytes. B cells are derived from the bone marrow. T lymphocytes also are formed from precursors in the bone marrow but undergo a period of differentiation in the thymus before seeding various lymphoid tissues. Both T and B cells express receptors on their cell surfaces that are specific for a particular antigen. For B cells, the antigen receptor is an immunoglobulin molecule, while for T cells, the receptor is a protein called the T cell receptor. Two types of T cells can be identified. Some T cells have a receptor made of an α- and β-subunit.

Table 9.2 Cells and soluble mediators of cell-mediated immune responses (adapted from Anderson and Hill, 1988)

Cell type	*Characteristics*	*Principal relevant soluble factors*
T lymphocytes	Found primarily in circulation and lymphoid tissues; will home to sites of foreign antigenic stimulus in response to bacterial and leukocytic chemotactic factors; may also be responsive to hormonal influences; recognize foreign antigens when presented with MHC class I or II membrane antigens; long-lived memory cells rapidly respond to specific foreign antigens to mount rapid effective secondary immune response; subsets with a variety of effector and immunoregulatory functions	Lymphokines (interleukin (IL)-2, IL-3, IL-4, IL-5, IL-6, γ-interferon (γ-IFN), colony-stimulating factor (CSF); prostaglandin E_2 (PGE_2), diamine oxidase, perforans
Monocyte	High phagocytic and pinocytic capacity; long life in tissue; capacity to differentiate locality; ability to interact specifically with lymphocytes to promote antigen-specific response; usually become prominent in inflammatory lesions after 8–12 h; have Fc receptors for IgG antibodies, use IgG to identify foreign antigens (antibody-dependent cellular cytotoxicity (ADCC)), opsinization mechanism)	Monokines (IL-1, tumor necrosis factor (TNF)); complement components (C1, C2, C3, C4, C5, factor B, properdin); PGE_2, PGF_2, leukotrienes B and C; peroxidase; superoxide, hydrogen peroxide, hydroxyl radicals; monohydroxy-eicosatetraenoic acids; prostacyclin; elastase collagenase, plasminogen activator, lysozyme, procoagulant activity (PCA) factor; fibronectin
Neutrophils	Rapid migration; available in large numbers; short life-span in tissues; high phagocytic capacity; rapid burst of oxidative metabolism after stimulation; potent repertoire of oxidative metabolites and digestive enzymes; major elements in acute inflammation; have Fc receptors for IgG subclass antibodies (IgG_1 and IgG_3 in humans) and participate in ADCC responses	Peroxidase, polymorphonuclear leukocytes elastase, collagenase, lysozyme, myeloperoxidase, lactoferrin, alkaline phosphatase, β-glucuronidase, acid glycerophosphatase, cathepsins, α-fucosidase, 5′-nucleotidase, β-galactosidase, arylsulfatase, *N*-acetyl-β-glucosaminidase, mucopolysaccharides, trypsin-like proteases, histamine-release inhibitors, histaminase, PGE_2, superoxide, hydrogen peroxide, hydroxyl radicals
Eosinophils	Frequently found in tissues infected with parasites or with high levels of IgE; cytotoxic activity directed toward parasites; surface receptors for IgG, IgE and complement components (providing recognition sites for cell activation and release of components)	Peroxidase, superoxide, hydrogen peroxide, PGE_2, leukotrienes B and C, diamine oxidase, kinase, lysophospholipase, arylsulfatase B, phospholipase D
Basophils	High-affinity receptors for IgE; degranulation triggered by IgE receptors cross-linking and also by some lymphokines; circulating cells, localize in tissue only under special circumstances; cutaneous basophil hypersensitivity reactions in response to soluble antigens, parasites, tumor cells or allogeneic cells; activated by soluble products of lymphocytes, polymorphonuclear leukocytes, macrophages	Histamine, serotonin, dopamine, plasminogen activator, heparin, diverse proteolytic enzymes, acidic proteoglycans, chemotactic factors for neutrophils, limited amount of classical lysosomal enzymes listed for neutrophils, peroxidase, superoxide, hydrogen peroxide
Mast cells	High-affinity receptors for IgE; sessile cells, located primarily in blood vessels, lymphatics and connective tissue; especially abundant in skin and mucosal tissues	Similar to those produced by basophils
Platelets	Circulating non-replicating cells derived from megakaryocytes; may undergo activation during immune reactions; activated platelets become sticky and aggregrate, trapping leukocytes in areas of inflammation and cell-mediated immunity reactions; secrete clotting and growth factors, vasoactive amines and lipids, neutral and acid hydrolases, which contribute to inflammatory responses	Platelet-derived growth factor, serotonin, catecholamines, fibrinogen, cathepsin, alkaline phosphatase, β-glucuronidase

(Continued)

Table 9.2 (Continued)

Cell type	*Characteristics*	*Principal relevant soluble factors*
Plasma cells	Cells of B lymphoid lineage that reside primarily in lymphoid tissues and at mucosal surfaces; presence in reproductive tissues may be hormonally controlled; are directed by specific antigen to any lymphokine to produce a variety of immunoglobulins, many of which bind to immunoglobulin in Fc receptors on macrophages, NK cells, and neutrophils and allow them to participate in ADCC cell-mediated immunity responses	Immunoglobulins (IgG, IgA, IgE, IgM)

These cells, called $\alpha\beta$T cells, predominate in lymphoid organs, such as the spleen and lymph node, and are the major cells in blood. Other lymphocytes have a T-cell receptor made of a γ- and δ-subunit. These $\gamma\delta$T cells are numerous in epithelia, such as the skin and the lining of the intestinal and reproductive tracts. One key feature of lymphocytes is their capacity for immunological memory. When a lymphocyte recognizes an antigen specific for its receptor, it undergoes a process called activation whereby the cell proliferates. Some of these daughter cells differentiate into effector cells that perform various activities, such as antibody production or lysis of target cells. Several diseases are associated with autoimmune responses (Table 9.3).

B lymphocytes

Immunity mediated by B lymphocytes is referred to as humoral immunity because transfer of immunity from one animal to the next can be achieved via transfer of blood plasma or serum. B cells inhibit microbial growth by secreting soluble proteins called antibodies that circulate in the blood and are present in extracellular fluids. Antibodies exert a variety of actions that inhibit microbial growth. Some activated B cells secrete antibody but persist in the animal for months or years. Thus, subsequent exposure to the same antigen can result in heightened immune response.

Structurally, antibodies are members of a family of proteins called immunoglobulins. Each immunoglobulin is made up of four separate protein subunits (two heavy chains and two light chains) organized to give the molecule two sites for binding antigen, and one site called the Fc portion that is involved in binding to specific cells and to complement (Figure 9.5). There are several types of immunoglobulin molecules secreted by B cells including IgG, IgM, IgA, IgD and IgE. Each activated B cell secretes only one immunoglobulin

Table 9.3 Classification of some human autoimmune diseases (adapted from Rao, 2002)

Disease	*Self-antigen*
Organ-specific autoimmune disease	
Hashimoto's thyroiditis	Thyroid proteins and cells
Autoimmune hemolytic anemia	RBC membrane proteins
Goodpasture's syndrome	Renal and lung basement membrane
Graves' disease	Thyroid-stimulating hormone receptor
Addison's disease	Adrenal cells
Idiopathic thrombocytopenic purpura	Platelet membrane proteins
Insulin-dependent diabetes mellitus	Pancreatic beta cells
Pernicious anemia	Gastric parietal cells
Myasthenia gravis	Acetylcholine receptors
Myocardial infarction	Heart
Post-streptococcal glomerulonephritis	Kidney
Spontaneous infertility	Sperm
Systemic autoimmune disease	
Multiple sclerosis	Brain or white matter
Rheumatoid arthritis	Connective tissue, IgG
Ankylosing spondylitis	Vertebrae
Scleroderma	Nuclei, heart, lung, kidney, gastrointestinal tract
Systemic lupus erythematosus	DNA, nuclear proteins, RBC and platelet membrane
Sjogren's syndrome	Salivary gland, liver, kidney, thyroid

RBC, red blood cell

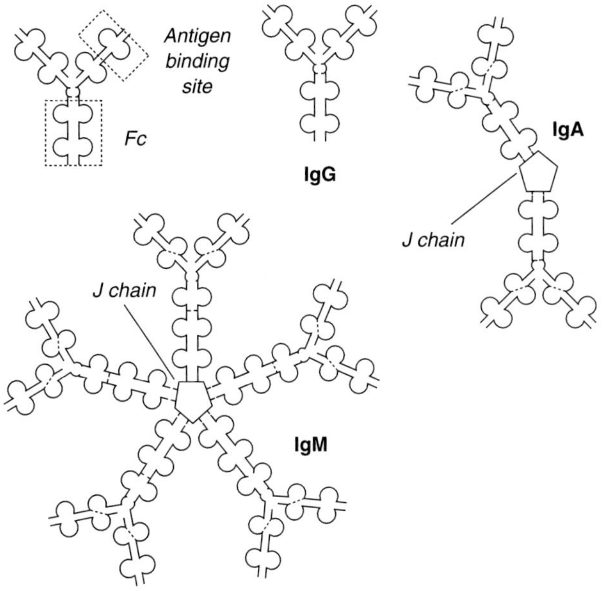

Figure 9.5 Schematic representations of the structure of IgG, IgA and IgM. Each immunoglobulin is formed by two heavy chain molecules and two light chain molecules held together by disulfide bonds (indicated by dashed lines). The loops in each chain are formed by intramolecular disulfide bonds. There are two antibody sites for each immunoglobulin monomer. The Fc portion of the protein is responsible for binding to complement and to immunoglobulin receptors on neutrophils, macrophages and other cells. IgG is secreted as a monomer, whereas IgA is a dimer and IgM exists as a pentamer. Multimeric forms of immunoglobulin are held together by a protein called J-chain. In addition, IgA secreted across epithelial surfaces (not shown here) contains another protein called secretory component. Adapted from Abbas *et al.*, 1997

type specific for one antigen. The most common immunoglobulin in blood is IgG. Another immunoglobulin molecule of particular interest for the reproductive tract is IgA, which is a major antibody in several mucosal sites, such as the gastrointestinal and reproductive tracts. Immunoglobulin A exists as two separate antibody molecules joined by a short protein called J-chain. In addition, IgA secreted across epithelia contains an additional protein, called secretory component, that is added as IgA crosses epithelial cells on its way to the mucosal surface.

Antibody binding to a microorganism can result in several actions that lead to the clearance of the microbe. For many microbes, successful colonization of a host requires binding of the microbe to cell membranes of the host. This can be made more difficult when the bacteria are coated with antibody. In addition, the Fc portion of IgG and IgA can be bound by specific receptors on macrophages and neutrophils, so that the rate of phagocytosis can be enhanced when bacteria are coated with antibody. Proteins of the complement system can also bind to the Fc portion of IgG and lead to complement-mediated lysis of the microbial cell. Cells infected with virus or bacteria can be destroyed in a process called antibody-dependent cell cytotoxicity, which occurs when NK cells or eosinophils release toxic granules upon binding of their surface Fc receptors to antibody attached to infected cells. Receptors for the Fc portion of immunoglobulins also exist on T and B cells, and this provides for additional regulation of lymphocyte function by antibody-bound particles.

Sperm immunology

Coitus is associated with microbial contamination because the penis, and sometimes the seminal plasma, contain microorganisms. Despite these microbial invasions, microorganisms can be rapidly removed from the reproductive tract and the tract usually remains free from infection. A sterile environment in the reproductive tract is maintained by the presence of an effective antimicrobial defense system that includes physical barriers, phagocytes that engulf and kill microorganisms, B lymphocytes that produce antibodies against invading microbes, and T lymphocytes that can kill virus- and bacteria-infected host cells (Hansen, 2000). Immune function in the reproductive tract is regulated by hormones to maximize antimicrobial function. The immune system consists of different cell types which prevent establishment of infection by microorganisms, and clear cancerous or damaged cells in the host. These cells are organized into specialized tissues such as the thymus, spleen and lymph nodes, circulate in the blood and are present in various tissues of the body, especially those in contact with the external environment.

Responses to sperm

Sperm are antigenic when injected subcutaneously into females. Therefore, mechanisms must be found to remove sperm from the reproductive tract following coitus in a way that will not lead to the development of humoral or cellular immunity to sperm. The main fate of sperm in the reproductive tract is phagocytosis by neutrophils; deposition of sperm induces an influx of phagocytic cells (neutrophils, macrophages and dendritic-like cells) into the reproductive tract. The lymphocytes in the lymph nodes draining the uterus can become activated by seminal plasma,

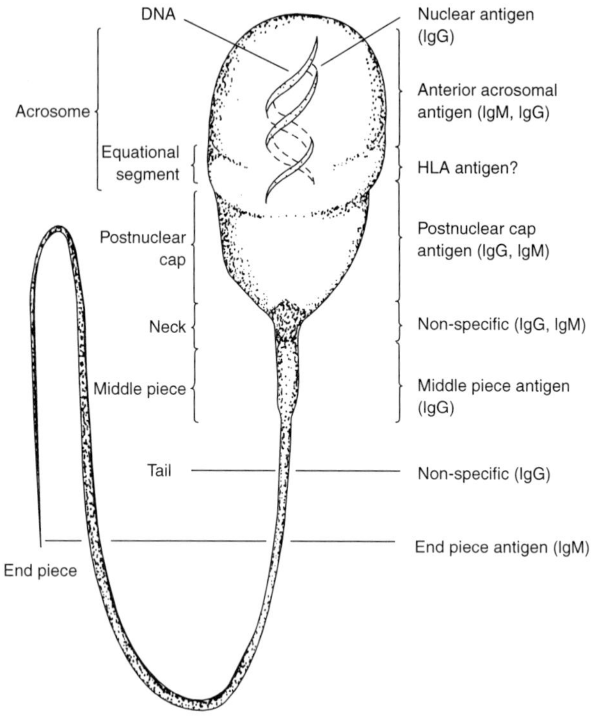

Figure 9.6 Distribution of DNA, IgM, IgG within the sperm

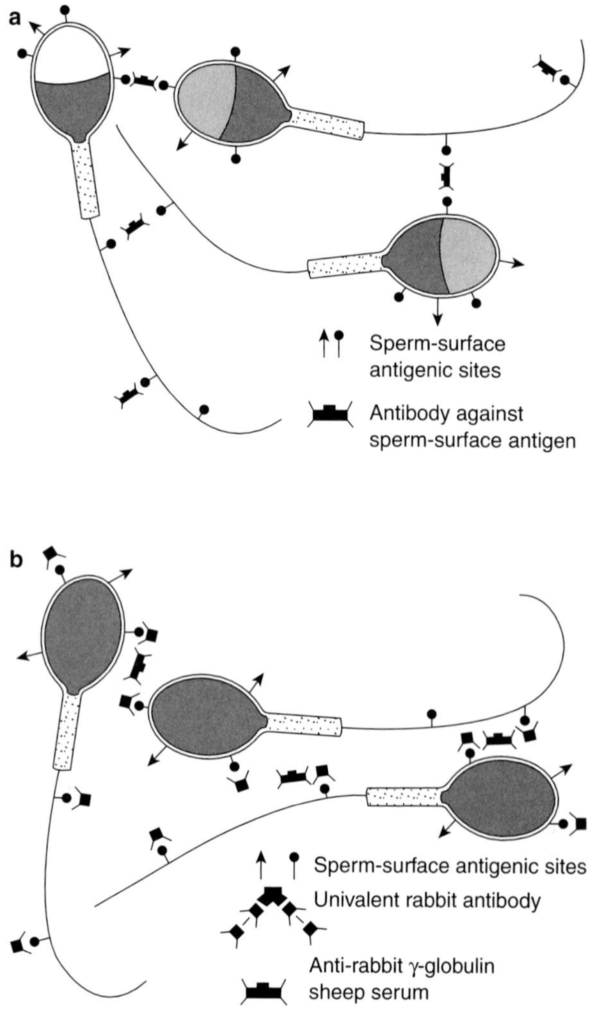

Figure 9.7 (**a**) Agglutination by antibody: when two sperm surface antigenic sites on separate cells are cross-linked by antibody, immunological agglutination occurs. (**b**) Antiglobulin agglutination occurs when sperm are secondarily cross-linked through antisperm by bivalent antiglobulin

perhaps because immunosuppresants are inactivated as sperm antigens reach the lymph nodes.

Despite the presence of mechanisms to prevent immune responses to sperm, females can develop antisperm immunity, and antibodies directed towards sperm can occasionally be recovered from the reproductive tract.

Sperm antibodies and autoimmune responses

Spermatozoa are capable of inducing an antibody response (Figures 9.6 and 9.7). Despite unsuccessful attempts to use immunity to sperm as a method of male contraception, sperm antibodies can cause reproductive failure. Immunopathological mechanisms of sperm antibodies cause autoimmune responses:

(1) Arming macrophages/enhancing of sperm from male genital tract;

(2) Mediating cytotoxic (immobilizing) effects on sperm in the presence of high titer of complement cascade components;

(3) Sperm unable to penetrate cervical mucus because of agglutination or related pathological mechanisms;

(4) Interfering with sperm capacitation, decapacitation and sperm hyperactivation;

(5) Influencing sperm selection within the female genital tract.

Several immunopathological markers can detect certain autoimmune responses. IgA sperm-specific antibodies are the main indicators of poor semen penetration (Figure 9.8). Antigenic components of semen originate in the testis, epididymis, vas deferens and accessory glands. They can be broadly classified as those in the seminal plasma and those that are sperm bound. Sperm carry a mixture of antigens, including sperm-specific antigens, histocompatibility antigens (i.e. those responsible for the rejection of

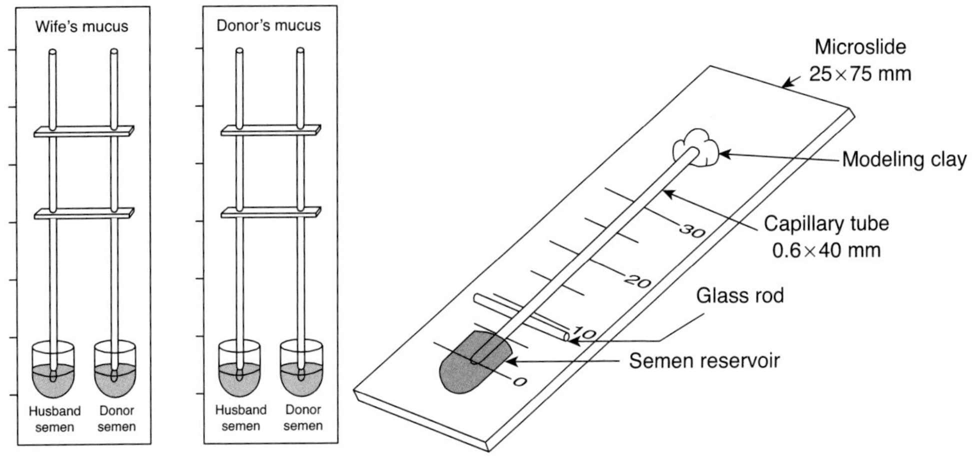

Figure 9.8 Capillary mucus penetration test (Kremer as modified by Fjallbrant). Cervical mucus is drawn up into capillary tubes (0.5 mm internal diameter, 40 mm long) and one end sealed with plasticine or modeling clay. The capillary tube is mounted on a special calibrated microslide with the open end placed into a chamber containing semen. The slide is placed into a humid chamber and incubated at 37°C for 1 h. The slide is examined under low-power microscopy to determine the furthest penetration of sperm. Donor semen and husband semen are tested against donor's mucus and wife's mucus. Penetration ratings: poor ≤ 5 mm; fair 6–19 mm; and good ≥ 20 mm. Sperm from men with circulating and seminal plasma antisperm antibodies show poor penetration

tissue grafts), blood group antigens and other somatic tissue antigens. Sperm antigens may be antigenic within the male (autoantigens) or the female (isoantigens) reproductive system. Of the sperm antigens, those on the surface of the plasma membrane are probably responsible for the reproductive failure. To be effective, antibodies against sperm must enter the seminal fluid or the cervical mucus following deposition in the female tract.

An autoimmune response is normally prevented by the relative isolation of the seminiferous tubules from the rest of the body by the blood–testis barrier. If the barrier is breached, antisperm antibodies are produced that might attack sperm. Autoantibodies against sperm are found in the serum of infertile men. Antisperm antibodies can prevent fertilization by immobilizing sperm, impairing sperm penetration of cervical mucus, inactivating acrosomal enzymes presumed essential for fertilization, inhibiting the attachment of sperm to the zona pellucida, or interfering with embryonic viability. This problem has been overcome by the development of monoclonal antibodies against sperm surface components.

10

Andropause and osteoporosis

There is no decline in men's fertility before the age of 35 years. However, there are normal-age related changes in the sexual response cycle in men (Tables 10.1 and 10.2). The man's age appears to affect conception if the woman is over 35. At the age of 40 men are 40% less likely to succeed in getting their partner pregnant within a month than when they were 35. The decline in fertility is not dramatic, but men are advised to deposit a frozen semen sample at age 35 in case they want to become fathers at a later age. The superfertile period (6 days preceding ovulation) remains the same for women of all ages. It was suspected that part of the reason why it is more difficult for older women to become pregnant could have been that their fertile period was shorter than that of younger women. Assuming that couples had sexual intercourse at the best time for conception – 2 days before ovulation – and assuming that the men were the same age as the women, women younger than 27 had a 50% chance of conceiving during that menstrual cycle.

Table 10.1 Physiological events during the male reproductive cycle

Stage of life cycle	*Age*	*Physioanatomical events*
Fetal differentiation (weeks of gestation)	5 (CRL 7)	Gonadal primordial germ cells appear
	6 (CRL 16)	Seminiferous cords develop
	7 (CRL 29)	Interstitial cells appear
	8 (CRL 40)	Müllerian ducts regress
	9 (CRL 50)	Wolffian ducts develop; urethral folds fuse into penis (first prostatic bud appears)
Adolescence (years)	12–17	Extensive development of Leydig cells
	11–12	Testicular spurt and fat spurt; seminiferous tubules differentiate (spermatozoid and primary spermatocyte)
	12–13	Straight pubic hair appears; Leydig cells differentiate; secondary spermatocytes appear: penis spurt and height spurt; wavy pubic hair appears
	13–14	Voice deepening; first ejaculation; circumanal hair
	15–17	Sperm appear; axillary hair; fat decreases; sweat and sebaceous glands are large
Reproductive senescence		Various testes size and firmness decreases; basement membrane and tunica propria of seminiferous tubules thicken; tubules decrease in diameter; degenerative changes in germinal epithelium; reduced sperm production; Sertoli cells obliterate, contain golden-brown pigment granules; progressive intertubular fibrosis causes separation of seminiferous tubules from blood supply; prostate gland enlarges, its contractions become weaker; number of coitus per year declines from 109 (35–44 years of age) to 81 (45–53 years) to 22 (65–74 years)

CRL, crown–rump length

Table 10.2 Normal age-related changes in the male sexual response cycle

Arousal
Lengthening of excitation phase – delayed erection
Lengthening of the plateau phase – longer interval to ejaculation
Less well-defined sense of impending orgasm – decreased penile rigidity
Orgasm
Shortening of the ejaculatory event
Fewer and less forceful expulsive contractions of the urethra
Increased incidence of resolution without ejaculation
Postorgasm
More rapid detumescence
Lengthening of refractory period

Sexuality and fertility in men are under the control of the hypothalamo-pituitary axis. Sexuality and aging, urological factors, androgen replacement therapy and clinical parameters of andropause are related to osteoporosis and osteoporotic fractures (Comhaire, 2000; Morales *et al.*, 2000; Olson, 2000; Schivi and Rehman, 1995; Stas *et al.*, 2003; Vermeulen, 2001; Wespes and Schulmann, 2000). Andropause is associated with major changes in hormone profile including testosterone, melatonin and growth hormone (GH). Symptoms of andropause include excessive height loss, curvature of the spine, chronic back or spinal pain, jaw shrinkage and loss of mobility. Bone mineral density (BMD) is used to diagnose osteoporosis. There are several risk factors for osteoporotic fracture: Caucasian, low BMD, prior fracture after age 50 and hypogonadism. Secondary causes of systemic andropause include endocrine profile, malignancy, gastrointestinal disorders, drugs, genetic factors and renal failure or acidosis (Table 10.3). Decline in androgen level is associated with changes in body composition and erectile dysfunction. There are several methods of administration of testosterone therapy for older men, including injectable, transdermal, scrotal patch, non-scrotal patches with or without enhancers, testosterone gel and orals.

BONE STRUCTURE AND OSTEOPOROSIS

Bones are made of calcium and phosphorus crystals, held by protein fibers (Figures 10.1 and 10.2). Calcium produces the strength and rigidity in bones, and protein allows flexibility. Other minerals that

Table 10.3 Parameters and factors affecting bone mineral density

General
Caucasian
Low bone density
Prior fracture after age 50
Hypogonadism
Alcoholism
Excess dietary protein
Family history
Inactivity
Smoking
Falls
Anticonvulsant therapy
Hyperthyroidism
Endocrinological
Hypogonadism
Cushing's syndrome
Hyperthyroidism
Type I diabetes
Hyperparathyroidism
Malignancy
Lymphoma
Leukemia
Multiple myeloma
Mastocytosis
Gastrointestinal
Anorexia nervosa
Gastrectomy
Lactase deficiency
Hepatic failure
Malabsorption
Celiac disease
Small bowel resection
Low vitamin D
Crohn's disease
Drugs
Methotrexate
Cyclosporin A
Alcohol
Anticonvulsants
Heparin
Glucocorticoids
FK 506
Thyroid suppression
Vitamin A excess
Genetic
Homocystinuria
Marfan's syndrome
Rheumatoid arthritis
Ehlers–Danlos syndrome
Renal
Renal failure
Idiopathic hypercalciuria

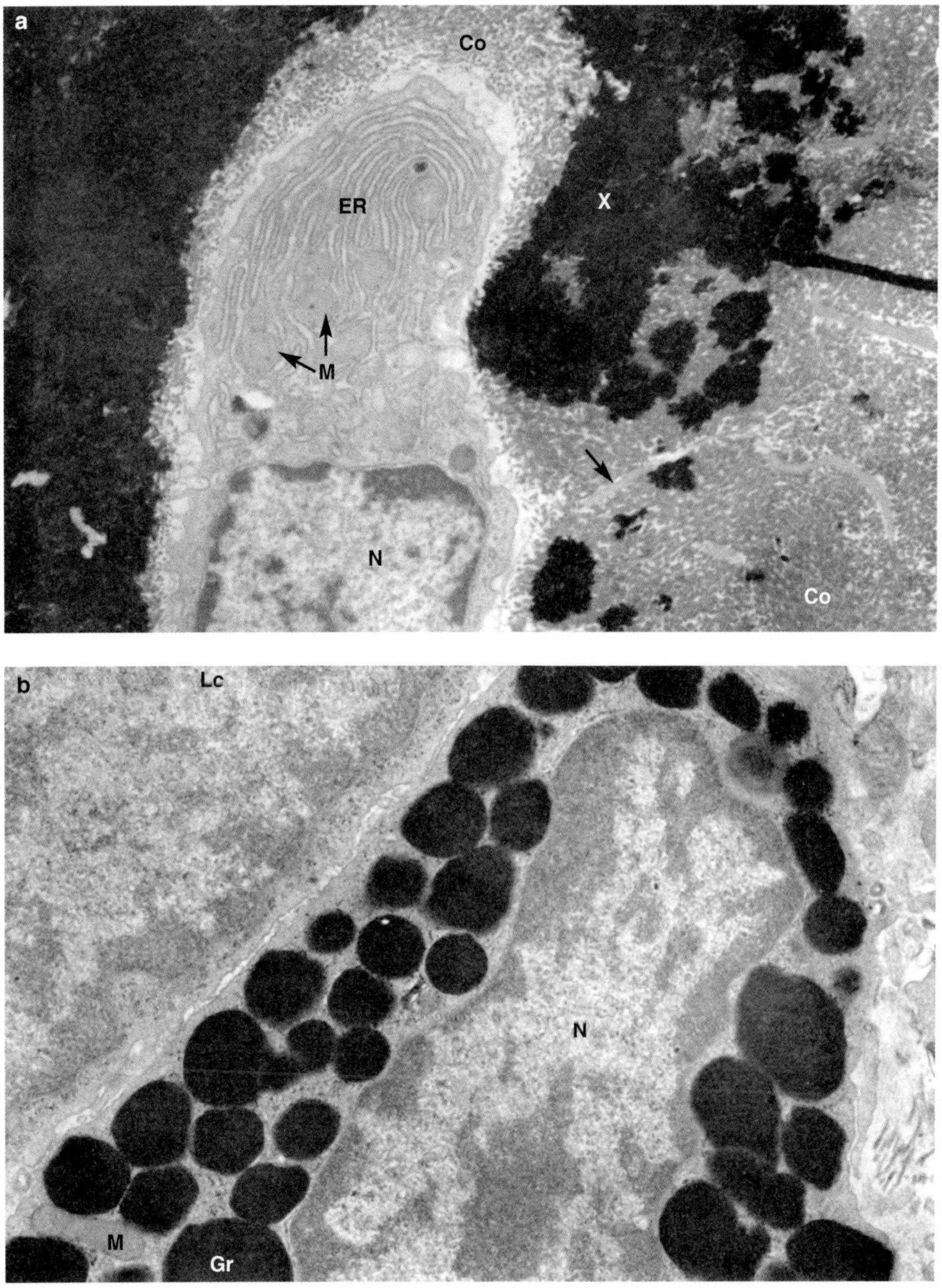

Figure 10.1 (**a**) Osteocyte and bone. (**b**) Master cell. Co, collagen fibrils; ER, endoplasmic reticulum; M, mitochondria; X, mineralized matrix; Gr, granule; Lc, lymphocyte; N, nucleus

help hold bone cells together are fluoride, sodium, potassium and magnesium. Bones are in a constant state of change and contain fluids. Bones continue to grow up to the age of 20 years, and then begin to increase in density. The bone mass of an individual depends not only on the amount of bone mass lost as a function of hormonal status and age, but also on the peak bone mass attained during growth and development (Figure 10.3). Thus, osteoporosis and attendant fractures can occur when either there is a failure to reach peak bone mass or resorption exceeds formation after peak bone mass is achieved (Eskin and Troen, 2003) (Figure 10.4). Osteoporosis results from abnormalities in bone remodeling, whereas osteomalacia results from defects in bone mineralization due to calcium deficiency.

Osteoporosis is a skeletal disorder in which bone strength is compromised due to loss of bone density and a decline in quality of bone. Osteoporosis is due, in large part, to an uncoupling of bone formation and resorption. While current diagnostic procedures can distinguish those at risk of fracture from those not at risk, there is a large overlap in bone density between men who fracture and those who do not. There is an

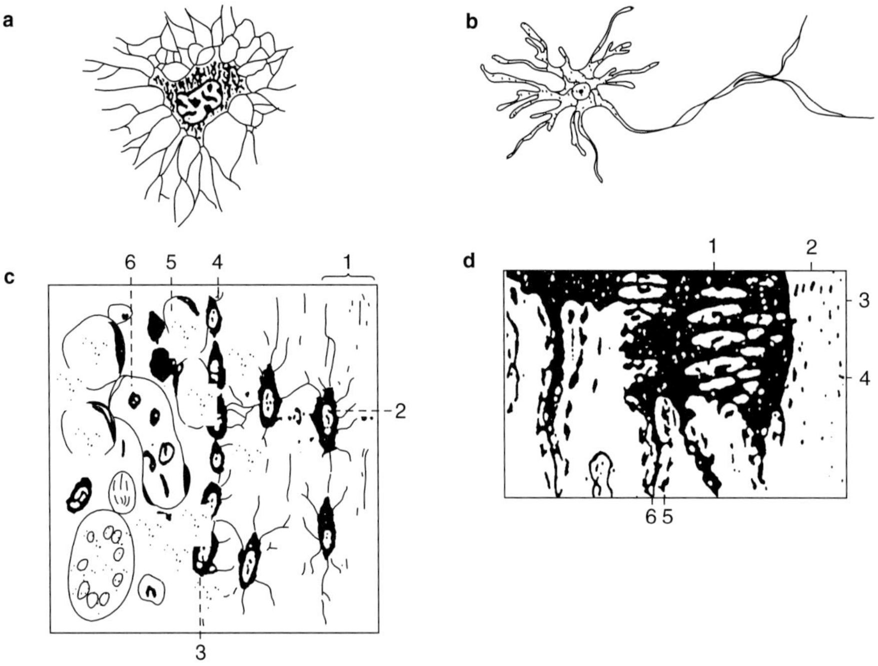

Figure 10.2 Functional ultrastructure/biodynamics of bone formation. (**a**) Bone cell within the Haversian system of a membrane bone. (**b**) Nerve cell with axon (the long branch) and dendrites (the short branches). (**c**) Secretion of bone and adjacent marrow: (1) bone lamella; (2) lacunae, i.e. osteocyte space and cell; (3) osteoblast cells; (4) endosteum; (5) fat cells in bone marrow; (6) blood vessels and various other cells of bone marrow. (**d**) Bone adjacent to spongiosa area: (1) eroded cartilage; (2) bone cortex; (3) periosteum; (4) osteocyte embedded; (5) osteoblast; (6) bone matrix

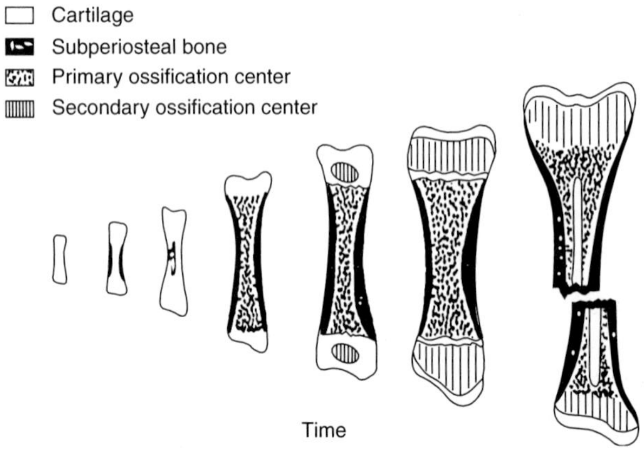

Figure 10.3 Developmental changes of long bones

absolute osteoclast overactivity (possibly with increased numbers of cells) in high-turnover osteoporosis. In senile osteoporosis bone formation lags behind resorption; hence the rate of resorption is relatively higher than that of formation, resulting in a net bone loss. Osteoporosis is characterized not only by low bone mass, but also by microarchitectural deterioration of bone tissue with a consequent increase in bone fragility and susceptibility to fractures (Eskin and Troen, 2003) (Figure 10.2).

Calcium in other body functions

Calcium is deposited in bones and withdrawn as needed. Calcium has other important functions besides building strong bones and teeth. It is important in brain and nerve functions, normal blood clotting, smooth muscle contraction and expansion, acting as glue that holds cells together, transportation of chemical ions across cell membranes, and lowering blood pressure/hypertension.

In all, 99% of the body's calcium is within bones. The average man, woman and child have sufficient calcium for their needs if they eat a balanced diet, with emphasis on the basic four food groups. Milk/milk products are the richest sources of calcium, and this type of calcium is easily absorbed by the body. Milk products, available almost everywhere, are relatively inexpensive and easy to use in almost any diet. However, not all milk products are rich in calcium. Cream cheese, coffee cream, whipped cream and butter are mostly fat, and contain little calcium. Adding more milk solids or cheese to foods prepared at home, such as puddings, custards, cream soups, bread products, pastas, casseroles and beverages, can increase the amount of calcium in the diet. Sardines and canned salmon are also good

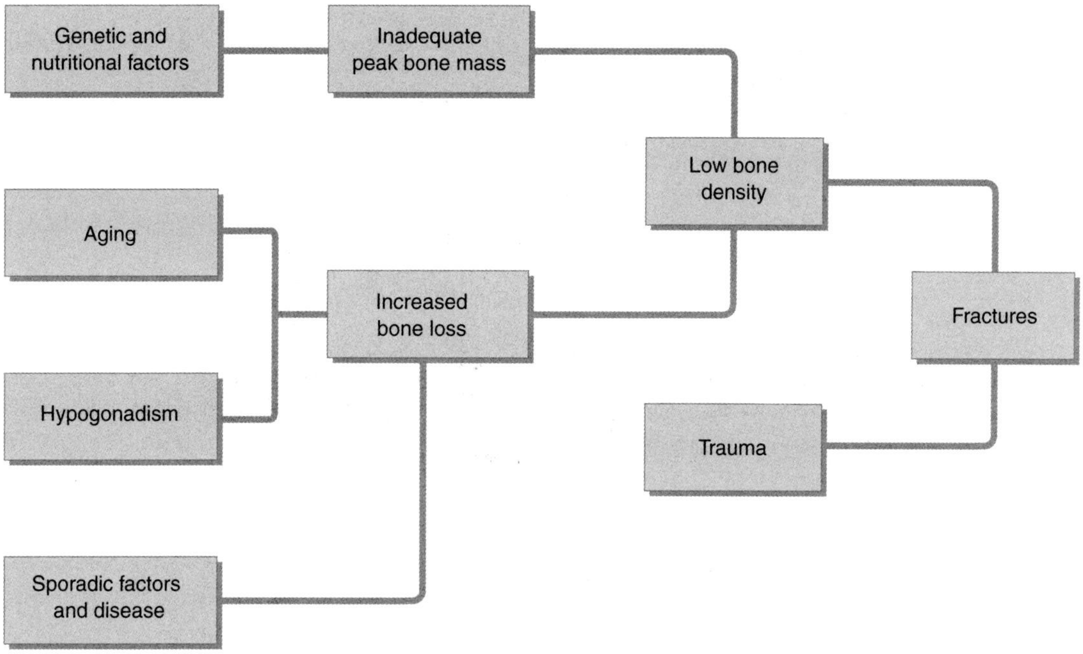

Figure 10.4 Pathophysiology of osteoporotic fractures (Olson, 2000)

sources of calcium, especially if the tender bones are eaten.

Red meat and poultry are not good calcium sources. Legumes, fruits and vegetables, cereals, grains, breads and pastas are all contributors to calcium intake. When lime is added to dry corn to make hominy, or to corn meal for tortillas and other southwestern delicacies, the calcium content of corn is increased. Fruit and vegetables are also a good source of boron, a mineral that, research indicates, assists calcium absorption and bone mineralization.

Assessment of bone mineral density

BMD (area density in g/cm^2) is measured using dual-energy X-ray absorptiometry, operating in fan beam mode. Quality control scans are performed daily using the manufacturer-supplied anthropomorphic spine phantom at various bone locations. The lumbar spine (LS), femoral neck (FN), Ward's triangle (WT) and trichinae (T) are assessed. LS is assessed from L2 to L4, in the anteroposterior view. At the upper left femur, hip BMD is measured at three regions of interest: FN, WT and T. Z score expresses the BMD in relation to the average value expected for that age and is presented in age-specific SD units, while T score expresses SD units in relation to a young, healthy population. The Z and T score values are calculated using the manufacturer's reference values, which were obtained from Greek subjects. The WHO diagnostic criteria for osteopenia and osteoporosis are used to define low bone density. According to WHO guidelines, osteoporosis is present if BMD is more than 2.5 SD below the peak bone mass reference standard for young adults (T score ≥ –2.5 SD) (Table 10.4).

Table 10.4 Diagnosis of osteoporosis based on bone mineral density

Diagnosis	*Bone mineral density (T score)*
Normal	≤–1 SD
Osteopenia	–1 to –2.5 SD
Osteoporosis	≥–2.5 SD with history of fragility fracture

ANDROPAUSE

With increasing life expectancy and decreasing reproduction rate, the population structure is changing. Extensive investigations have been conducted on the biology of andropause in men (Tables 10.5–10.7). In aging men the typical patterns of daily rhythmicity become less distinct. This is part of a very complex picture in which not only isolated hormones are involved, but also interactions between hormones. Many factors from the external and internal environment mediated by neurotransmitters constantly

Table 10.5 Physiopathology of andropause: testosterone levels, changes in body composition, erectile dysfunction (ED) and future research (Comhaire, 2000; Morales *et al.*, 2000; Stas *et al.*, 2003; Vermeulen, 2001; Wespes and Schulmann, 2000)

Testosterone levels
Subtle, non-specific, frequently not acknowledged symptoms. Only 1% of plasma testosterone is free. About 11–59% is weakly bound to albumin and 40–88% is tightly bound to sex hormone-binding globulin (SHBG). Bioavailable testosterone refers to albumin-bound plus free testosterone. Both total and free testosterone decline with aging. As a result of the age-related increase in SHBG concentration, the decline in free testosterone is more profound than that of total testosterone
Decline
Involves hypothalamic–pituitary–gonadal axis associated with decline/alteration in number of Leydig cells. Failure to increase LH levels in response to the hypoandrogenic state results in a relative hypogonadotropic hypogonadism. Other factors involved are hereditary factors, obesity, diet, stress depression, chronic diseases such as diabetes mellitus, coronary arteriosclerosis, chronic renal failure, chronic liver disease, sleep apnea syndrome and rheumatoid arthritis, and medications, such as glucorticoids, smoking and alcohol intake
Changes in body composition
Testosterone leads to a decrease in body fat, increase in lean body mass and changes in muscle strength. Bone density may be increased in elderly men undergoing testosterone therapy, although additional longer-term data are needed to confirm that androgen replacement can sustain a stabilization or reversal of bone loss
Andropause/erectile dysfunction
Androgen deficiency, especially in elderly men, is not the most common cause of ED. Other common vascular, neurological and psychological iatrogenic factors are very likely to co-exist with androgen deficiency
Future research
Long-term effects of androgen replacement therapy on prostate
Role of androgens in pathogenesis of benign prostatic hyperplasia (BPH) and prostate cancer
Effects of testosterone therapy on BPH or prostate cancer
Effects of testosterone therapy on an existing cancer
How PSA levels are affected by androgen deficiency and androgen replacement
Large-scale, long-term clinical studies are needed to resolve the issues related to andropause and to assess the long-term risk versus benefit profile of androgen replacement therapy

LH, luteinizing hormone; PSA, prostate-specific antigen

Table 10.6 Major changes in hormone profile during andropause

Decline in free total testosterone, about 1% decline/year; no prescribed specific threshold level for testosterone deficiency, according to age, because some androgen responsive organs are more or less sensitive during andropause
Unknown preferred forms of replacement: tablets, plaster, ointments, depots, selectively acting androgens, androgens, selective androgen receptor modulators (SARMs), α-reductase blocker(s)
Testosterone substitution may have the risk of aggravating an asymptomatic prostate cancer. As men grow older, the percentage of detected carcinomas rises, as do the cases of symptomatic BPH irrespective of any hormonal intervention
Side-effects of testosterone replacement therapy are limited and predictable as long as PSA levels are controlled
Benefits for bone and body composition may have a positive effect on myocardial infarction, stroke and other unwanted reactions: liquid retention, sleep apnea and stimulation of undiagnosed BPH
Decreased secretions and circadian periodicity, and increased sleep disorders, affect growth hormones (GH) which occurs with 'deep sleep' (slow-wave sleep). Melatonin 'sleep hormone' cannot generate sleep, but initiates it and modulates its quality
Decline in GH. During slow-wave sleep men produce, in contrast to women, the major proportion of GH. Sleeping disturbances cause GH deficiency, aggravated by obesity and inactivity

BPH, benign prostatic hyperplasia; PSA, prostate-specific antigen

Table 10.7 Classification of human 'androgenic' diseases

High plasma androgen levels
Idiopathic precocious puberty in boys and girls
Hirsutism in adult females
Male pattern baldness in adult females
All signs of virilization in females, e.g. those due to civilizing tumors or the administration of androgens
Probably normal plasma androgen levels
Hypersexuality and 'aggressive states' in adult males
Acne and seborrhea in juveniles and young adults of both sexes
Baldness in adult males in genetically susceptible individuals
Benign prostatic hypertrophy; androgen-dependent cancer, e.g. prostatic carcinoma

Table 10.8 Testosterone replacement for older men

Preparation	*Dose and frequency of administration*
Injectable	
Testosterone-enanthate/ cypionate	100–200 mg every 2 weeks
Transdermal	
Scrotal patch	6 mg/day
Non-scrotal patches with enhancers	5 mg/day
Non-scrotal patches without enhancers	5 mg/day
Testosterone gel	5–10 mg/day (5–10 g of gel)
Oral	
Testosterone undecanoate (not available in USA)	80 mg bid or tid

affect the highly sensitive hormonal balance. Therefore, aging has also been defined as 'the gradual dysfunction of homeostatic processes'.

Declining testosterone levels are involved in 'andropausal' symptoms in men: loss of libido, erectile dysfunction, insulin receptor resistance, obesity, osteoporosis, disturbances of lipid metabolism, myocardial and circulatory disturbances, and impaired well-being and mood. Data have been derived from studies in hypogonadal men treated by testosterone replacement. In such patients libido increases, fat mass decreases, and muscle strength, BMD and erythropoiesis increase. Atherosclerotic plaque size is reduced after estrogen injections in cholesterol-fed rabbits. Phytoestrogen-fed monkeys had lower total cholesterol and low-density lipoprotein (LDL) cholesterol and higher high-density lipoprotein (HDL) cholesterol. Apart from atherosclerotic lesions, coronary artery vascular reactivity is improved.

Testosterone supplements

The delivery systems of testosterone supplements include: DPT (Depo®-testosterone, 400 mg intramuscularly every 2–3 weeks), TSD (Testoderm® scrotal patches, 4–6 mg/24 h and TTS (Testoderm® non-scrotal patches, 5 mg/24 h) (Table 10.8).

OSTEOPOROSIS

Osteoporosis is one of the commonest metabolic bone diseases, and its prevalence is expected to rise as the population grows older. Although osteoporosis is less prevalent in men than in women, the morbidity and mortality associated with male osteoporosis is greater. Severe osteoporosis in non-elderly men is usually associated with conditions involving bone loss, such as hypogonadism, hypercorticolism, hyperthyroidism and excessive alcohol intake (Table 10.6). If no known cause of bone disease can be identified it is termed idiopathic. Idiopathic osteoporosis (IO) is more commonly encountered in men than in women. The lack of identifiable causes of reduced bone density in men with IO has led to the suggestion that this disorder is the result of major abnormalities in bone-cell function or of the hormonal or paracrine pathways that regulate bone-cell metabolism. Growth hormone (GH), insulin- like growth factor I (IGF-I) and its major binding protein insulin-like growth factor binding protein-3 (IGFBP-3) could be major causes.

Symptoms, diagnosis and risk factors of osteoporosis

Symptoms of osteoporosis include:

(1) Excessive height loss (loss of ≥6 inches in height);

(2) Curvature of the spine – sign of vertebrae collapsing, distinctive hump below shoulders in severe cases;

(3) Chronic back or spinal pain, due to bone degeneration;

Table 10.9 Pharmacotherapy in older men: comparison of selected medications

Drug	*Advantages*	*Disadvantages*
Tricyclic antidepressants	Inexpensive, once daily dosing	Anticholinergic side-effects, multiple
		Drug interactions
Desipramine		Delirium
Nortriptyline		Radiotoxic
Protriptyline		
Amoxapine		
Selective serotonin reuptake inhibitors	Safer in overdosage, once daily dosing	Sexual dysfunction, nausea
Sertraline		Seizures
Paroxetine		Headache
Fluoxetine		Cytochrome P450 interactions
Citalopram		
Serotonin antagonist reuptake inhibitors	Few drug interactions, once daily dosing	Sexual dysfunction, priapism
Trazodone		Possible cardiotoxicity
Nefazodone		
Serotonin-norepinephrine reuptake inhibitors	Favorable side-effect profile	Hypertension, sexual dysfunction
Venlafaxine		Hyperlipidemia, multiple daily dosing
Mirtazapine	Appetite stimulant	Sexual dysfunction, blood dyscrasias, dependence potential
Dopamine reuptake inhibitors	Safer in overdose, minimal cardiotoxicity	Seizures
Bupropion		
Alternative therapy	Favorable side-effect profile	Lack of regulatory standardization, insufficient objective data
St John's wort		

(4) Jaw shrinkage – demineralization of jaw bone and teeth, dentures become less secure and need to be replaced;

(5) Loss of mobility – decreased flexibility, becoming severe and appearing earlier when the effects of osteoporosis, restricted body movement, leads to insecurity.

Treatment and therapy

Regular daily exercise should become a lifetime habit. Persons not already involved in regular exercise programs should consult a doctor before starting. Consuming 1500 mg of calcium in the diet every day protects most menopausal women. Younger women should take 1000 mg of calcium daily. Greater amounts of calcium should be taken only under direction of a doctor. Those who cannot digest milk may tolerate yogurt or buttermilk because both already contain lactase. Lactase, in the form of Lact-AID, is available at drugstores, and can be added to milk products to aid digestion. Calcitonin, a thyroid gland hormone, is prescribed to slow bone breakdown. Estrogen helps calcium retention and maintains healthy bones, and is sometimes prescribed for postmenopausal women. Any hormone therapy should be considered carefully, prescribed and periodically monitored by a doctor.

11

Prostate pathophysiology

Extensive investigations have been conducted on the pathophysiology of the prostate (Altman, 1993; Bostwick *et al.*, 1999; Fahmy and Bissada, 2003; Gronberg *et al.*, 1997; Habuchi *et al.*, 2000; Hardy *et al.*, 1996; Irvine *et al.*, 1995; Marks, 1999; Meyer and Nash, 1994; Miller, 1993; Montie and Pienta, 1994; Trent and Issacs 1996).

The prostate, which is partly glandular and partly muscular, is situated immediately below the internal urethral orifice at around the commencement of the urethra. It is located in the pelvic cavity, below the caudal part of the symphysis pubis, above the deep layer of the urogenital diaphragm. It is positioned ventral to the rectum, through which it may be palpated, especially when enlarged. The human prostate is 4 cm transversely at the base, 2 cm in anteroposterior diameter and 3 cm in vertical diameter, and weighs approximately 20 g. It is held in position by puboprostatic ligaments; by the deep layer of the urogenital diaphragm, which invests the prostate and the commencement of the membranous portion of the urethra; and by the anterior portions of the levatores ani, which pass backward from the pubis and hold the sides of the prostate. These portions of levatores ani, called levatores prostatae, support the prostate.

The prostate is enveloped by a thin but firm fibrous capsule, distinct from that derived from the subserous fascia, and separated from it by a plexus of veins. This capsule adheres firmly to the prostate and is structurally continuous with the stroma of the gland, being composed of the same tissues: non-striped muscle and fibrous tissues (Figures 11.1–11.5).

Muscular tissue constitutes the main prostatic stroma with scanty connective tissue between the muscular fibers forming thin trabeculae in which vessels/nerves of the gland ramify. Muscular tissue is arranged so that immediately beneath the fibrous capsule is a dense layer that forms an investing sheath for the gland. Around the urethra as it lies in the

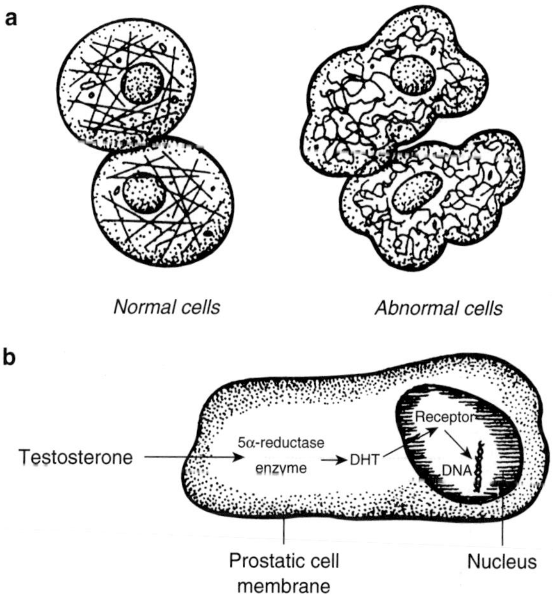

Figure 11.1 Left (**a**) Cell structure: normal body cells have an organized and regular skeleton made up of microscopic tubules that allow for normal growth. Cancer cells have lost this organized pattern, with distortion of the normal microtubules and loss of the normal cell shape and growth patterns. (**b**) Testosterone is important to the prostate, but not in its original form; it must be transformed to an active form. Testosterone is converted by an enzyme called 5α-reductase to dihydrotestosterone (DHT), the major androgen or male hormone inside the prostate cell. Testosterone circulates in the blood; it enters cells in the prostate by diffusion, like water through a tea bag, and is soon transformed into DHT. DHT hooks up chemically with a specific protein, moves to the cellular seat of power – the nucleus – and quickly becomes a powerful force in transmission of genetic information (DNA) from prostate cells

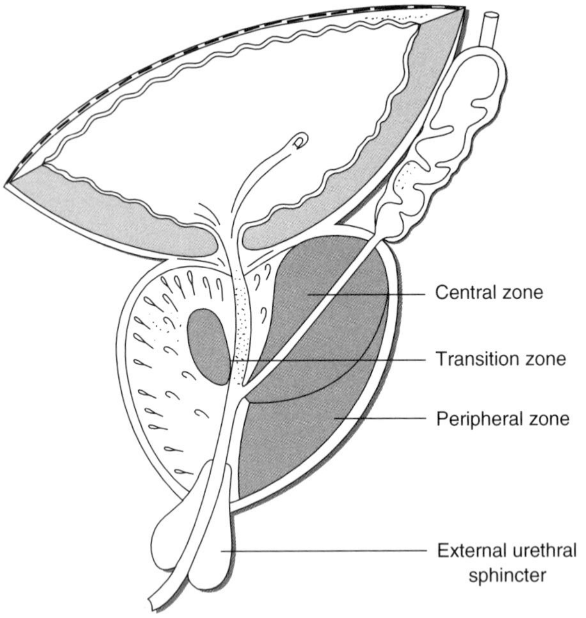

Figure 11.2 The three zones of the prostate (sagittal view)

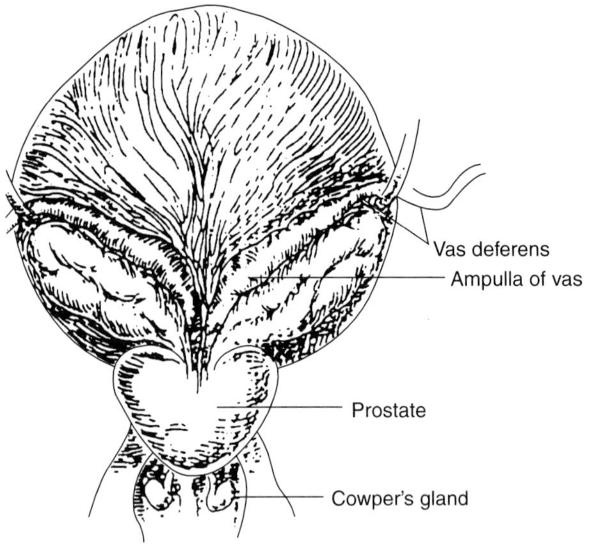

Figure 11.3 Anterior view of the human prostate/prostatic urethra. The anterior walls of the left ampulla, left seminal vesicle, have been cut away

prostate is another dense layer of circular fibers that is continuous above with the internal layer of the muscular coat of the bladder, and blends below with fibers surrounding the membranous portion of the urethra. In the part of the gland situated in front of the urethra the muscular tissue is dense, with no glandular tissue, while in the part that is behind the urethra, the muscular tissue has a wide-meshed structure, which is densest at the base of the gland (near bladder), becoming looser and more sponge-like towards the apex of the organ.

The glandular tissue of the prostate is composed of several follicular pouches with papillary elevation of lining follicles opening into elongated canals which join to form 12–20 excretory ducts. The ducts are connected by areolar tissue, supported by prolongations from the fibrous capsule and muscular stroma, and enclosed in a delicate capillary plexus. Columnar epithelium lines the canals and terminal vesicles. The prostatic ducts open into the floor of the prostatic portion of the urethra and are lined with two layers of epithelium, the inner layer consisting of columnar and the outer of small cubical cells. Colloid masses, known as amyloid bodies, are often found in gland tubes.

Arteries supplying the prostate are derived from internal pudendal, inferior vesical and middle rectal arteries. Veins form the prostatic plexus, which surrounds the sides and base of the gland. The plexus receives the dorsal vein of the penis and empties into the internal iliac veins and anastomotic connections with the vertebral system of veins, through which metastases of carcinoma may reach the bones or even the brain. Nerves are derived from pelvic plexus.

The prostate is perforated by the urethra and ejaculatory ducts. The urethra lies along the junction of its anterior with its middle third. The ejaculatory ducts pass obliquely through the posterior part of the prostate and open into the prostatic portion of the urethra.

The prostate has a base, an apex, a posterior, an anterior and two lateral surfaces. The base is close to the caudal surface of the bladder. The greater part of this surface is directly continuous with the bladder wall; the urethra penetrates it nearer to its ventral than its dorsal border. The lateral surface of the prostate is prominent, covered by the ventral portions of the levatores ani and separated from the gland by a plexus of veins. Caudally it is in contact with the deep layer of the urogenital diaphragm. The posterior surfaces (dorsal and rectal surfaces) are flattened from side to side and slightly convex craniocaudally; they are separated from the rectum by its sheath and important recto-vesical fascia. Near its cranial border is a depression through which the two ejaculatory ducts enter the prostate. This depression divides the posterior surface into a lower larger and an upper smaller part. The cranial smaller part constitutes the middle lobe of the prostate and intervenes between the ejaculatory ducts and the urethra; it varies greatly in size. The caudal larger portion can have a shallow median furrow, which imperfectly separates it into a right and a left lateral lobe. These form the main mass of the gland and are directly continuous

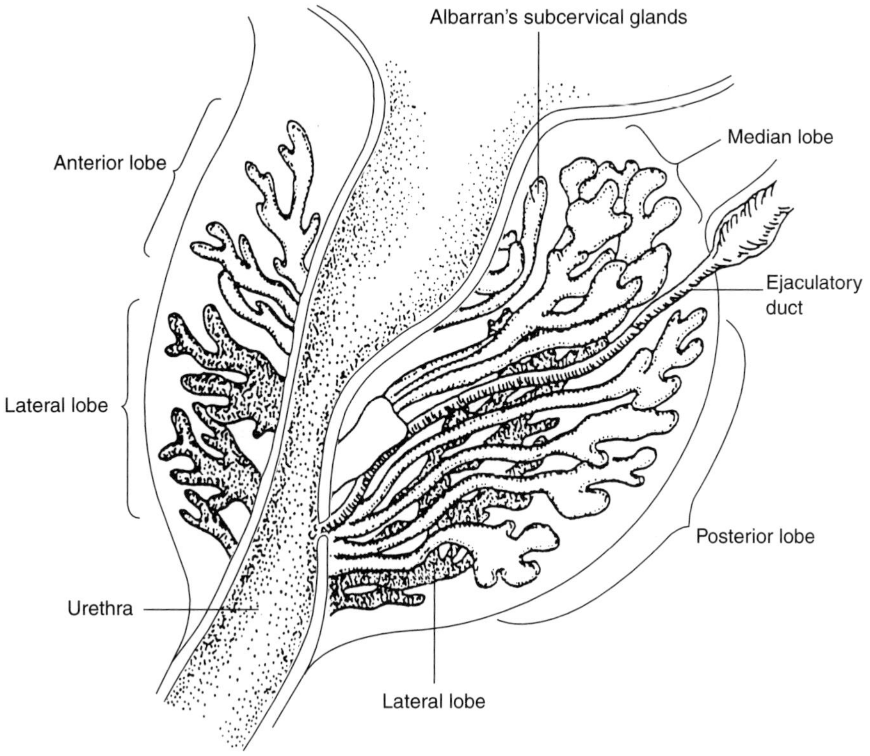

Figure 11.4 Detailed view of urethra and the orifices of the prostatic/ejaculatory ducts

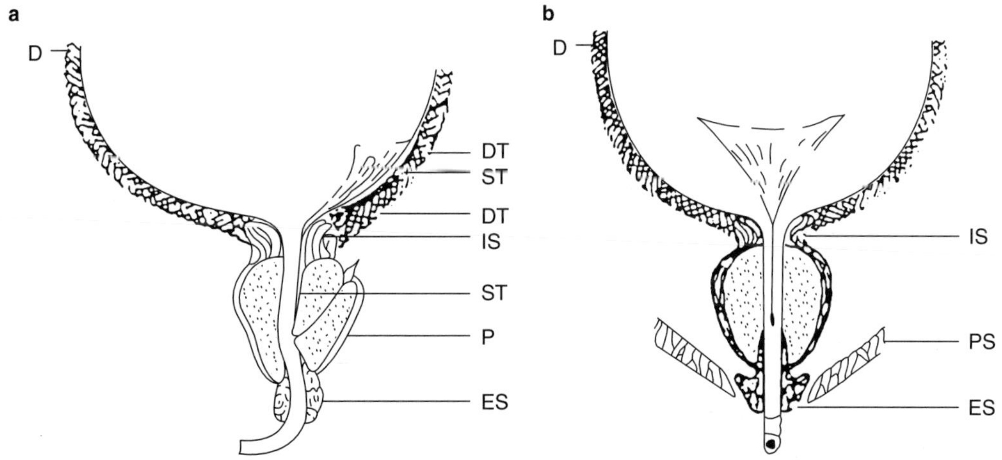

Figure 11.5 (**a**) A midline section through the male lower urinary tract, the lumen of the bladder and urethra is dilated and the right half of the trigone is indicated as a surface feature. The detrusor muscle (D) is in direct continuity with the morphologically identical deep trigone (DT). The superficial trigone (ST) extends inferiorly as far as the verumontanum. The smooth muscle of the bladder neck forms the internal urethral sphincter (IS) and is continuous with the prostatic capsule (P). The distal or external urethral sphincter (ES) is shown surrounding the membranous urethra. (**b**) Viewed from the front, the trigone is represented as a surface feature on the luminal aspect of the trigonal detrusor. PS, per urethral striated muscle

with each other dorsal to the urethra. Cranial to the urethra the lobes are connected by a band, the isthmus, which consists of the same tissues as the capsule and is devoid of glandular substance.

The urethra emerges from the anterior surface of the prostate a little cranial and ventral to the apex of the gland.

Enlargement of the prostate can cause obstruction of urinary flow through the urethra; this condition is more common in older men. Multiple ducts from the gland empty directly into the urethra. The prostate is a nodular gland with two narrow lobes connected by a thin transverse isthmus. The prostate secretes a thin, milky fluid containing calcium, citrate ions, phosphate ions, a clotting enzyme and a profibrinolysin. During emission the prostatic capsule contracts simultaneously with the contraction of the vas deferens; therefore the milky fluid may be quite important for successful fertilization, since the fluid of the vas deferens is relatively acidic owing to the presence of citric acid and metabolic end products of sperm (pH 3.5–4.0). Sperm do not become optimally motile until the pH of the surrounding fluids rises to 6.0–6.5. The slightly alkaline prostatic fluid seems to neutralize the acidity of other seminal fluids during ejaculation to enhance sperm motility and fertilizability. The clotting enzyme from prostatic fluid causes the fibrinogen of the seminal vesicle fluid to form a weak fibrin coagulum that holds the semen in the deeper regions of the vagina at the cervix. The coagulum then dissolves within 15–30 min because of lysis by fibrinolysin from the prostate.

PROSTATE CANCER

Physiopathology

The ductal epithelium of the prostate is surrounded by a sleeve of stromal cells, which consists primarily of smooth muscle cells that are involved in muscle contraction and innervation. The stroma contains fibroblasts, neuroendocrine cells and blood vessels. The structure and function of the prostate are dependent on androgens, particularly 5α-dihydrostestosterone (DHT), which preferentially binds to the androgen receptor. The reduction in prostate size that occurs after castration is primarily owing to the selective loss of the androgen-dependent secretory epithelial cells which undergo apoptosis. Prostate cancer is a disease of the aging male, and response to androgens, or androgen withdrawal, may be significantly influenced by age. Several antioxidant enzymes cause lobe-specific age-related decreases in the prostate: catalase, superoxide dismutase, glutathione peroxides and glutathione reductase. Normal body cells have an organized and regular skeleton composed of microscopic tubules that allow for normal growth. Cancer cells have lost this organized pattern, which causes the distortion of the normal microtubules and loss of the normal cell shape and growth patterns.

Incidence

The incidence of prostate cancer varies dramatically from country to country as well as between racial and ethnic groups. The age-matched rates for prostate cancer among American blacks and whites nearly tripled between 1973 and 1992. In the USA, 244 000 new cases of prostate cancer were estimated to be diagnosed in men over 50 years of age in 1995. This means an increase of 44 000 new cases being diagnosed within 1 year alone, as compared with 200 000 new cases in 1994. The lowest incidence rates have been observed in Asian populations: about 6/100 000 in Japan and less than 2/100 000 in China. The rates in Asians increase after immigration to the USA.

The pattern of prostate cancer parallels that of breast cancer in the female, and colon and pancreatic cancer in both sexes. Worldwide the incidence of mortality is unequally distributed, occurring more frequently in North America and northern Europe, and less frequently in Asia. Although the rate of prostate cancer in Japan is much less than that in the USA, it is continuously increasing; this may be due to a westernized diet, widespread environmental contamination and improved screening by prostate-specific antigen (PSA).

Endocrine parameters

Testosterone is important to the prostate, but not in its original form; it must be transformed into an active form. Testosterone is converted by the enzyme 5α-reductase to DHT; DHT is the major androgen, or male hormone, in the prostate. Testosterone circulates in the blood. It enters cells in the prostate by diffusion, like water through a tea bag, and is soon transformed into DHT. DHT binds with a specific protein, moves to the nucleus, and quickly becomes a powerful force in the transmission of genetic information (DNA) from prostate cells.

The estrogen : androgen ratio increases with aging because of the gradual decline in androgen levels. The relative decrease of androgens compared with estrogens is an initiating factor for benign prostatic hyperplasia (BPH). Strong correlation occurs between prostate cancer risk and high normal testosterone levels. Racial variation in the incidence may be explained by differences in testosterone biosynthesis and metabolism. Other initiating factors include androgen tissue concentrations, rate of testosterone reduction to DHT and sensitivity of androgen receptors. Prostate cancer is commonly multifocal, with an average of five apparently independent foci at the time of diagnosis. BPH is not prostatic carcinoma and is not related to family history.

Of testosterone in plasma 98% is bound to protein as testosterone binding globulin (TBG). Testosterone in the prostate is converted to DHT by the enzyme 5α-reductase. The inhibitor 'Proscar' inhibits the growth of BPH. A prospective study is under way by the Southwest Oncology Group on the preventive effect of Proscar in prostate cancer. Androgenic hormone depreciation in prostate cancer is accomplished by various methods.

Screening and testing

Screening should be initiated among men at high risk for prostate cancer before the age of 45 years. Screening in families with hereditary cancer is initiated at least 5 years before the earliest age at diagnosis in the family, and at least 10 years before the age at which metastatic disease appeared. PSA screening is terminated at the age of 70 years for men with consistently normal levels, since the risk of dying of prostate cancer is low. Men with PSA ≥3 ng/ml should undergo biopsy, and if the results are negative they should undergo repeat biopsy or re-examination at short time intervals. Men from families with hereditary prostate cancer (HPC) are concerned about their increased risk, and it is of psychological importance to these individuals that something be done to reduce their risk of dying of cancer. The risk of false-positive PSA tests should be discussed with the patient before he is offered regular screening.

PSA levels change with age, prostate volume and prostate cancer. Untreated hypogonadal men can have lower serum PSA concentrations than controls; absence of testosterone does not change PSA levels in eugonadal men, and patients with prostate cancer and low serum testosterone concentrations have lower serum PSA levels than those with normal serum testosterone levels. A prostate biopsy should be performed only if abnormalities are detected by digital rectal examination (DRE) or if PSA levels are rapidly increasing during testosterone therapy (an increase of 1.5 ng/ml or greater). Castration causes an 85% and 81% decrease in the total epithelial weight and total ventral prostate lobe weight, respectively; hypogonadal men have a reduced total prostate volume compared with eugonadal men. Non-obstructive BPH is not a contraindication to testosterone therapy. However, prostate cancer is an absolute contraindication to testosterone therapy, because testosterone administration may promote the growth of subclinical prostate cancer. DRE and serum PSA measurement should be performed before testosterone treatment, at 3 and 6 months, and yearly thereafter. PSA should be measured 1 month after initiation of therapy to detect any patient with previously undiagnosed prostate cancer that may behave in a very aggressive fashion after testosterone replacement therapy. Testosterone may be administered using a gel or patch to achieve a physiological pattern.

Testing is performed on leukocyte DNA from ordinary blood samples. Presymptomatic genetic testing has important psychological, medicolegal and ethical consequences. Testing should always be preceded by thorough education and counseling, and written informed consent. There should be active follow-up after counseling for genetic testing, regardless of whether testing was actually performed. The large number of genes involved in prostate cancer susceptibility, and the probable importance of environmental and additional genetic factors that modify cancer risk, make genetic analyses complicated.

The incidence of prostate cancer being detected at autopsy in older men is very high and increases steadily with age. However, the vast majority of these cancers remain insignificant. The progression to clinically detectable and/or lethal cancer varies in different geographic locations and ethnic populations. Patients with localized prostate cancer can be cured of their cancer. However, not all require a curative treatment with its attendant morbidity. Patients with limited life expectancy who have prostate cancer with good characteristics (low volume, low grade) do well for many years with expectant management (watchful waiting). Many elderly patients will die of competing causes long before prostate cancer progression. However, patients who have a long life expectancy and localized prostate cancer will eventually have disease progression causing significant morbidity and mortality. Unfortunately, patients with poor disease characteristics (large volume, non-organ confined and high grade) often do poorly despite therapeutic intervention. The majority of patients have intermediate disease characteristics and their prognosis is less predictable.

HEREDITARY PROSTATE CANCER

There is no difference between patients with HPC and those with sporadic prostate cancer regarding tumor grade and pathological stage at diagnosis. The clinical characteristics of cancer depend on which susceptibility gene is involved in a family HPC. Between 5 and 10% of prostate cancer is caused by dominantly inherited genes. HPC is diagnosed at a comparatively early age of onset. Patients from families with HPC are diagnosed 6–7 years earlier than those with sporadic disease. HPC may account for one-third of prostate

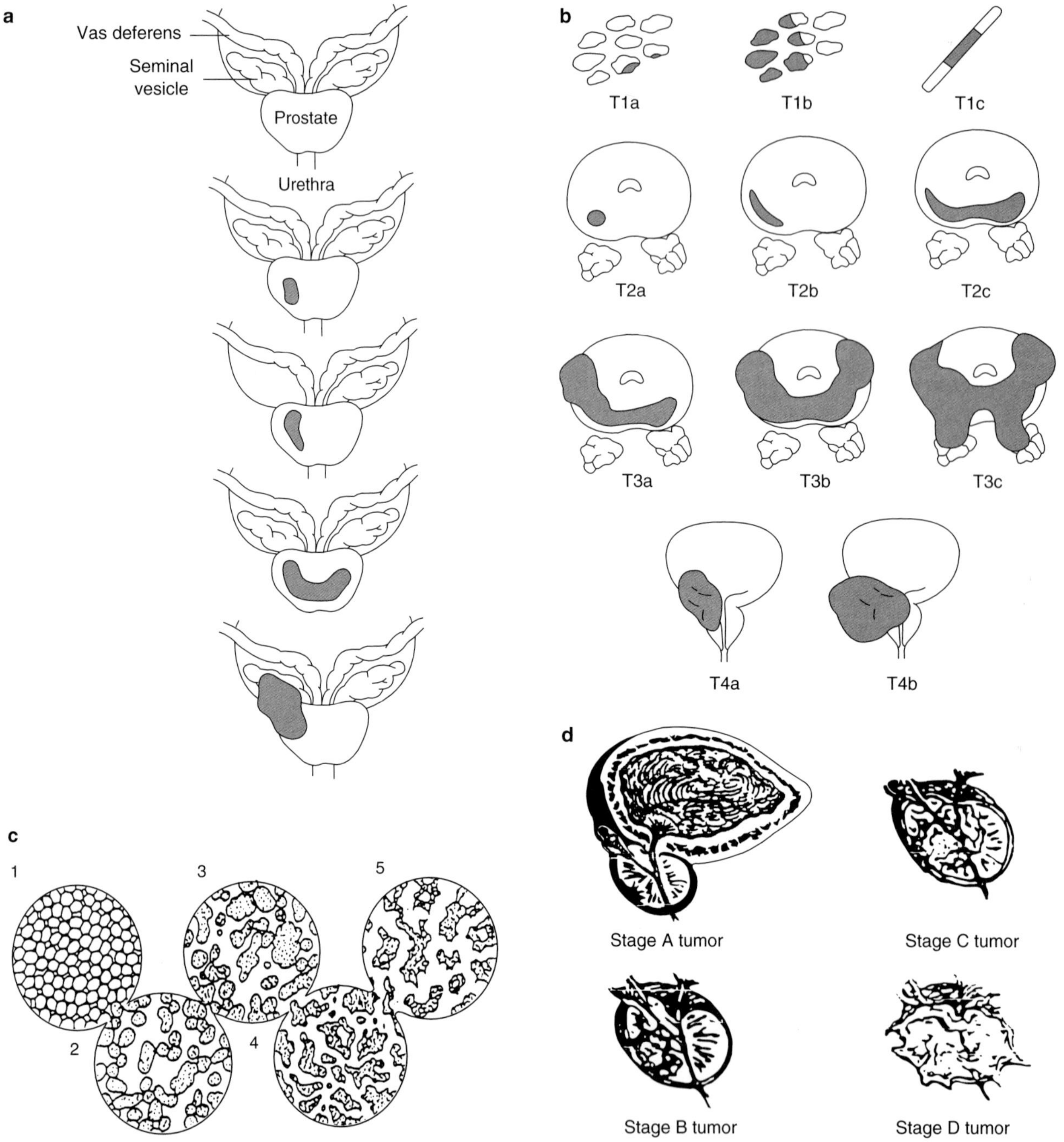

Figure 11.6 Manifestation and grades of prostate carcinoma. (**a**) Stages of prostate cancer using both the TNM (tumor nodes metastases) and the Whitmore–Jewett system. (**b**) Extent of prostate cancer according to the TNM staging system. (**c**) Histological grades of adenocarcinoma showing appearance of cancer cells according to the Gleason grade (Bostwick *et al.*, 1996). (**d**) The four stages of prostate cancer

cancer cases diagnosed before age 60, and more than 40% of those diagnosed before age 55. HPC should not be treated differently from the sporadic disease, other than that watchful waiting might be a less suitable option for men who have had the painful experience of having a close relative die of the disease. Men concerned about a possible hereditary predisposition to prostate cancer should be offered basic genetic counseling: explanation of the genetic mechanisms of autonomic dominant and X-linked traits, and notification of the risk in absolute and relative terms (Figure 11.6 and Table 11.1).

Genome-wide search with linkage analysis resulted in mapping the prostate cancer susceptibility gene to chromosome 1q24–25; this gene named HPC is linked to prostate cancer in 33% of patients. Linkage to HPC1 was mainly found in families with male-to-male germline transmission of early-onset disease diagnosed in five or more family members, with 29% of the families fulfilling these three linked criteria. A second gene has been located on the long arm of chromosome 1 (1q42.2–43) based on a linkage analysis susceptibility gene located on the X (Xq27–28). Less common genes include: HPCX on chromosome Xq27–28, CAPB on chromosome 1p36, HPC2 on chromosome 17p12 and HPC20 on chromosome 20q13.

Table 11.1 Effect of family history of prostate cancer on lifetime risk of clinical prostate cancer

Family history	*Relative risk*	*% Absolute risk*
Negative	1	8
Father affected at age 60 or older	1.5	12
One brother affected at age 60 or older	2	15
Father affected before age 60	2.5	20
One brother affected before age 60	3	25
Two affected male relatives*	4	30
Three or more affected male relatives†	5	35–45

*Father and brother, or two brothers, or a brother and a maternal grandfather or uncle, or a father and a paternal grandfather or uncle. †The absolute lifetime risk for mutation carriers is probably 70–90% for high penetrance genes such as HPC1

Unaffected men in families with HPC overestimate their lifetime risk of the disease. Thus, such information will often reduce concerns about cancer risk. For members of families with HPC who experience close relatives dying of cancer, often at an early age, causing anxiety or depression, psychological aspects of cancer predisposition should be addressed at counseling. The onset of HPC, which is associated with higher mortality, increases the potential gain in survival by curative treatments and decreases the proportion of men treated for tumors that would not have progressed to symptomatic systemic disease within their lifetime.

The positive predictive value of PSA varies with the prevalence of prostate cancer in the screened population. The higher is the prevalence, the higher the positive predictive value. Thus, the risk of prostate cancer for men with a slightly to moderately elevated PSA is much higher for those with a positive family history than for those with no affected relatives. The urologist should therefore decide whether to perform prostatic biopsies in men with a PSA of 3–10 ng/ml, considering family history and other established factors, such as the ratio of free-to-total PSA, PSA density and patient age. In some families there is X-linked inheritance as well as recessive inheritance.

Of patients having a relative with prostate cancer 40% had a positive biopsy compared with 29% of patients with a negative family history.

Table 11.2 Therapeutic approaches to prostate cancer

Surgery

Bilateral orchiectomy or daily administration of 203 mg of diethylstilbestrol

Antiandrogens

Ketoconazole: inhibits testicular and adrenal steroidogenesis, androgen level drops to castration levels within 24 h

Aminogluthemide block, 20, 24–desmolase inhibits conversion of cholesterol to pregnenolone

Non-steroid antiandrogens

Mostly used as combination therapy

Flutomide

Third generatioin bicalutamide 'Casodex'

RH agonists

Action: overwhelms hypothalamic–pituitary axis and initially testosterone production; increases then complete blockade of pituitary–gonadal axis results in androgen hormone levels dropping to castration levels

Decapitates include Luparan®/Depo Luparan, Zoladex®, newer product Viadure® 'subcutaneous cylinder implant', Abarelix®, Cetrolix® 'without initial androgenic surge'

Steroids

Antiandrogen: megestrol acetate 250 mg/day mostly used for severe hot flushes of GnRH agonist

GnRH, gonadotropin releasing hormone

Table 11.3 Effects of testosterone therapy on prostate specific antigen (PSA) levels and prostate volume in hypogonadal men

Duration (months)	Administration route	Effects	
		PSA	*Prostate volume*
41.5 ± 36.2	Oral, TTS, IM	NS	NS
18	Anabolic steroid abusers	NS	TPV: NS; CPV: 20%
Up to 12	IM, TTS	NS	NS
12–36	TTS	NS	NS
32	Implants, IM	NS	TPV: NS; CPV: NS

IM, intramuscularly; TTS, transdermal therapeutic system; TPV, total prostate volume; NS, not significant; CPV, central prostate volume

Prophylactic radical prostatectomy might be an option when presymptomatic genetic testing becomes feasible and gene carriers with extremely high risk (70–90%) of prostate cancer can be identified. Mutation carriers should be identified and offered prophylactic treatment or intensive surveillance. HPC carriers can be assured that their cancer risk is not higher than that of the general population. Hereditary cancer susceptibility is caused by germline mutations.

Most genes involved in hereditary susceptibility to prostate cancer are relatively site specific. The small difference in age at onset between hereditary and sporadic prostate cancer (6–7 years compared with 20 years in breast, ovarian and colorectal cancers) implies that environmental factors may be of importance in many families with HPC.

Little is known about the genes that modify the expression or penetrance of the prostate cancer, which could partly explain the difficulties in confirming and cloning the mapped genes. Most cases of prostate cancer seem to occur in a genetically predisposed minority of the population. This could form the basis of a future selective screening strategy.

Protooncogenes

Mechanisms involved in oncogenesis include protooncogene activation, mutation or loss of tumor-suppressor genes, activation of antiapoptotic genes or loss of proapoptotic genes. The effect of genes that enhance a process is shown as +, whereas the effect of genes that suppress a process is shown as –. Cell division and proliferation are stimulated (+) by the products of protooncogenes. Some tumor-suppressor genes directly regulate protooncogene function (gate keepers); others act more indirectly by maintaining genome integrity and correcting mutations during DNA replication and cell division (caretakers). Activation of antiapoptotic genes has the same effect. Activation of oncogenes or antiapoptotic genes is dominant and requires only a single mutant allele. The action of tumor-suppressor genes is recessive; when both alleles are mutated or lost, cell growth is unregulated or genomic integrity is compromised. Loss of proapoptotic genes may occur through loss of both alleles or through a dominant negative mutation in one allele.

THERAPEUTIC APPROACHES

Management of hormone refractory prostate cancer (Table 11.2)

Prostate cancer that is progressive despite the maintenance of castration levels of testosterone is generally referred to as hormone refractory or androgen-independent prostate cancer. These terms, however, are misnomers, as most progressive cancers remain sensitive to androgens and some may respond to alternative hormonal manipulations. Development of hormone refractory prostate cancer is a significant clinical finding which usually has a median survival of 9–12 months.

Hormone refractory prostate cancer is a heterogenous disease and prognosis may vary among different subgroups of patients. Patients may present only with a rising PSA without significant disease-related symptoms, or they may present with multiple osseous metastases, a declining performance status and severe pain. Mechanisms implicated in the development of androgen independence may include androgen receptor mutations and expression of antiapopotic protein, bcl-2. Assessing disease response to treatment has been a barrier in development of new treatments, as about 60% of patients will have disease confined to bone, which is not amenable to classic response criteria (Figures 11.7 and 11.8).

Chemotherapy has been extensively evaluated in the management of patients with hormone refractory prostate cancer. In a randomized trail, combination of mitoxantrone and prednisone was shown to be superior to prednisone alone, primarily with regard to palliation of symptoms (Pilepich *et al.*, 1995; Soloway *et al.*, 1995).

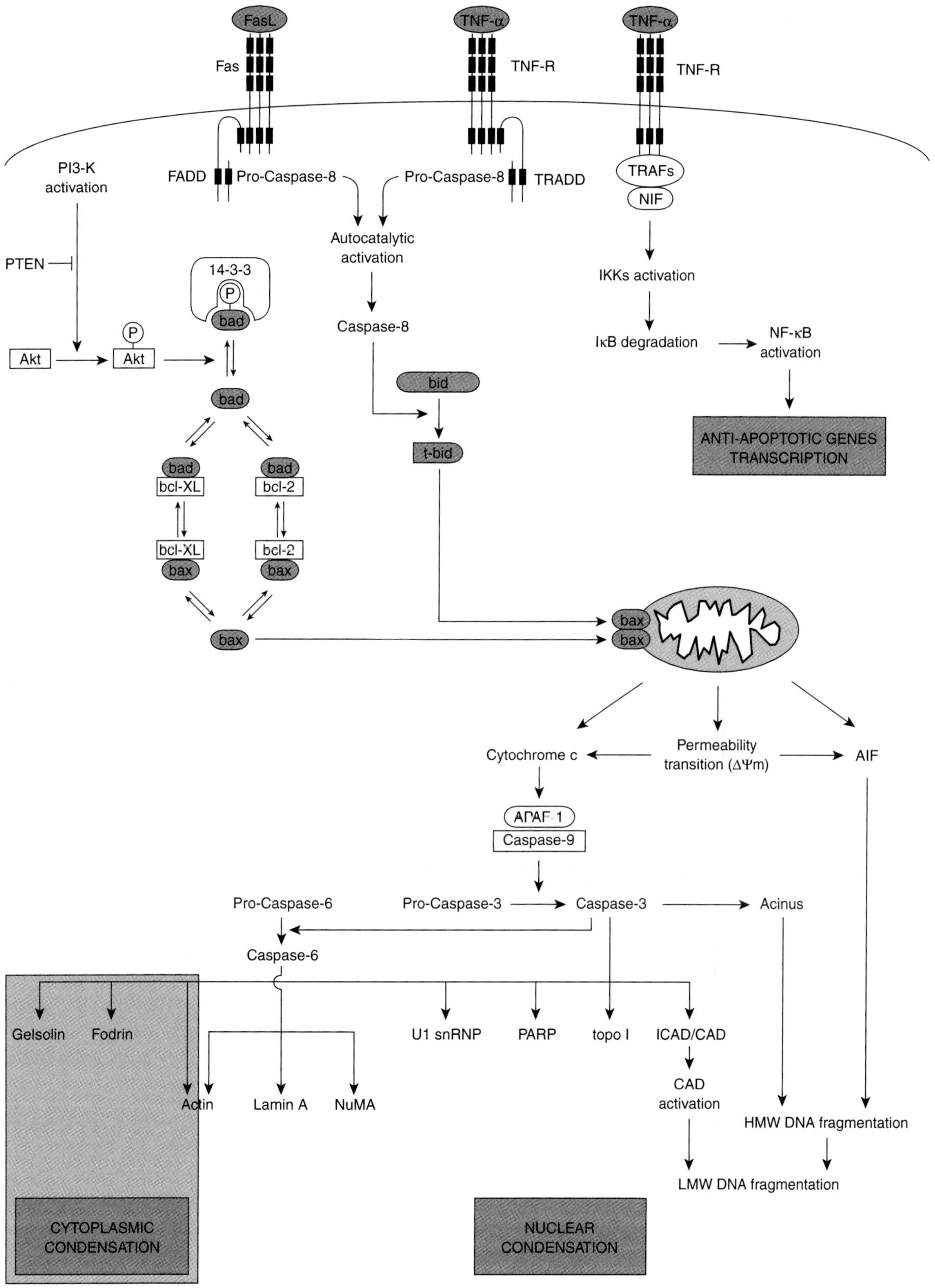

Figure 11.7 Role of the mitochondrion and Bcl-2 family proteins in programming cell death. From Lee and Tenniswood, 2003, with permission. Fash, Fas ligand; FADD, Fas-associated death domain; TNF, tumor necrosis factor; R, receptor; TRAF, tumor necrosis factor receptor-associated factor; TRADD, TNF receptor-associated death domain; NIF, neutrophil inhibitory factor; PTEN, phosphatase and tensin homolog; IKK, IκB kinase; NF, nuclear factor; AIF, apoptosis-inducing factor; APAF, apoptotic protease-activating factor; NUMA, nuclear mitotic apparatus; snRNP, small nuclear riboproteins; ICAD, inhibitor of caspase-activated DNase

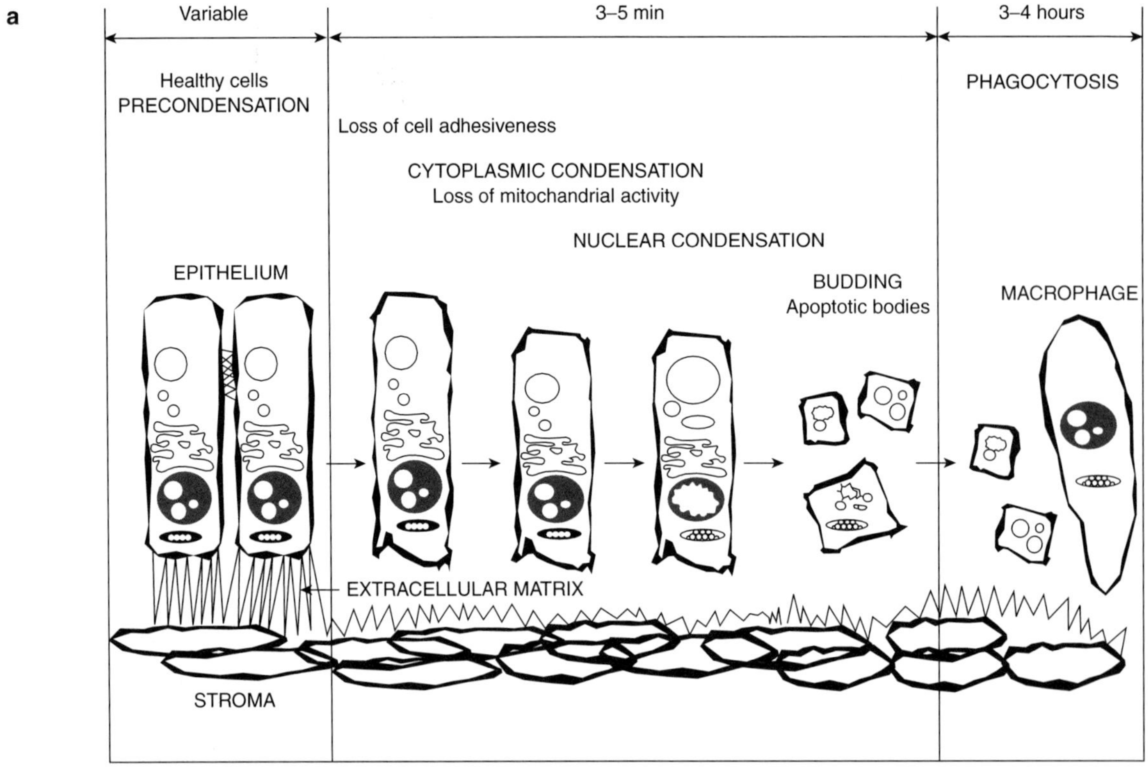

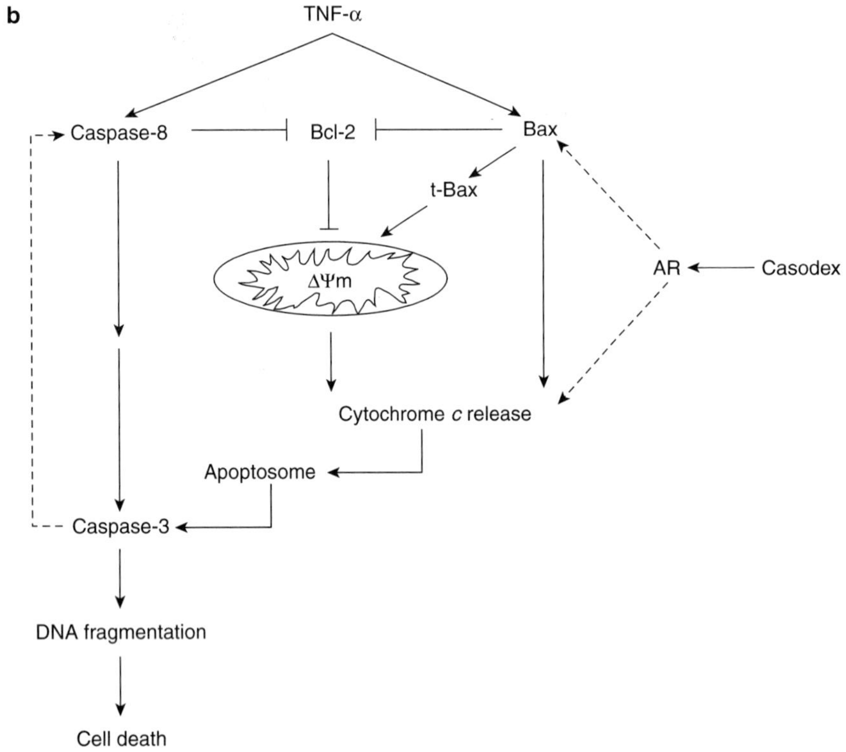

Figure 11.8 (**a**) Schematic representation of the stages of apoptosis in individual glandular epithelial cells. Approximate time line is shown. (**b**) Schematic model of the proposed mechanism of Casodex®-induced cell death in human prostate cancer. TNF-α, tumor necrosis factor-α; AR, androgen receptor. From Lee and Tenniswood, 2003, with permission

Synthetic non-steroids

A new family of synthetic non-steroidal molecules displays selective preferential activities for androgen receptors in certain tissues such as muscle, bone and the central nervous system. Specific androgen receptor modulators are not substrates of the 5α-reductase enzyme and are therefore not converted to DHT. Consequently, they do not have proliferating activity in the prostate (Negro-Vilar, 1999).

Non-steroidal antiandrogens

These include flutamide, bicalutamide (Casodex) and nilutamide. They have been used for long- or short-term combined androgen blockade (in conjunction with luteinizing hormone releasing hormone (LHRH) agonists) and as single agents. Currently, antiandrogen monotherapy is not considered to be as effective as surgical or medical castration in the initial management of advanced prostate cancer. However, they may have a role in combined androgen blockade. Furthermore, they are used during the transitional phase of hormone refractory prostate cancer at which time patients may still respond to secondary hormonal management, e.g. by use of high-dose bicalutamide, estrogen therapy or other steroid antiandrogens such as ketoconazole. The timing of androgen withdrawal is not strictly defined. All symptomatic patients and those with evidence of skeletal metastases clearly benefit from androgen deprivation. Furthermore, patients with pelvic lymph node metastases also benefit from early androgen deprivation.

Radioactive seed implants

Interstitial radioactive seed implantation for prostate cancer offers another viable treatment option for patients with prostate cancer. The advantages over surgery are the avoidance of a major surgical procedure, less incidence of significant complications, such as incontinence, and the rapidity with which normal functions can begin. Erectile dysfunction continues to be a concern. Most feel that the true rate of erectile dysfunction after Brach therapy is approximately 50%. The major advantages over external beam radiotherapy involve the time commitment by the patient. Modern external beam radiotherapy is a 7–8-week treatment course, whereas Brach therapy is now largely an outpatient procedure. Longer follow-up is needed adequately to evaluate how successful Brach therapy will be for the treatment of localized prostate cancer (Pollack and Zagars, 1997; Roach *et al.*, 1996).

External beam management with high-dose conformal radiotherapy

External beam radiotherapy has been used for the curative treatment of prostate cancer for many years. The problems with traditional means of treating prostate cancer with radiotherapy have been a less than optimal cure rate and an unacceptable frequency of unpleasant adverse effects, most notably intestinal problems.

Angiogenesis and survival period of cancer patients

'Angiogenesis' cutting off a tumor's blood supply improves cancer survival, but does not cure the disease. Treatment with angiogenesis is based on the drug Avastin™, which acts against vascular endothelial growth factor, one of the more than 20 chemicals that help the blood vessels of the tumor to grow and survive.

In a recent study at Duke University, 923 colon cancer patients all received a standard chemotherapy cocktail of irinotecan, 5-fluorouracil and leucovorin. They were also randomly given either Avastin or placebo. Those on Avastin survived an average of 20 months, compared with almost 16 months in those receiving only standard treatment (personal communication). The results are a surprise, since an earlier study found no benefit of Avastin against breast cancer.

Nutrition

Nutritional recommendations for patients with prostate cancer emphasize the role of a healthy diet, low in fat and high in fruit, vegetables and grains. Fat intake should be <40 g (and preferably <33 g). Consumption of adequate amounts of vegetables and fruit is recommended including cooked tomatoes and berries. The role of nutritional supplements, vitamin E, selenium, lycopenes, ellagic acid and some soy components is being studied.

Molecular parameters

Extensive investigation has been conducted on the molecular mechanisms of cell death in human prostate cancer (Lee and Tenniswood, 2003). Emphasis was placed on the role of mitochondria and Bcl-2 family proteins in programmed cell death and the stages of apoptosis in individual glandular epithelial cells (Figures 11.7 and 11.8).

Recommended research

Recommended future research includes investigation of the:

(1) Long-term effects of androgen replacement therapy on the prostate;

(2) Role of androgens in pathogenesis of benign prostatic hyperplasia (BPH) and prostate cancer;

(3) Effects of testosterone therapy on BPH or prostate cancer;

(4) Effects of testosterone therapy on an existing cancer;

(5) How PSA levels are affected by androgen deficiency and androgen replacement.

Large-scale, long-term clinical studies are needed to resolve the issues related to andropause and assess the long-term risk versus benefit profile of androgen replacement therapy.

12

Cardiovascular anomalies, infections and infectious diseases

CARDIOVASCULAR ANOMALIES

Heart disease

Heart disease is an inclusive term for a variety of disorders of the heart itself as well as a network of blood vessels throughout the body that distribute nutrients and oxygen in arteries and collect waste in veins. The arteries branch into smaller arterioles and then into still smaller capillaries, vessels which are less than one-tenth the thickness of a human hair.

One-fifth of the US population already have one or more forms of heart disease; millions more are at risk. The cardiovascular disease death toll exceeds the combined total of deaths attributable to cancer, accidents and infections. Men are three times more at risk for heart disease than women. Heart disease causes suffering and sorrow for the victims and their families; however, it also has an impact on the economic health of a nation. The total cost of heart-related hospitalizations, doctors' bills, nursing home services, medication and lost productivity are estimated to be $200 billion per annum in the USA. Men over 60 years of age are recommended to have their blood pressure checked regularly as a preventive measure. Blood pressure measurement is expressed as the systolic over the diastolic blood pressure, with 120 over 80 as the normal adult level, 140 over 90 as borderline high blood pressure and 160 over 95 as a cause for concern.

Ischemic heart disease, characterized by reduced blood supply to the heart, is the most common cause of death in most western countries. Ischemia means 'reduced blood supply'. The coronary arteries supply blood to the heart muscle and no alternative blood supply exists; thus, a blockage in the coronary arteries reduces the supply of blood to the heart muscle. Most ischemic heart disease is caused by atherosclerosis. Initially there is narrowing of coronary arteries causing angina. The narrowing is mainly caused by fatty plaques lining the wall of the artery. A fatty plaque may rupture leading to a heart attack. (Heart attacks caused by simple narrowing are relatively uncommon.) A heart attack causes damage to heart muscle by cutting off its blood supply.

Complications of a heart attack include temporary damage and pain (ischemia), loss of muscle activity (acute heart failure), permanent heart muscle damage (acute myocardial infarction/infarct), long-term loss of heart muscle activity (chronic heart failure), cardiac arrhythmia (irregular heartbeat which can be fatal) and other structural damage to the heart including damaged heart valves, actual perforation of the heart and a thin-walled fibrous floppy heart.

Preventive measures, including not smoking, treatment of hypertension, regular exercise and diet, are easy to achieve. Obesity exerts unnecessary strain on the heart and increases serum cholesterol and triglyceride levels. Excess saturated fat in the diet should be avoided. Some unsaturated fats may be beneficial in reducing the risk of heart disease when consumed in moderation. Dietary cholesterol has a modest effect on serum cholesterol. Cholesterol-reducing drugs are recommended.

Specialized coronary care can include cardiopulmonary resuscitation (heart massage), defibrillation to revert cardiac arrhythmias, fitting of an artificial pacemaker to prevent cardiac arrhythmias, treatment with drugs such as adrenaline to increase the heart rate, administration of thrombolytic agents to clear away the causative blood clot, anticoagulation therapy

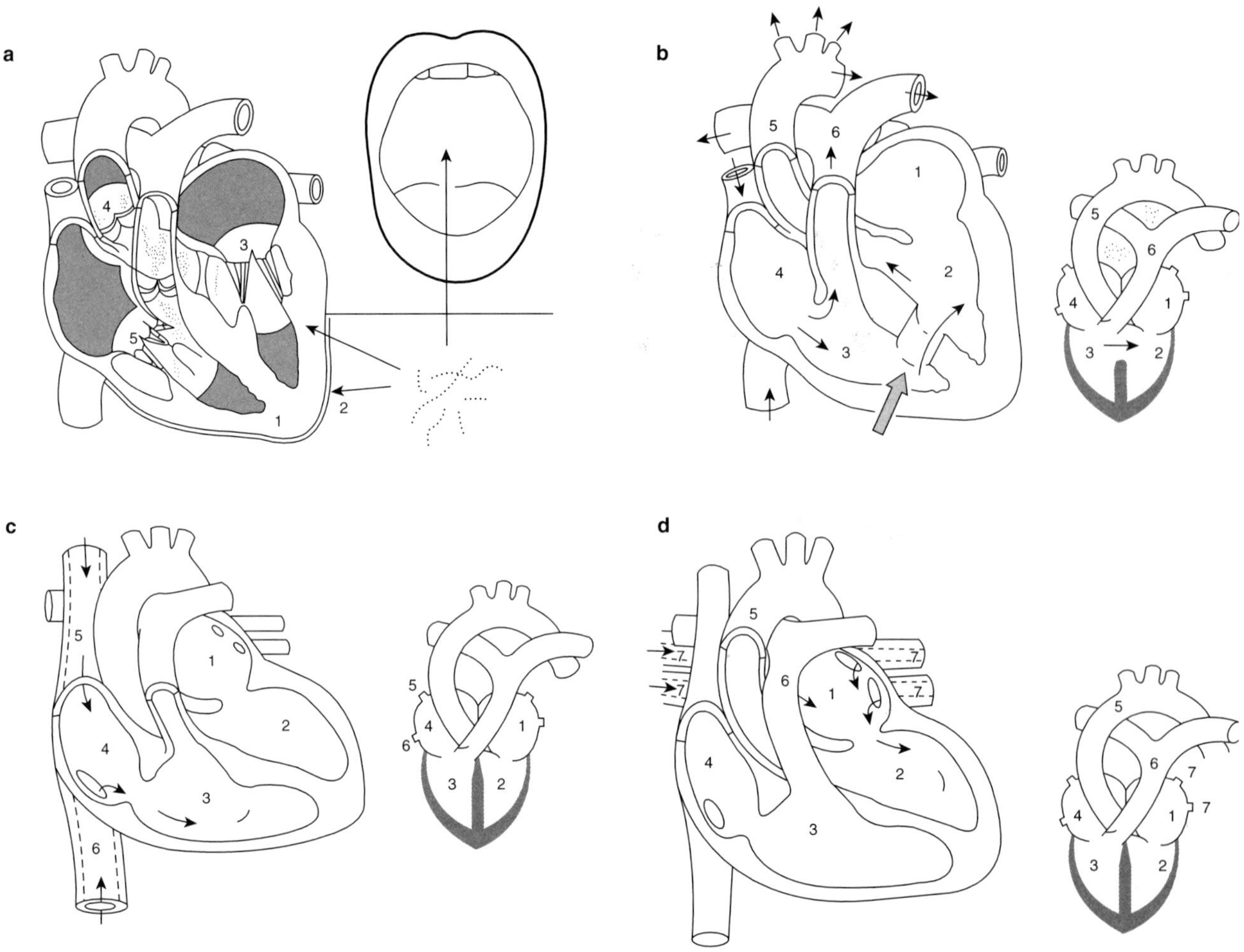

Figure 12.1 Major anatomical anomalies of the heart. (**a**) Rheumatic fever is apparently a sequela of a streptococcal infection, characteristically originating as a respiratory infection with a sore throat. Involved cardiac areas can include the heart muscle (1), the pericardial sac around the heart (2) and, most frequently, the mitral (3) and aortic (4) valves, and, rarely, the tricuspid valve (5). (**b**) Interventricular septal defect (abnormal opening between ventricles). Returned venous blood from right ventricle (3) is shunted to left ventricle (2), causing oxygenated and unoxygenated blood to mix. This imposes an increased workload on both ventricles. (**c**) Congestive failure of right heart. Normal circulation shown in small drawing. In right heart failure, the right ventricle (3) has difficulty in delivering venous blood to the lungs. Blood backs up in the atrium (4) and the superior (5) and inferior vena cava (6) causing dilatation, with a back-up of blood, increased pressure in the veins in the upper and lower parts of the blood and in the liver. (**d**) Congestive failure of left heart. In contrast to normal circulation (small drawing), ineffective discharge of the left ventricle (2) causes back pressure in the left atrium (1), enlargement of pulmonary veins (7) and increased pressure in lung vessels. Dotted lines show normal size of pulmonary veins

to prevent additional blood clots, treatment with isotropic drugs to raise blood pressure, and unblocking of arteries with surgery or angioplasty ('balloon angioplasty').

Preventive therapy after a heart attack can include cardiac surgery, regular administration of anticoagulants to prevent further arrhythmias and of drugs to control heart rhythm, and physical exercise within safe limits to train the heart.

Some major anatomical anomalies of the heart are shown in Figure 12.1.

Pulmonary embolism/deep vein thrombosis

The heart pumps oxygen-rich blood through the arteries to the rest of the body. Veins carry the blood back to the lungs for re-oxygenation. Fighting gravity to push blood up from the legs is difficult and can be complicated by illness, injury or prolonged inactivity. Deep vein thrombosis occurs when a dangerous blood clot forms deep in the leg muscles. The clot can float to the lungs, causing sudden death. Almost 2 million Americans suffer from deep vein thrombosis each year.

Such clots have made headlines when seemingly healthy people collapse after long airplane flights overseas. Most clots actually occur when people are hospitalized for surgery, trauma or some other reason.

A clot moving to the lungs causes pulmonary embolism. Some 80 000 patients suffering from pulmonary embolism die as a result. The following are risk factors:

(1) Hospitalization for a serious illness or surgery;
(2) Other immobility, such as paralysis or long-distance travel by plane, train or car;
(3) Chronic diseases such as high blood pressure, heart disease or cancer;
(4) An inherited tendency for sticky clot-prone blood;
(5) Excess estrogen during pregnancy, from birth control pills or hormone therapy;
(6) Aged over 40 years;
(7) Smoking;
(8) Obesity.

The Centers for Disease Control and Prevention and the American Public Health Association are co-ordinating extensive investigations in an attempt to prevent these clots and to screen all hospital patients.

SEMEN INFECTIONS

Herpes simplex virus infection

Seventy-five per cent of male infertility is idiopathic, whereas <5% is due to endocrine disorders, spermatic duct obstruction, antisperm antibodies, toxins, drugs, cryptorchidism, infection, sexual dysfunction and ejaculatory failure. Herpes simplex virus (HSV) DNA has been detected by polymerase chain reaction (PCR) in the sperm of men with genital HSV infection and is associated with infertility. HSV DNA is also localized within the sperm. The virus seems to play a significant role in male infertility, and its early detection by the nested PCR enables successful antiviral therapy to be administered, thus increasing the possibility of restoration of fertility and long-term protection of sperm quality (Kapranos *et al.*, 2003). The detection of herpes viruses within semen facilitates better control of the transmission.

Ralstonia picketti infection of semen

Ralstonia picketti, a rare infection of semen, is usually transmitted through topical saline solutions resulting in infection within the respiratory and gastrointestinal tract. Cytolysosomes are autosomes, or secondary lysosomes, which are specialized for the removal of cellular debris and organelles. These structures, found in various cell types, are activated in response to system stress such as bacterial infection, and seem to be derived from neutrophils and are produced in response to reproductive tract infection with *R. picketti* (Carrell *et al.*, 2003). It is not known whether this infection is related to sperm phagocytes in the epididymis.

Viral infection of semen

Viral infection of semen occurs with HIV, murine retroviruses, cytomegalovirus (CMV) C and hepatitis B. In HIV infection, and to a lesser extent in CMV and hepatitis B, infected semen appears to be important in disease transmission. Infected semen has also been implicated in the horizontal transmission of murine retroviruses. The transmission of viral, as well as non-viral, agents via this route in man can be almost completely eliminated through the use of condoms.

Sperm washing

Elegant techniques have been developed to eliminate seminal plasma, viral particles, non-spermatic cells and non-motile sperm from semen and to select sperm with the best motility.

In hepatitis C virus (HCV) and HIV seropositive males sperm washing involves the following steps:

(1) Removal of seminal plasma:
    (a) dilution of sperm in fresh media;
    (b) centrifugation at 400 *g* for 10 min;
    (c) resuspension in sperm media.
(2) First purification of non-spermatic cells and abnormal non-motile sperm:
    (a) centrifugation at 300 *g* for 20 min;
    (b) first wash with PureSperm 45%;
    (c) resuspension in 2 ml of media.
(3) Selection of sperm with best motility:
    (a) centrifugation at 200 *g* for 10 min;
    (b) collection of 0.35 ml of deposit;
    (c) incubation at 37°C in 5% CO_2;
    (d) resuspension in 0.5 ml.

After washing sperm are stored in cryotubes at –80°C (Garrido, 2004).

If washed samples are to be used for ART, viral presence should be tested after washing. The introduction of diagnostic PCR improved detection techniques and the safety of ART. Samples that are HIV negative after washing could still be HCV positive. Garrido *et al.* (2004) found five out of 41 samples (fraction of motile sperm after washing) were positive for HIV (12%) and five out of 21 were positive for HCV (24%) after washing. The presence of HIV and HCV was lower than 200 IU/ml and 600 IU/ml for HIV and HCV, respectively. Molecular tests are necessary to confirm sperm washing success. Motile sperm can be selected from hemophilic HIV-1 positive patients by discontinuous Percoll gradient centrifugation followed by 'swim-up'. Semen washing before use may reduce the risk of HIV transmission from an infected man to an uninfected woman. However, an evaluation of the viral presence after washing is required (Garrido, 2004).

VIRAL INFECTIONS

There are several viral infections of the urogenital tract including papilloma viruses (genital types), herpes viruses (herpes simplex 2) and retroviruses (HTLV-III). Sexual intercourse may induce tears or abrasions in the vaginal epithelium or trauma to the urethra allowing viral entry via the genitourinary route. Sexually transmitted viruses in man include HIV, herpes simplex and human papilloma viruses 11, 16 and 18 (responsible for genital warts or condyloma acuminata). Acute hemorrhagic cystitis in young boys is associated with adenovirus 11 and 21. Other viruses, including polyoma viruses, can produce viruria; however, this is generally not associated with symptomatic disease. The biophysical characteristics of cervical mucus, the pH of vaginal secretions and the chemical composition of urine play a role in host defense against infection.

Human T cell leukemia virus

Adult T cell leukemia (ATL) is caused by a retrovirus, human T cell leukemia virus (HTLV), associated with various diseases including neurological disorders 'tropical spastic paraparesis' (TSP) or HTLV-1-associated myelopathy (HAM).

The transmission of HTLV occurs through one of three different modes:

(1) Male to female transmission during sexual intercourse via HTLV-1-infected cells in semen;

(2) Transplacental passage of infected maternal lymphocytes or through infected lymphocytes in breast milk;

(3) Blood products; however, unlike HIV, only blood products that involve passage of whole cells from donor to recipient can transmit the virus. The virus is transmitted among intravenous drug abusers, presumably through passage of infected blood lymphocytes in shared needles.

Thus, the overall mode of HTLV-1 transmission is similar to that of HIV, with the exception that the virus is apparently not readily transmitted by cell-free body fluids.

Gender differences in viral infection rate

The rates of rhinovirus infection for young adult females are higher than those for males of similar age. A greater exposure to young children is thought to account for this difference. Rhinovirus illness rates are also highest for small children and decrease with increasing age. Estimates of rates for families in Seattle, USA, were almost 0.8 per person year for young children and 0.54 for mothers. The illness rates for mothers are greater than those for young adult males. Compensation for this higher illness rate among young adult females in early adult years appears to ensue in later years when illness rates are higher among males. Respiratory syncytial virus (RSV), responsible for serious lower respiratory tract disease, occurs 30% more often in males than in females. In US urban centers the various forms of lower respiratory disease associated with RSV infection are more frequent in white than in black infants.

Viral infections associated with bird population

In 1999 and 2002, several people in the US died from West Nile virus, which is indigenous to the Middle East. Feathered birds, which make long-distance journeys at specific times each year, spread West Nile virus along their migration routes. Mosquitoes, which may bite infected birds, are the only creature that transmits the virus. Caged birds catch the virus from each other; when one bird is infected, all the cage mates die from the virus. Some species succumb after drinking water containing the virus or feeding on a bird that had West Nile virus.

The disease has been confirmed in more than 110 North American species ranging from bald eagles to ruby-throated hummingbirds, Carolina wrens to Canada geese and mockingbirds to purple martins. The virus may have a very large impact on bird populations since thousands of birds have become seropositive, estimated to be more than 15 000 in October 2002. Currently, virologists are studying whether eagles, hawks and owls can transmit the virus to each other. The strain of virus circulating in the USA is also found in Israel, where West Nile was first reported to be killing birds. The USA is being swept with a bird-virulent strain of West Nile virus, in which birds are killed before the virus is picked up in mosquitoes and people. Birds are very sensitive and several thousands of crows have died in the eastern part of the USA; 30–50% of species such as robins and catbirds have antibodies to the virus, indicating that they have had West Nile but survived. Birds in captivity with the disease die within 6 days.

After the West Nile outbreak in New York, one-third of the healthy birds tested had antibodies, showing that they had contracted the virus and recovered. Birds shed a large amount of virus in feces and from their mouths in the case of crows. In the laboratory, house finches and common grackles contracted West Nile fever after drinking water containing the virus. Great horned owls and house sparrows developed it after feeding on infected animals. Oral transmission from bird to bird is quite common. Most birds that die from the virus will not be found because other wildlife eats the carcasses or they decompose. Some 90% of bird carcasses are scavenged within 24 hours.

Of all wildlife, probably no species travels more or farther than birds. Some nest in the Arctic and winter in the tropics. In the fall many eastern birds take a coastal route along South Carolina. Birds from West Nile hotspots, like South Carolina, will pass through or settle there for the winter. Birds that have died of West Nile in North American zoos tend to be species from Central and South America, where loss of habitat puts pressure on many birds. Birds infected in the USA could carry the virus to the tropics. Mosquitoes could feed on the birds then on people from countries where West Nile has not been reported. West Nile virus was not predicted to spread as quickly as it has done. The virus spread from New York to Montana in 3 years. By October 2002 there were 954 confirmed human cases nationwide, and 43 confirmed deaths.

Table 12.1 HIV/AIDS statistics in India (United Nations, 2001)

Total population	1027 million (2001)
Cumulative AIDS cases	25 497 (males)
	8297 (females)
Adults living with HIV/AIDS (15–49 years) (1999)	3 500 000 (0.7%)
AIDS deaths	310 000 (1999)
AIDS orphans	558 000 (1999)
Life expectancy at birth with HIV	64 years (2000–2005)
Life expectancy at birth without HIV	65 years (2000–2005)
Condom usage	3%
Transmission/risk categories	
Sexual	28 630 cases (84.72%)
Injectable drug users	1092 (3.23%)
Blood/blood products	1070 (3.17%)
Perinatal transmission	792 (2.34%)
Unavailable history	2210 (6.54%)

HIV/AIDS INFECTIONS

Around 42 million people are currently living with HIV; this amounts to 0.7% of the world population. Of those infected almost 70% live in sub-Saharan Africa, with more than 50% being women and young people aged 15–24 years. In 2001, 1.07 million adults and children were newly infected with HIV in Asia and the Pacific, bringing the total number of people living with HIV/AIDS (PLWHA) in the region to 7.1 million. At the end of 2001, the national adult HIV prevalence rate in India was under 1%, with an estimated 3.97 million PLWHA (Table 12.1). To aggravate the problem, HIV fuels the TB epidemic, which is a particular threat in Asia and the Pacific, where there is more than 60% of the world's TB burden.

Sperm surface in HIV patients

In the initial stages of HIV infection, the patient may ejaculate motile (and fertile) sperm. Some patients undergoing highly active antiretroviral therapy (HAART) produce active sperm with normal motility. Antiviral regimens affect lymphocytes, sperm chromosomes and morphology, and semen quality in HIV patients. HIV particles are present on the sperm membrane as determined by labeling with monoclonal/polyclonal anti-HIV antibodies. Atomic force microscopy (AFM) is a powerful technique to evaluate any alterations in the sperm of HIV patients, and the effects of HAART including minute details, e.g. viral particles on sperm membrane. AFM, unlike electron microscopy, permits virions to be imaged in their nearly natural environment and detects any possible penetration into the membrane or any budding (Joshi *et al.*, 2000, 2001a, 2001b). An AFM unit attached to a conventional Olympus microscope (BX 60) is employed for the investigation. The system 'SIS ultra objective' is obtained from Surface Imaging Systems GmbH (Germany).

In 2003 half of world's HIV cases were women

For the first time in the 20-year history of the AIDS epidemic, as many women as men are infected with HIV. The virus is spreading most rapidly in eastern Europe, where nearly every country is experiencing a major outbreak. It has also marched swiftly across Central Asia and into China, where it was almost non-existent a few years ago. However, there are a number of countries where there is strong empirical evidence that rates of infection are declining, and in each case they are declining among young people. In South Africa HIV infections among pregnant teenage girls fell 25% between 1998 and 2001. In Uganda, the number of new HIV infections has been dropping every year for the past 10 years. This positive trend is the first sign that prevention and education programs are making an impact.

Overall, there is an increase in the sheer number of people being infected; however, there is also an increase in the number of countries now facing epidemics. For example, 10 years ago HIV was confined to small areas of eastern Europe. Today, every country in the region has an HIV problem. No society is immune; although HIV was quite well established in many Asian countries very early on, a very stable low rate of infection persisted in a number of countries. In Indonesia, after many years of silence, an epidemic is growing. As Schwartlander said, 'Of course HIV was there, but it did not really lead to major epidemics. It was just over the past two years that massive spread of HIV has begun, initially in injecting drug users'. In China, where HIV was 'virtually non-existent' a few years ago, there are now 1 million people with HIV, and the number could well rise to 10 million by the end of the decade; again, drug use is a major factor.

Sub-Saharan Africa is still by far the worst-affected region. The situation there also reflects the spread of HIV among women, with about twice as many young women as men being infected. In 2001, 6–11% of women aged 15–24 years had HIV compared with 3–6% of men in the same age group. It is particularly difficult for women in this region to take precautions against HIV because of their subordinate position in society. Rape is common in some countries. The phenomenon of intergenerational sex is also driving much of the epidemic in southern Africa, where between one-quarter and one-third of older men are HIV positive. For example, in Zimbabwe many adolescent girls have sex with men in return for clothes and money for school fees. This shift towards more women being infected will ultimately exacerbate the spread of HIV, because the virus can be spread not only through sex, but also through nursing and childbirth.

Anti-HIV treatment (to prevent virus invading blood cells)

The role of dendritic cells in the initial stages of infection is illustrated in Figure 12.2. Cytokine networks regulate HIV replication (Figure 12.3).

Some 850 000–950 000 people in the USA are infected with HIV and there are about 40 000 new infections each year. Today's typical HIV therapy cocktail costs about $15 000 a year.

Fuzeon® (enfuviritide) helps to reverse one of the three steps that HIV takes to penetrate immune cells. Fuzeon is difficult to manufacture. Furthermore, it must be taken by injection twice a day, rotating between the abdomen, thigh and upper arm. Other current anti-HIV drugs come in pill form. Fuzeon works for people who have become resistant to other HIV treatments, and as many as 100 000 patients in the USA could benefit. The drug is expected to cost about $20 000 per year. The FDA approved the drug on an accelerated basis, meaning that long-term data on the drug's effectiveness are not yet available. Fuzeon, a fusion inhibitor, fights HIV in a completely new way. It works by preventing the HIV from invading the white blood cells, which are its primary targets. In contrast, current AIDS drugs all work after the virus has already invaded the cells, by blocking either of two substances that HIV uses to reproduce and spread. The accelerated approval of this new drug should provide new hope for those suffering from advanced HIV infection.

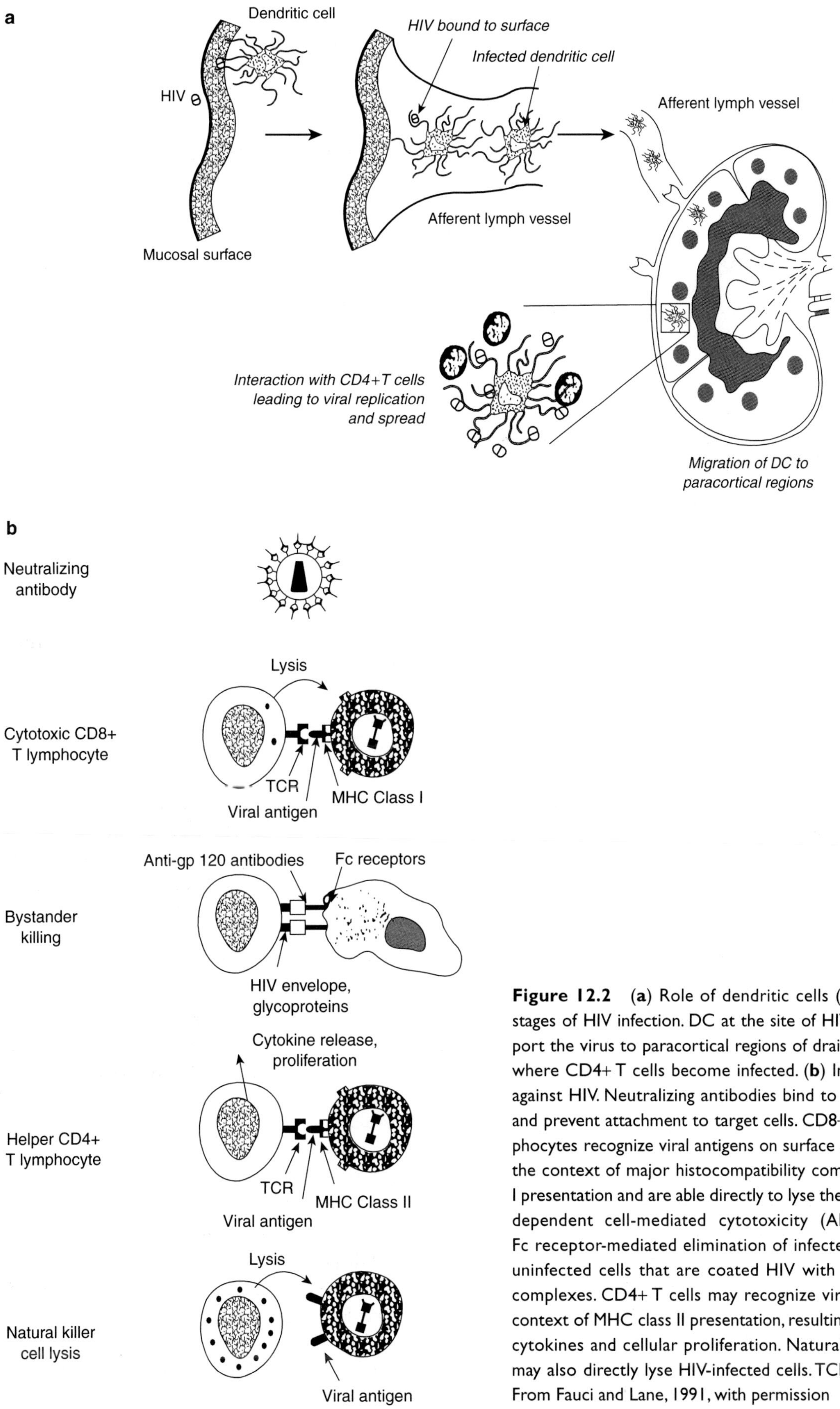

Figure 12.2 (**a**) Role of dendritic cells (DC) in the initial stages of HIV infection. DC at the site of HIV exposure transport the virus to paracortical regions of draining lymph nodes, where CD4+ T cells become infected. (**b**) Immune responses against HIV. Neutralizing antibodies bind to viral components and prevent attachment to target cells. CD8+ cytotoxic T lymphocytes recognize viral antigens on surface of infected cells in the context of major histocompatibility complex (MHC) class I presentation and are able directly to lyse these cells. Antibody-dependent cell-mediated cytotoxicity (ADCC) results in Fc receptor-mediated elimination of infected cells as well as uninfected cells that are coated HIV with antigen–antibody complexes. CD4+ T cells may recognize viral antigens in the context of MHC class II presentation, resulting in the release of cytokines and cellular proliferation. Natural killer (NK) cells may also directly lyse HIV-infected cells. TCR, T cell receptor. From Fauci and Lane, 1991, with permission

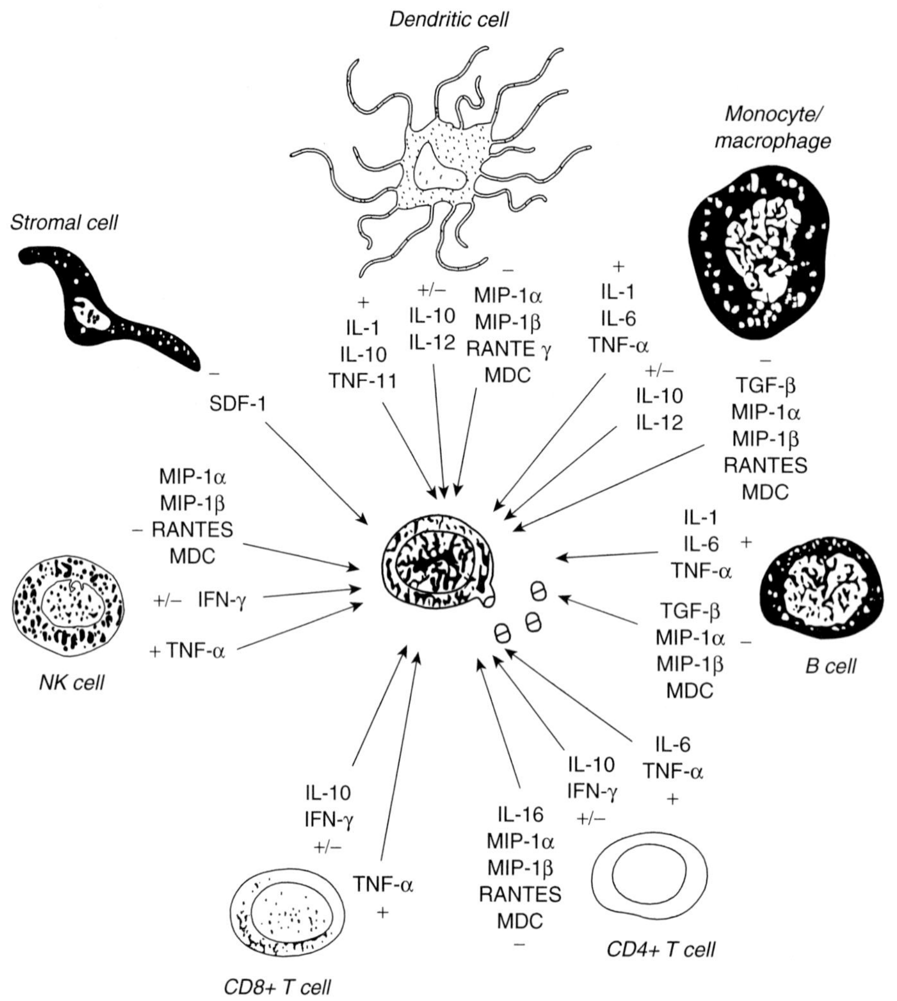

Figure 12.3 Cytokine networks that regulate HIV replication. Cytokines that enhance viral replication (+), inhibit viral replication (–) and enhance or inhibit viral replication depending upon the conditions (+/–) are shown. IL, interleukin; MIP, macrophage inflammatory protein; DFS, stromal cell-derived factor; MDC, macrophage-derived chemokine; TNF, tumor necrosis factor; TGF, transforming growth factor; IFN, interferon; NK, natural killer. From Cohen and Fauci, 2001, with permission

Superinfection

Since AIDS was first recognized about 20 years ago, 26 million people have died – 95% of them in the developing world. About 45 million people worldwide are infected with HIV. About 30 million live in poor countries; more than 6 million of these are in immediate need of HIV drugs, and economists estimate that it would cost $10 billion a year to bring treatment to half of these people by 2005. Superinfection with more than one strain of HIV may be more common than previously thought, and may complicate efforts to make a vaccine. Most cases of 'superinfections' are transient and are not detected. Genetic tests on a superinfected woman showed that the two viruses had mixed and produced a hybrid that replaced the original virus.

Sexual transmission of HIV and hepatitis C virus

HIV is detected in both RNA and DNA in different fractions of semen, although their presence in the motile sperm is controversial. Viral DNA in the testicular tissue of men with HIV-1 infection is localized to the spermatozoid, spermatocytes and, rarely, the spermatids. Low numbers of macrophages are infected mainly in the prostate; however, they are not detected in the prostate, epididymis, seminal vesicles or penis. HIV-1 selective infectivity explains venereal spread of the virus. HIV-1 destroys carrier cells causing dramatic impairment of spermatogenesis and atrophy of the testes in men with AIDS. In semen cell subpopulations isolated by immunomagnetic bead techniques, T cells are most commonly infected with

HIV (75% of samples), followed by macrophages (38% of samples); however, HIV is never detected in motile sperm or immature germ cells, supporting that both T cells and macrophages, but not germ cells, are the cellular vectors of HIV transmission in semen.

Semen is a relevant vector of HIV transmission to the female partner and progeny. Hepatitis C virus (HCV) is transmissible but to a several times lesser extent than HIV. Serodiscordant couples where the man is infected can bear children with an insignificant risk of infection transmission if adequate methodologies are employed to both sperm cleaning of the virus and the subsequent confirmation of its absence. Sperm washing with density gradients followed by swim-up is the method of choice, with nested PCR to detect any remaining viral sequence (Garrido *et al.*, 2004).

The prevalence of HCV infection in high-risk groups is much lower than that of other sexually transmitted infections, and the risk of apparently sexually transmitted HCV infection does not always correlate with the intensity and duration of sexual exposure. Persons living in long-standing monogamous relationships are at a lower risk of acquiring HCV compared with those having several partners or those constantly exposed to sexually transmitted diseases (STD), possibly due to sexual risk-taking behaviors, although differences in rates of exposure to non-sexual sources are not ruled out. In heterosexual relationships, hepatitis B is readily transmitted sexually and hepatitis C and D are not as easily transmissible via sexual intercourse. The prevalence of HCV infection increases in groups with a high risk of exposure to sexually transmitted viral infections. In drug addicts, HCV RNA is found in almost all serum samples tested. However, Garrido *et al.* reported that only in one semen sample was there no correlation between CD4 counts, stage of HIV infection, liver damage and HCV RNA in serum or semen. Anti-HCV positive drug users infected with HIV tested for HCV, hepatitis G virus and GB virus-C RNAs by PCR assay hybridization and sequence analysis were HCV viremic; however, HCV RNA was not identified in the semen, but PCR inhibitors were found.

Some European countries have prohibited assisted reproduction protocols in serodiscordant couples with infected men, but have allowed centers to perform semen washing and artificial reproductive techniques (ART).

Although HCV is present at low concentrations in the semen of a few HCV positive patients, Garrido *et al.* (2004) found no purified sperm fraction used in ART was HCV positive and no seroconversion was observed in women and newborns, thereby suggesting a very low risk of virus transmission. HCV presence in semen implies a possible risk of nosocomial contamination; therefore, safety regulations must be strictly applied by laboratories.

Detection of HCV after extensive sperm washing with a modified RNA extraction protocol demonstrated that even semen treatment in the laboratory is insufficient to eliminate viral presence, and that molecular confirmation is needed before employing semen samples from HCV seropositive patients in ART; there is no correlation between serological status in terms of viral blood levels and positive results after washing.

Semen and blood can be compartmentalized as having different characteristics. Thus, a good post-wash detection technique, including positive and negative controls of each step (RNA extraction, reverse transcription (RT) and PCR), must be included. Detection is performed with RT-PCR dependent methods, which have good sensitivity; however, the relevant presence of polymerase inhibitors interferes with the results, and yields a high number of false negatives. Given the low transmissibility, linked with the sperm washing treatments for HIV, this is not sufficient to ensure that HCV is not present in the semen of HCV positive males, and even in sperm.

Recurrence of HCV after liver transplantation is associated with high blood levels of HCV RNA. Higher blood levels of HCV may promote bodily fluid expression of the virus. Detection of HCV RNA presence in several bodily fluids including seminal plasma is performed by nested PCR; the amplified product is confirmed by Southern blot hybridization and restriction end nuclease digestion. Potential infectivity of bodily fluids in patients testing negative for serum HCV RNA has been discounted. The presence of HCV RNA in saliva and seminal fluid of patients positive for serum HCV RNA has also been discounted. However, the presence of HCV RNA in saliva and seminal fluid of patients positive for serum HCV RNA suggests sexual and household contact as likely modes of no parental transmission of type C hepatitis.

Motility, concentration and morphology of sperm from HIV and HCV patients are comparable, except for the most severe cases, when AIDS is developed. Semen from seropositive men has fewer motile sperm, more round cells and is more viscous than that of controls; there is correlation between the proportion of motile sperm and the percentage of CD4+ lymphocytes in peripheral blood, and no deleterious effect is caused by AZT (zidovudine) administration.

HIV-1 seropositive men at various stages of the disease, without zidovudine therapy and in early-stage disease maintained normal semen parameters, while untreated men with advanced disease had significant reductions in sperm concentration, total sperm count and normal sperm forms.

Men receiving zidovudine, regardless of disease stage, had normal semen parameters similar to those of untreated patients with early-stage disease. Men with AIDS presented pyospermia and abnormal sperm. Fertile men had a greater volume of sperm, higher sperm concentration, per cent motility, per cent rapid and linear motility, and total strictly normal sperm than HIV seropositive men. HIV affects fertility only at the most advanced stages of the disease, and the fertility of asymptomatic or mild symptomatic males is not initially affected by the disease.

INFECTIOUS DISEASES: FROM DIPHTHERIA AND SCARLET FEVER TO AIDS AND SARS

In 1968 many scientists considered infectious diseases to be yesterday's problem. With the development of antibiotics from the 1940s onwards, diseases such as diphtheria and scarlet fever went from being life-threatening afflictions to treatable infections. Jonas Salk's vaccine took the fear out of polio, and the tuberculosis sanatoriums were being emptied. Euphoria governed medical science. Researchers liked to think that they were on the crest of a wave sweeping away the threat from parasites, viruses and bacteria. In the 1980s infectious diseases reappeared; however, drugs were not effective as they had been. With increased and sometimes incorrect use, resistance to antibiotics has grown, breathing new life into some old pests. In the late 1980s, patients presented at New York hospitals with new strains of tuberculosis that did not respond to drugs. In the 1990s these swept through Russia. Furthermore, there have been new and frightening diseases. In Zaire in the mid-1970s, a man walked in from the jungle with a severe fever that made him vomit black blood. He died shortly afterwards. Within days many of the nuns who took him in had also fallen ill with Ebola, one of the most easily transmissible viruses. Viruses continued to reappear and to cross from one species to another, including humans, and often the new host has little immunity. Every year brings a different strain of influenza, many of the strains originating in China.

Infectious disease outbreaks coincide with chaotic economic development. Teeming new cities with poor sanitation that lack strong health systems, rapid migration of populations from country to city, changing sexual habits and the breakdown in traditional family structures all provide fertile ground for the spread of new diseases. Foreign travel exacerbates the problem, quickly transferring a virus from a small African village to a large, western city. The microbes that caused the 1918 Spanish flu were transported around the world by boat; today, they would catch a plane. Then there is HIV/AIDS. Since HIV was first identified, more than 20 million people have died from AIDS. By 2010, the total number of infected people is expected to reach 105 million, most of them in poor countries. It is the biggest public health disaster since the Black Death in the 14th century.

Medical science still has its Utopian streak, these days in the form of genetics. The decoding of the human genome has raised hopes of large advances in the understanding and treatment of diseases. Some researchers talk of an era of 'personalized medicine', with each patient walking around with a card that shows his or her genetic make-up so that treatments can be tailored specifically. These advances will generate some useful tools for the study of infectious disease. Researchers were able, for example, to pin down the genetic make-up of the severe acute respiratory syndrome (SARS) virus within weeks of its appearance.

Common diseases and related STD in man are shown in Tables 12.2 and 12.3.

CLINICAL APPLICATIONS

Anthrax may be treated and detected by lysin

A novel agent that could help to detect an anthrax attack and serve as an antidote to the deadly disease has been developed. The agent was isolated from a virus that preys on the anthrax bacterium and replicates inside it. When the virus particles need to escape, they order the synthesis of a special enzyme, 'lysin', that chews through the bacterium's cell wall. Although designed to pierce the wall from the inside, the lysin

Table 12.2 Common diseases and related sexually transmitted disease

Disease	*Characteristics*
Chancroid	
Description	A sexually transmitted disease characterized by painful genital ulceration and inflammatory inguinal adenopathy. It is uncommon in the US but found worldwide. Chancroid is endemic and a cofactor for HIV transmission
Symptoms	Tender genital papule that ulcerates after 24 h Irregular edged, painful ulcer(s) Ulcers may be 1–5 cm in size Ulcers may occur on the shaft of the penis, glans and meatus in men Ulcers in women are most commonly occur in labia majora but are also seen in labia minora, perineum, thigh and cervix Painful inguinal adenopathy with abscess (bubo) formation in 30% of patients Atypical presentations include folliculitis and foreskin abcess
Causes	*Haemophilus ducreyi* (gram negative bacterium)
Risk factors	Multiple sexual partners Uncircumcised males Prostitutes often are carriers
Medication	Azithromycin 1 g po single dose (more expensive than other treatments) Ceftriaxone 250 mg IM single dose Ciprofloxacin 500 mg po bid for 3 days or other quinolone Erthromycin base 500 mg qid for 7 days
Epididymitis	
Description	Inflammation of epididymis resulting in scrotal pain, swelling/induration of posterior-lying epididmis/eventual scrotal wall edema, involvement of adjacent testicle/hydrocele formation
Symptoms	Scrotal pain, sometimes extending to the groin region, may begin relatively acutely over several hours Urethral discharge or symptoms of urinary tract infection, such as frequency of urination, dysuria, cloudy urine or hematuria Initially only posterior-lying epididymis, usually lowermost tail section, will be very tender/indurate Elevation of testes/epididymis improves discomfort Entire hemiscrotum becomes swollen, testis becomes indistinguishable from epididymis/scrotal wall becomes thick/indurate, reactive hydrocele may occur Fever/chills occur with severe infection/abscess formation
Causes	Younger than age 35 usually chlamydial or *Neisseria gonorrhoea* look for serous urethral discharge (clamydia) or purulent discharge (gonorrhea) Older than age 35 coliform bacteria usually but sometimes *Staphylococcus aureus* or *S. epidermidis* often associated with distal urinary tract obstruction tuberculosis, if sterile pyuria/modularity of vas deferens sterile urine reflux after transurethral prostatectomy granulomatous reaction following bacillus Calmette–Guerin (BCG) intravesical therapy for superficial bladder cancer Prepubertal boys usually coliform bacteria evaluate for underlying congenital abnormalities, such as vesicoureteral reflux or ectopic ureter

(Continued)

Table 12.2 (Continued)

Disease	Characteristics
	At any age amiodarone, an antiarrhythmic agent, may cause a non-infectious epididymitis, that resolves with decreasing drug use
Herpes simplex	
Description	Viral disease with many manifestations, painful vesicles in clusters on skin, cornea or mucous membranes; may occur as encephalitis, pneumonia or disseminated infection. Course of primary disease is 2 weeks; duration of recurrence varies; viral shedding in recurrence is briefer than with primary disease. Newborns or individuals with immune compromise are at risk for major morbidity or mortality
Symptoms	Vesicles cluster and open as painful ulcerated lesions, often with erythematous base Herpetic whitlow: localized primary, a finger with intense itching and pain, followed by vesicles that may coalesce with swelling, erythematic, and may mimic pyogenic paronychia; neuralgia and axillary adenopathy sometimes; heals over 2–3 weeks without incision Primary herpetic gingivostomatitis/pharyngitis: first infection with HSV-1 usually in early childhood; incubation from 2 to 12 days, then fever, sore throat, pharyngeal edema and erythematic; small vesicles develop on pharyngeal/oral mucosa, rapidly ulcerate/increase in number to involve soft palate, buccal mucosa, tongue, floor of mouth, lips/cheeks; tender gums may bleed; fetid breath, cervical adenopathy; fever, general toxicity, poor oral intake/drooling Primary herpes keratoconjunctivitis: by HSV-1 usually; can present as unilateral conjunctivitis with regional adenopathy, as blepharitis with vesicles on lid margin
Medication	Acyclovir primary genital herpes: 400 mg po tid or 200 mg po × 5 doses daily for 7–10 days recurrent genital herpes: 800 mg bid or 200 mg po × 5 doses daily for 5 days for chronic suppression in persons with frequent recurrences: 400 mg bid primary herpes gingivostomatitis, recurrent herpes labialis and other HSV skin infections: 200 mg po q4 h × 5 doses daily for 10 days Penciclovir (Denavir®) oroherpes recurrence: 1% cream q2 h while awake for 4 days Valacyclovir (Valtrex®) better bioavailability orally than cycloid, is converted to cycloid; indicated for use only in immunocompetent primary genital herpes: 1 g po bid for 7–10 days recurrent genital herpes: 500 mg po bid for 3–5 days, chronic suppression 1 g po q/day (10 or more recurrences per year) or 500 mg po q/day (9 or less recurrences per year)
Condyloma acuminata	
Description	Condyloma acuminata are soft, skin colored, fleshy warts that are caused by the HPV (human papilloma virus). There are at least 70 known types of HPV and types 6, 11, 16, 18, 31, 33, 35 have been associated with condyloma acuminata. The disease is highly contagious, can appear singly or in groups, small or large. They appear in the vagina, or the cervix, around the external genitalia and rectum, the urethra, anus, also conjunctival, nasal, oral and laryngeal warts and occasionally the throat. The incubation period may be from 1 to 60 months
Symptoms	Tumors, soft, sessile Surface smooth to very rough Multiple finger-like projections Perianal condylomata acuminata usually rough and cauliflower-like Penile lesions often smooth and popular Penile lesions often occur in groups of three or four Male sites – frenulum, corona, glans, prepuce, meatus, shaft, scrotum
Causes	Human papillomaviruses. These are circular double-stranded DNA molecules. There are over 70 HPV subtypes. The causes of common venereal warts are types 6 and 11. Cervical dysplasia and carcinoma *in situ* are likely caused by types 16, 18, 31, 33, 35

Table 12.2 (Continued)

Disease	*Characteristics*
Diagnosis	Lichen planus Normal sebaceous glands Seborrheic keratosis Molluscum contagious Keratomas Scabies Crohn's disease Skin tags Melanocytic nevi Vulva intraepithelial neoplasia
Medication	Imiquimod (Aldara®) 5% cream applied overnight 3 times weekly until warts clear for up to 16 weeks Cryotherapy: liquid nitrogen is applied to warts in 5–10 s bursts. Requires 2–3 weekly sessions Podophyllin in tincture of benzoin. Apply directly to warts, leave on 104h, then wash off. Repeat treatment every 7 days until gone Podofilox (Condylox®) for external warts. Apply to external warts every 12h (allowing to dry) for 3 consecutive days, may repeat after 4 days Topical cidofovir gel undergoing trials; applied once daily for 5 days every other week for maximum of 6 cycles

Table 12.3 Sexually transmitted diseases (STD)

Symptoms of STD
Chronic pain, strictures and infertility
Increased risk of acquiring or transmitting HIV
Transmission of STD to female partners in whom chronic complications and adverse sequelae are more common
Sequelae of untreated or mistreated STD
Urethral discharge: *Chlamydia trachomatis, Neisseria gonorrhoea*
Scrotal swelling: *C. trachomatis, N. gonorrhoea*
Genital ulcer disease: *Treponema pallidum* (syphilis), *Haemophilus ducreyi* (chancroid), herpes simplex virus
Inguinal bubo: *C. trachomatis* (lymphogranuloma venereum)
Other common sexually transmitted infections include genital warts (caused by the human papilloma virus (HPV), HIV and the hepatitis B virus (found more commonly in men)

enzyme can also crumble it from outside. Doses of lysin injected into mice infected with a close relative of anthrax saved most of the animals from a certain death. Lysin can be used like an antibiotic to treat people who may have been exposed to spores in an anthrax attack. If injected quickly enough, the lysin would destroy the anthrax bacteria in the bloodstream before they had multiplied and released overwhelming amounts of toxin. Attack strains of anthrax can be made resistant to antibiotics, but not to lysin. Future research is required before the enzyme could be used as a drug.

Scientists have a prototype of a lysin-based anthrax detector. An important feature of lysin is that it attacks only anthrax and a rare strain of a closely related bacterium. This allows the lysin to be a quick and sensitive detector for anthrax spores that might be used in an attack.

A hand-held detection device has been developed that would accept an air filtrate or environmental sample. Initially, any anthrax spores are made to germinate from their protective coat. Lysin is applied to the emerging bacteria, making their contents spill out. An antibody-based anthrax detector is already in use, but antibodies are difficult to manufacture and variable in quality. A faster and more sensitive device should be developed. The lysin-based method can detect a sample of 2500 spores in 10 min or as few as 100 spores after an hour's reaction time. Lysins for other dangerous microbes could be added to the sensitive devices. Scientists are already experimenting on lysins from viruses that attack cholera and *Yersinia pestis*, the agent of plaque. This would work for many other species of bacteria, because each has its own set of viruses that produce lysins specific for their target bacteria. Lysins could thus provide a whole new class of antibiotics to which bacteria could not develop resistance. Resistance is a matter of particular concern to biological warfare experts who fear that attack microbes could be made more lethal by first

Table 12.4 Disorders of male reproductive organs

Syndrome	*Causes*	*Lesions*	*Changes in semen*
Testicular degeneration	Thermal, localized or systemic infections; nutrition (vitamin A); vascular lesions; aging; obstructive lesions of the head of epididymis; noxious agents; hormonal factors	Testicular size reduced; fibrosis; disturbances in spermatogenesis; seminiferous tubules destroyed some cases	Increase in immature/abnormal sperm with normal motility; ejaculate is thin/watery due to reduction in sperm concentration; giant cells; azoospermia or necrozoospermia
Orchitis	Brucellosis, tuberculosis	Inflammatory changes in testes leading to degeneration of seminiferous tubules	Asthenozoospermia; oligozoospermia; teratozoospermia: giant cells; erythrocytes/ leukocytes; normal semen volume
Epididymitis	Brucellosis viral infections	Inflammation of epididymis; infiltration of lymphocytes/ neutrophils; dead sperm/giant cells	Poor semen characteristics, contaminated by inflammatory exudates
Seminal vesiculates	Brucellosis	Unilateral inflammation of seminal vesicles; glands enlarged/fibrosed	Purulent exudates in semen; normozoospermia; asthenozoospermia

making them resistant to common antibiotics. The anthrax strain used in past attacks was virulent but susceptible to the usual antibiotics. A resistant strain would probably have caused many casualties.

Possible adverse effects on humans of meat from antibiotic-fed livestock

Antibiotics used to feed and treat livestock may contribute to adverse after-effects in consumers eating meats and meat products from such animals. The FDA is attempting to limit the extensive use of such antibiotics. FDA regulations released in September 2002 require the maker of a proposed animal antibiotic to assess whether it could encourage the growth of disease-causing bacteria that are resistant to antibiotics used in human medicine. If the drug were too similar to an important antibiotic for people, for instance, it could be kept off the market. Currently, the drug maker has only to show that it does not leave any dangerous residue in meat. Resistant pathogens do form in treated animals and can be transmitted to humans through food. From a public health perspective, the risk must be minimized.

It has long been known that the overuse of antibiotics by doctors and their patients has reduced the ability of the drugs to cure infections. Giving animals antibiotics in their feed can also cause microbes in the livestock to become resistant to the drugs, and people can become infected with the resistant bacteria. The FDA action is part of a contentious worldwide debate over the long-term use of antibiotics in raising livestock. Public health advocates estimate that 70% of antibiotic use in USA occurs on the farm, some to treat sick animals but also to promote growth of flocks and herds. The European Union has banned some animal antibiotics, and farmers in Denmark have stopped using antibiotics to promote growth. The Animal Health Institute, which represents animal drug makers, indicates that advocates exaggerate the hazards of animal antibiotics to human medicine. Animal antibiotics are a tiny part of the problem, and many animal antibiotics are not closely related to those used for humans. Antibiotics can help farmers produce more healthy animals and cheaper meat.

Nasal-mist flu vaccine

Influenza is the cause of 36 000 deaths annually in the USA. Most of the victims are patients with other health problems, children aged under 2 years and people over 65 years. The FDA has approved a nasal-mist flu vaccine FluMist™ to replace the annual injected vaccine, for healthy people aged 5–59 years. FluMist would not be appropriate for people who most need vaccine protection, such as toddlers, the elderly and people with asthma and other chronic diseases. For children from 5 to 8 years, the approval requires two doses of FluMist 6 weeks apart. Patients aged 9–49 years only require one dose. The safety and effectiveness of FluMist has not been proven for people 50 and over. The FDA encourages people over 50 to have the injected flu vaccine.

FluMist contains each of the three live influenza virus strains expected to be active during the flu season. In the 2003–2004 season, these included two types of influenza A, which cause severe illness, and one type of influenza B, which causes a milder form of the disease. The live virus in the vaccine has been modified and weakened so that it produces immunity without causing illness. In the past there have been vaccine shortages at the beginning of some flu seasons because there are few manufacturers of the drug and the formula must be changed each year to match the changes in the circulating virus. FluMist is manufactured by MedImmune Vaccines Inc. (Gaithersburg, MD). Some 4–6 million doses were to be available by October, the start of the flu season. Each dose of FluMist costs $46, more than twice the typical cost of injected flu vaccine.

FUNGI AND BACTERIA

Aspergillus and its conidia formation

Aspergillus is a genus of fungi including some common molds which grow on foods. A few species are known to contain toxic substances and, when eaten, may cause severe intoxication. Molds of this group growing on stored cereals and producing powerful toxins have caused serious social problems. Furthermore, aspergillus fungi, when they occasionally become rampant within the human body, may cause aspergillosis, which has recently increased in occurrence.

Staphylococci

Staphylococci are a group of microbes widely distributed in nature. In human and animal bodies they are found on the skin, in the nasal and oral cavities, and in the digestive tract. They occur abundantly in suppurative foci. *Staphylococcus aureus* is particularly pathogenic; it is common in the human upper respiratory tract. The cocci growing in the nasal vestibulum are directly involved in infection. This group of microbes has recently attracted attention with regard to hospital-acquired infection and the occurrence of strains resistant to antibiotics. The term staphylococcus comes from its grape-like appearance under the light microscope (staphyle: a bunch of grapes).

Candida albicans

Candida, formerly called monilia, is a genus of yeast-like fungi forming smooth, white colonies on solid media (candidus: glowing shite; monilia: necklace). Among the large number of species, only *Candida albicans* causes the human infection moniliasis. C. *albicans* infests the mouth, bronchi, lungs, intestines and vagina as well as the skin and nails. Occasionally sepsis, severe general infection and meningitis may occur. C. *albicans*, when cultured on an appropriate solid medium, forms cream-like colonies composed of densely grown threads called hyphae.

Section IV Assisted Reproductive Technology

13

Genetic andrology and genetic engineering

Several abnormalities of the reproductive system are known to be of genetic origin, but only some specific types of reproductive anomalies are really characterized as genetic anomalies. Some of these include cryptorchidism and testicular hypoplasia. There are some basic genetic concepts that must be recognized before particular genetic factors can be determined to lead to abnormalities in the structures and functions of the reproductive system.

BASIC GENETIC CONCEPTS

Chromosomes

The total number of chromosomes is constant in all normal individuals within a particular species, and when arranged in pairs the chromosomes are identical for all members of that species. The paired chromosomes in mammalian somatic cells are called autosomes. The sex chromosomes are not autosomes; they are paired in mammalian females (XX; homogametic sex) and unpaired in males (XY; heterogametic sex). The mammalian X chromosome is usually larger than the Y chromosome. In birds, however, the female is the heterogametic sex (ZW) and the male is homogametic (ZZ). Thus, unlike in mammals, the female bird determines the sex of the offspring.

The normal chromosome number for a somatic cell is called the diploid number ($2n$) and is constant in normal individuals within a species. However, the gamete has one-half the diploid number of chromosomes and this is known as the haploid number (n). When a male and a female gamete unite at fertilization, the diploid number is restored.

The complete set of chromosomes is called the karyotype. The karyotype can be displayed by photographing, cutting out and arranging the chromosomes systematically according to cytogenetic conventions. Chromosomes can be classified according to the length of the chromosome and the position of the centromere seen at the metaphase stage. The centromere is a heterochromatic region (non-staining), which tends to constrict the chromosome at a specific

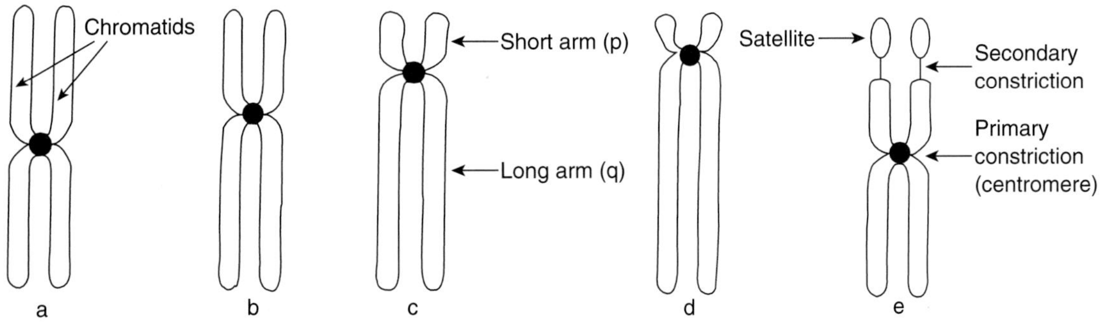

Figure 13.1 Types of chromosomes based on centromeric position: (a) metacentric; (b) submetacentric; (c) acrocentric; (d) telocentric; (e) metacentric with satellite arms. Metacentric and submetacentric are so-called biarmed chromosomes

position (primary constriction). If the centromere is situated halfway between the chromosome arms it is known as metacentric, and when located towards one end of the chromosome it is called submetacentric. However, if the centromere is located at the very end, the chromosome is referred to as acrocentric (Figure 13.1).

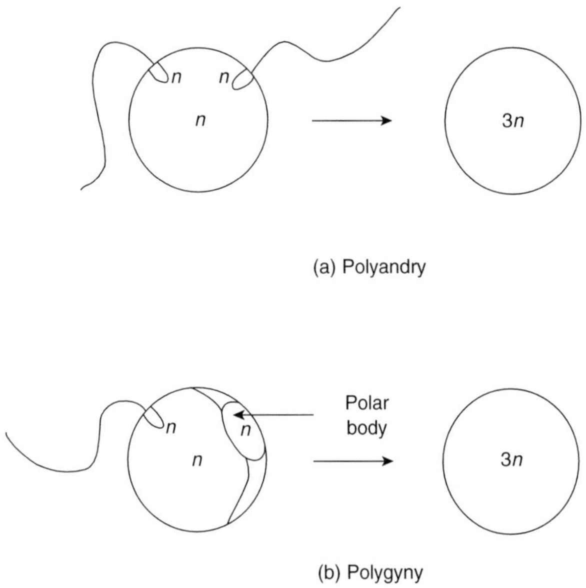

Figure 13.2 Mechanisms resulting in triploidy by (a) polyandry and (b) polygyny

Figures 13.2 and 13.3 show different mechanisms resulting in triploidy by polyandry and polygyny, and mechanisms of non-disjunction and anaphase chromosome lag leading to aneuploidy. Figure 13.4 illustrates a map of imprinted regions in the human genome.

Genes and patterns of inheritance

Genes, located in a fixed position (locus) on a chromosome, are the basic units of inheritance. Each gene governs a specific trait (phenotype) and is recognized by alteration (mutation) of that particular gene which changes the phenotype of an individual who carries the mutant gene. Genes which control the alternative expression for specific traits are called alleles. Thus, the genotype of an animal is its complete set of genes, and the phenotype is the expression of these genes, whether as physical, biochemical or physiological traits.

A trait determined by a gene can be inherited either as an autosomal or sex-linked trait, and can also be either dominant or recessive. Traits that are governed by dominant genes express themselves when these genes are present on both chromosomes of a homologous pair (homozygous condition), or on only one of the chromosome pair (heterozygous condition). On the other hand, a recessive trait

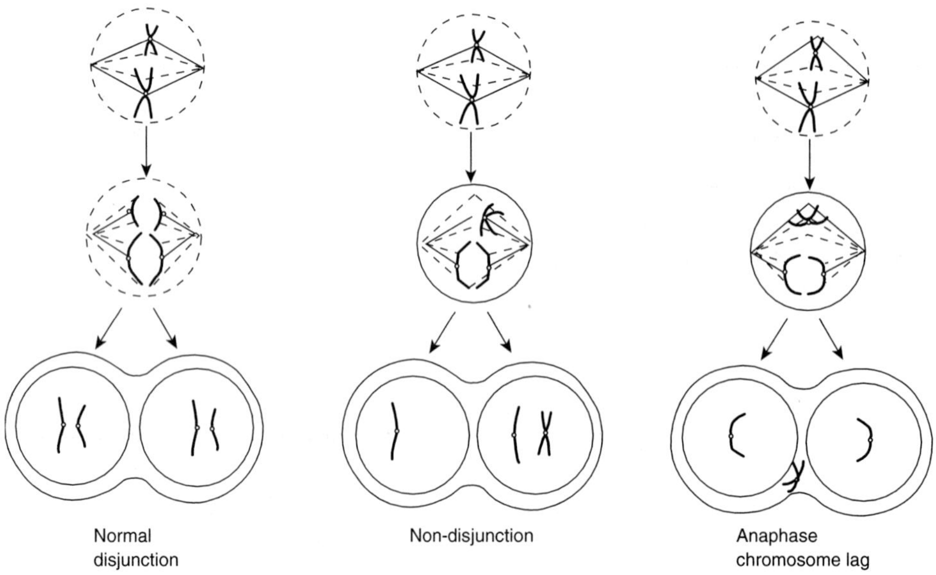

Figure 13.3 Diagrammatic illustration of the mechanisms of non-disjunction and anaphase chromosome lag leading to aneuploidy

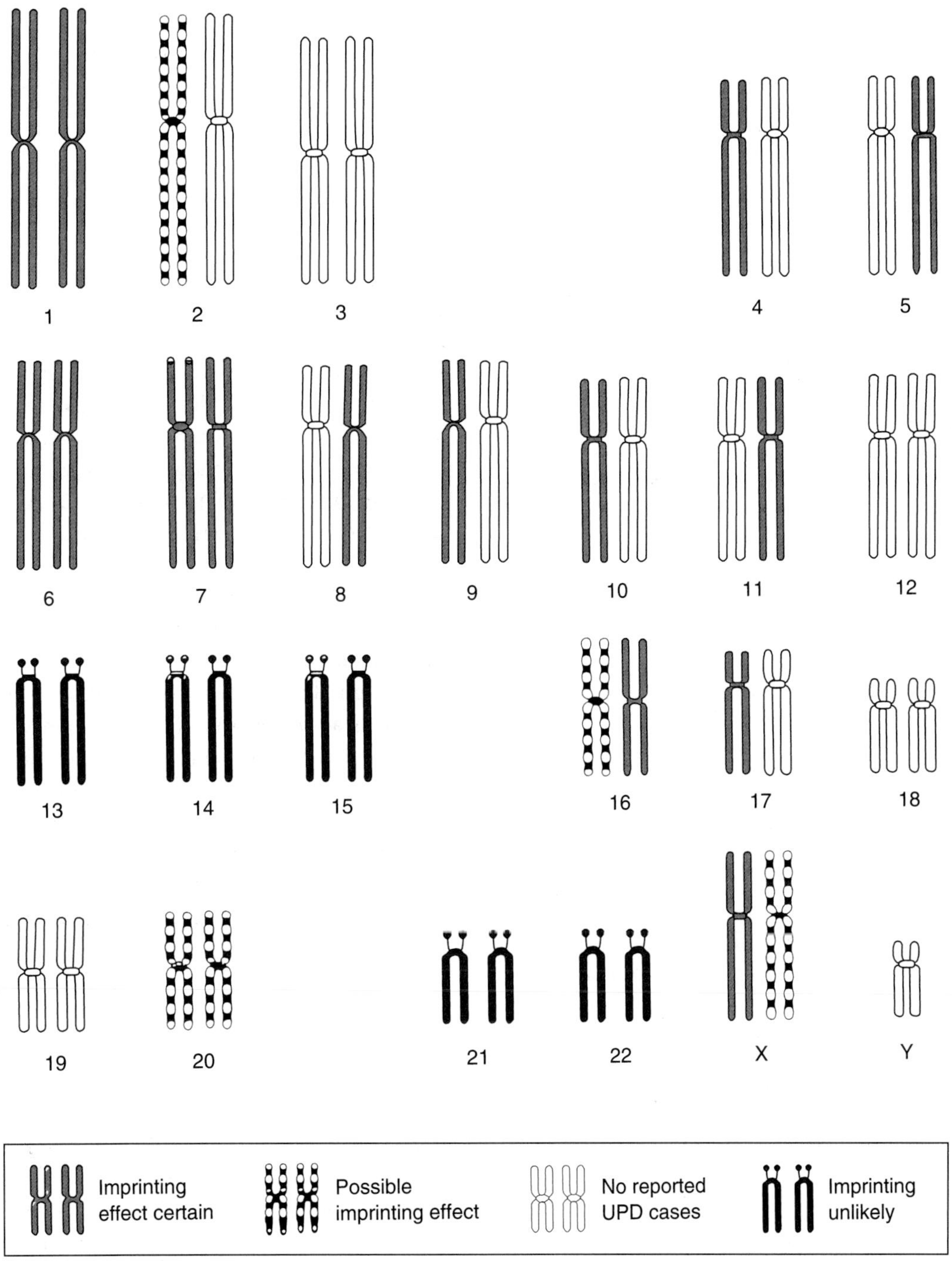

Figure 13.4 Map of imprinted regions in the human genome, based on phenotypes detected in cases of non-apparent disomy involving the maternally inherited homolog (left chromosome in each pair) or the paternally inherited homolog (right chromosome in each pair). UPD, uniparental disomy. Revised from Ledbetter and Engel (1995)

may only be expressed when both parents have contributed the mutant genes.

Autosomal dominant traits affect both males and females. They tend to vary considerably in their severity (expressivity), and rarely skip a generation (non-penetrance).

Abnormalities of both structure and function of the reproductive system may be genetically determined. As most anomalies are the result of an interaction between environment and genotype, it is difficult to classify them strictly into inherited or acquired disorders. Most inherited abnormalities follow simple Mendelian inheritance, a few are acquired as sex-linked, and others as polygenic traits.

CHROMOSOME ANOMALIES (FIGURES 13.5–13.7)

Chromosomal arrangements occur during mitosis and meiosis. Normally the ovum (X) is fertilized by sperm X or sperm Y. In abnormal cases of non-disjunction of oogenesis or spermatogenesis, fertilization may occur between an abnormal sperm and/or an abnormal egg, resulting in various chromosomal anomalies. Structural anomalies of the chromosomes include translocation, deletions, rings and inversions of chromosomes during either mitosis or meiosis (Figure 13.5). Such anomalies affect individual autosomes or sex chromosomes. The animal cell comprises a nucleus, protein-manufacturing units and energy-production points. Spiraling double strands of atoms are the DNA, the master chemical of genes. The sequence or layout of these atoms contains all the instructions the cell needs to function.

Aberration of chromosome number

Aberrations of chromosome structure and number are important because of their association with reproductive problems such as birth defects and embryonic or fetal death. Changes in chromosomes may be alteration in the total number of chromosomes, involving either addition to or loss of one or more chromosomes or set of chromosomes. Changes may also be structural, associated with rearrangement of chromosome segments within a chromosome or between two chromosomes. Modification of the chromosome number may affect a whole set of chromosomes such that, instead of the normal diploid ($2n$) number of chromosomes, triploid ($3n$), tetraploid ($4n$) or even pentaploid ($5n$) animals may result. This condition is known as polyploidy.

There are various mechanisms leading to these numerical changes. Mechanisms resulting in polyploidy include errors during meiosis (failure in the reduction of chromosome number) or at the time of fertilization (polyandry or polygyny), and abnormalities of the mitotic spindles at critical stages during fetal development.

Aberration of chromosome structure

A change in the structure of a chromosome is a result of one or more segmental breaks on that chromosome, with or without reunion of the broken segments. These can be divided into four major categories: deletion, duplication, inversion and translocation. In addition to these, misdivision of the centromere may occur occasionally, leading to the formation of an isochromosome (Table 13.1).

Deletion

Chromosomal deletion is a consequence of one or two breaks and the loss of a chromosome segment, and may be either terminal or intercalary. A terminal deletion occurs when there is a break and the loss of the terminal segment, or two breaks and the reunion of the broken ends to form a ring. On the other hand, intercalary (or interstitial) deletions involve the loss of a chromosome segment between two breaks. A chromosome segment devoid of a centromere (acentric fragment) is lost during cell division because it is unable to orient itself on the mitotic spindle. Deletions involving large chromosome segments are not seen in animals, because cells from which the chromosome segments are deleted are not viable. Nevertheless, if the segment deleted is small or genetically inactive (heterochromatic), the cell with the deletion may be maintained. For instance, a cell containing a deleted chromosome may be viable and capable of reproduction. However, its phenotype (or tissues containing cells with deletions) may be adversely affected. In a majority of cases, deletions can be identified using banding techniques, which enable segmental delineation of the chromosome.

Y chromosome microdeletion The prevalence of Y microdeletions is about 7% with a range of 1–35% depending on the patients selected for study and study techniques. Most Y chromosome microdeletions occur on the long arm (q) and are subdivided into three azoospermic factor (AZF) regions: a, b and c (Figure 13.6). Genes encoded in the AZF regions may be important in spermatogenesis. However, a small portion (up to 2%) of the fertile male population may also harbor very small microdeletions of the Y chromosome, probably involving non-coding regions. Before the advent of *in vitro* fertilization (IVF) with intracytoplasmic sperm injection (ICSI) and sperm retrieval techniques, such as testicular sperm extraction (TESE), many men affected by Y chromosome microdeletions could not reproduce. Choi *et al.* (2004) reported successful pregnancies with the use of sperm from Y microdeleted men and ICSI.

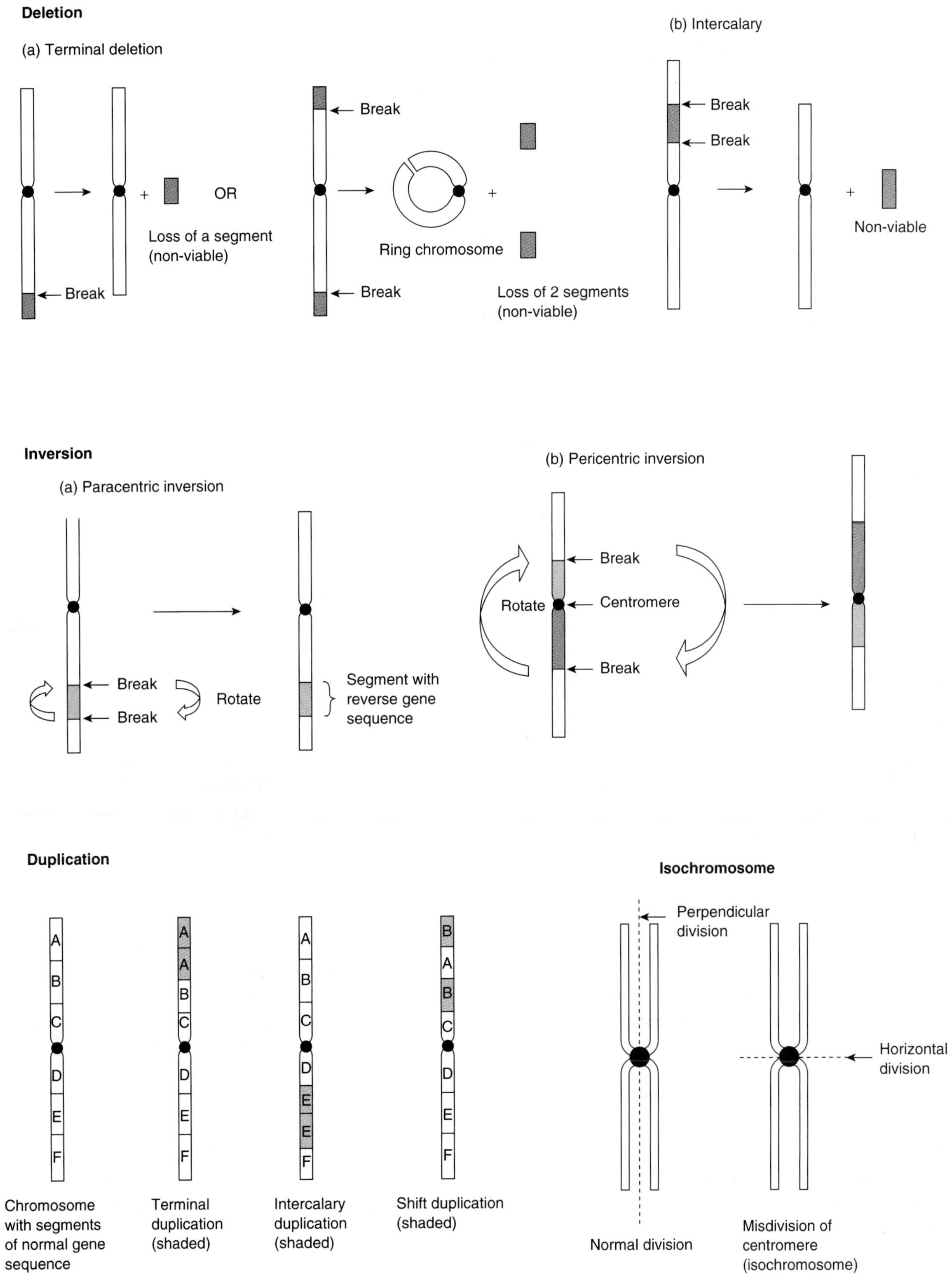

Figure 13.5 Diagrammatic illustrations of various structural aberrations: deletion, inversion, duplication and isochromosome

Table 13.1 Basic types of chromosomal alterations

Type of alteration	*Definition*	*Example*
Numerical	Alteration in chromosome number	
Aneuploidy	Inexact multiples of haploid number eggs, e.g. $2n \pm 1$; $2n \pm 2$	39,XXY, Klinefelter-like syndrome 63,XO, Turner-like syndrome
Euploidy (polyploidy)	Exact multiples of the haploid number, e.g. $3n$, $4n$, $5n$	180,XY
Mosaic	An animal with two or more cell populations (different karyotypes) derived from a single zygote which differ in chromosome number and/or structure	60,XY/59,XY,rob (1,29)
Chimera	An animal or its tissues having two or more populations of cells derived from two or more zygotes	60,XX/60,XY
Structural	Alteration in structure of the chromosome	
Deficiency	A segment of a chromosome is lost	38,XY,t (7q−;11q+)
Duplication	A chromosome segment exists in excess of the normal	
Inversion	A segment is in a reverse sequence	
Translocation	A segment or a whole arm of one chromosome is transposed to another chromosome	59,XY,rob (1,29) 38,XY,rcp (13q−;14q+)

Duplication

Duplications involve addition of an extra segment to a chromosome, through abnormal replication or unequal crossing over in meiotic cells of the parent. A duplicated segment can be terminal or intercalary, and at times shifted to another region. However, duplications are more common and less harmful than deletions. Instead, duplications of genes and segments of chromosomes are considered to be more important in evolution as they are believed to provide potential material for new gene combinations.

Inversion

Inversion involves two breaks on a chromosome and the rotation of the broken segment prior to reunion of the broken ends, resulting in the reversal of the gene sequence. Inversions can be either pericentric or paracentric. In pericentric inversion, the centromere is included in the inverted segment; however, for a paracentric inversion the centromere is not involved and it is confined to only one arm of the chromosome. Paracentric and pericentric inversions interfere with gametogenesis.

(1) Isochromosomes represent misdivision of the centromere and are always metacentric with identical but reversed gene sequence. For example, the metacentric bovine X chromosome when misdivided would give rise to a long and a short chromosome, each with two identical arms, that would actually be two chromatids.

(2) Translocation occurs when a portion of one chromosome is attached to a non-homologous chromosome. It often involves a reciprocal exchange of a segment between chromosomes. Reciprocal translocation is a result of an exchange between a segment of one chromosome and a segment of another. Translocation is relatively rare in humans and domestic animals.

(3) Interchange between segments of different chromosomes involving small segments of autosomes will be overlooked in farm animals such as cattle and goats, since the autosomes are all acrocentric in these species. Thus, the identification of translocated chromosomes is only possible with the aid of techniques such as banding.

In non-disjunction, both chromosomes move to the same pole, resulting in both daughter cells becoming aneuploid, since one of them will have a chromosome in excess of normal ($2n+1$) while the other will have one less than normal ($2n-1$). In anaphase lag, one of the chromosomes falls behind and, thus, fails to be included into the nucleus of the daughter cells. This results in only one of the daughter cells being aneuploid.

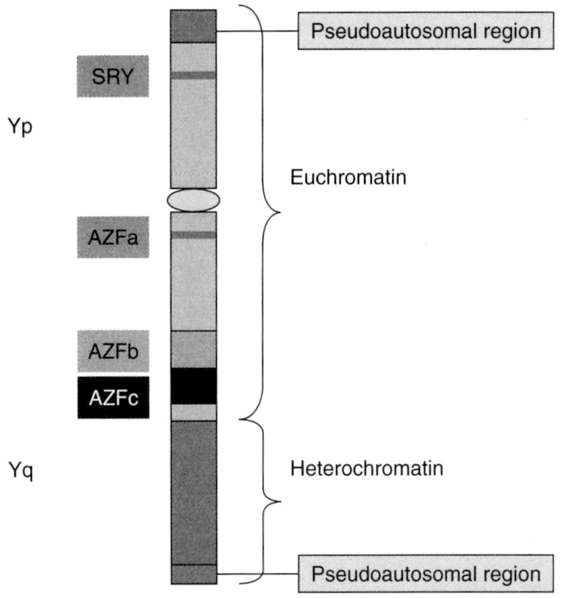

Figure 13.6 Diagram of the Y chromosome depicting the location of azoospermic factor (AZF) regions a, b and c. SRY, sex-determining region of the Y chromosome. From Choi *et al.*, 2004, with permission

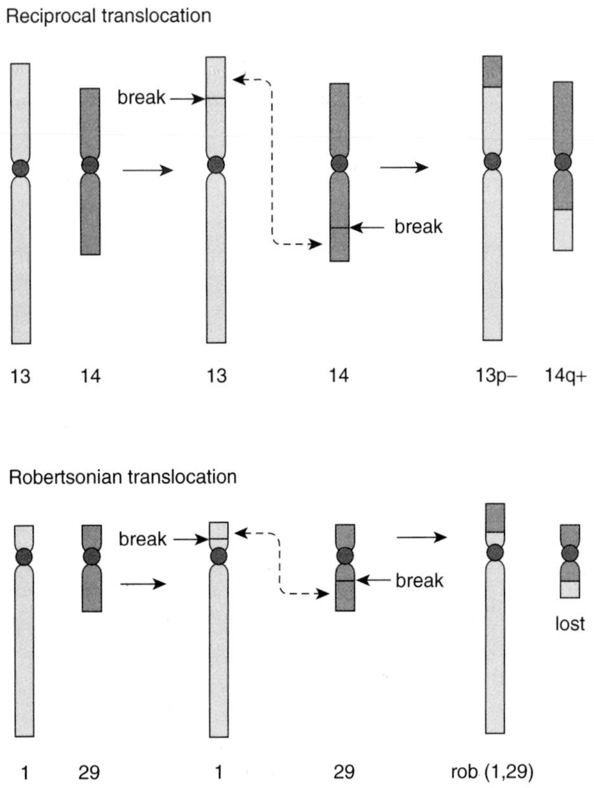

Figure 13.7 Diagrammatic illustrations of reciprocal translocation and Robertsonian translocation

In general, lacking a chromosome in the whole complement set is incompatible with life, while the presence of an extra chromosome disrupts the normal process of embryogenesis. When a large chromosome is associated in aneuploidy, the conceptus dies at an early embryonic stage of fetal development, regardless of the type of aneuploidy involved. However, an exception to this rule is X chromosome aneuploidy.

Abnormal spermiogenesis

A high incidence of abnormal sperm is linked with testicular hypoplasia. Testes of abnormal size, which exhibit inadequate growth and development, are considered to be hypoplastic. Although cryptorchid testes are hypoplastic, testicular hypoplasia also occurs with normal descended testes. Abnormal spermiogenesis may also cause sperm anomalies (Table 13.2).

X AND Y CHROMOSOME-BEARING SPERM

Female animals have two similar sex chromosomes (X and X), whereas males have two different sex chromosomes (one X chromosome and one smaller Y chromosome). The gametes (egg and sperm) are haploid cells and contain either an X or a Y chromosome (Table 13.3). Diploid somatic cells of females (homogametic sex) contain a pair of X chromosomes, but somatic cells of males (heterogametic sex) have X and Y sex chromosomes. The genetic sex is determined in the oviduct at the time of fertilization, and the sex of the offspring is determined by the sex chromosome within the sperm.

Extensive investigations have been carried out for preselection and complete separation of X and Y sperm before artificial insemination. Sex of the offspring can also be predetermined in embryos arising from diploid or haploid nuclear transplantation into recipient ova, parthenogenetic activation of ova, or fusion of two oocytes. Different cytogenetic and cytological techniques are used to examine the diploid cells at an appropriate stage of fertilization to diagnose the genetic sex of the embryo. For example, fluorescence microscopy is used to detect the presence of a Y chromosome. Chromosome analysis is performed by culturing leukocytes or fetal cells to study the individual chromosomes using karyotyping procedures, which involve four concepts:

(1) Morphological, physiological, biophysical and immunological differences between X and Y sperm;

(2) Factors affecting the primary and secondary sex ratio;

(3) Techniques for separation of X and Y sperm based on valid statistical evaluation of the results;

(4) Attempts to alter the sex ratio by the use of 'sexed' sperm.

Molecular biology of sperm

When sperm are transported through the female reproductive tract, they undergo capacitation to acquire their fertilizing potential. Sperm release and/or acquire various micro- and macromolecules on their plasmalemma as they migrate through the vaginal secretions, cervical mucus, endometrial secretions, oviductal fluid and peritoneal fluid.

The degree of maturation and age of sperm in an ejaculate can influence density. Packed cell volume of bovine sperm is markedly affected by the osmolality of the medium. Live bull sperm placed in a hypo-osmotic saline solution swell to three times their normal size. Dead sperm do not swell or react osmotically. Live sperm placed in hyperosmotic media shrank from a volume of about 25 μm^3 to 20 μm^3.

Cytogenetics of X and Y sperm

There are many potential differences between sperm containing an X or a Y chromosome (Table 13.3). Sex chromosomes are responsible for any differences in DNA content. The presence of an X or a Y chromosome could cause a difference in the size, shape, weight, density, motility (type and velocity), surface charge, and surface biochemistry or internal biochemistry of sperm (Table 13.3). The degree of difference may also be affected by other factors such as the age of semen, repeat breeding (possible differential embryo mortality) and use of bulls that had been born as co-twins with heifers (and have circulating XX leukocytes).

There are species variations in the mass difference between X and Y chromosomes. The presence of large X chromosomes could result in greater weight and density of the X-containing sperm, if the size and other constituents are the same.

Table 13.2 Some inherited sperm defects affecting fertility

Defect	*Description*	*Fertility*
Knobbed sperm	Acentric thickening of acrosome	Sterility
Decapitated	Head and tail separated at the neck region	Sterility
Dag defect	Folding of tail over the middle piece of sperm, giving an impression of a swollen middle piece	Infertility
Pseudodroplet	Rounded or elongated thickening of the middle piece	Sterility
Corkscrew	Tail defect	Infertility
Diadem effect	Nuclear pouch formation	Infertility
Sterilizing tail stump	Tail defect	Sterility

Table 13.3 Some differences between X- and Y-bearing sperm

Parameter	*Difference*	*Evaluation*
DNA size	Less in Y sperm	Measurable and accepted
	X sperm is larger	Y sperm measured may or may not be representative of random sperm population
Identify motility	Y chromosome fluoresces	Species specific
	Y sperm faster	Evidence primarily dependent on accuracy of F-body staining technique
Surface charge	X sperm migrate to cathode	No charge difference between X and Y sperm

F, fluorescent

Sperm plasmalemma

The external plasmalemma has different characteristics in different parts of the sperm. X and Y sperm have different surface characteristics at spermiation from the germinal epithelium. If ejaculated, such differences would be masked by components that are absorbed from the seminal plasma.

Karyotyping of sperm

The distinction between X and Y sperm based on the fluorescence of the Y chromosome is facilitated by quinacrine staining of sperm, which causes fluorescence of the long arm of the Y chromosome, and a fluorescent spot (F body), which appears in 39–47% of sperm in smears stained with quinacrine. Banding techniques such as G-band and Q-band methods are recommended. Such procedures permit the accurate identification of individual chromosomes. Staining of chromosomes is carried out using a Giemsa dye mixture.

Technology to separate X and Y chromosome-bearing sperm

Extensive investigations have been conducted on X and Y chromosome-bearing sperm (Tables 13.3 and 13.4). Ten methods have been applied using: sedimentation of immobilized sperm in media; skim-milk powder, glycine, sodium citrate, glycerol; albumin column; velocity sedimentation; centrifugation through density gradients; motility and electrophoretic separation; isoelectric focusing; HY antigens; flow sorting by DNA content; and Sephadex column (Beernink, 1984; Bennet and Boyce, 1973; Bhattacharya *et al.*, 1966; Corson *et al.*, 1984; Ericsson and Glass, 1982; Hafs and Boyd, 1971; James, 1980; Meisstrich, 1982; Moore and Hibbitt, 1975; Pinkel and Gledhill, 1982; Sherbet *et al.*, 1972).

Most of the techniques employed for sperm separation are based on non-equilibrium sedimentation (based on velocity of fall) or on equilibrium sedimentation on a density gradient (sedimentation to the level where specific gravities of sperm and the medium are equal). These techniques use simple gravity or centrifugation and are based on Stokes' law of sedimentation of a rigid sphere through an incompressible, viscous fluid at a low Reynolds number (non-turbulent conditions). Aggregation of cells in the buffer is evaluated, and a concentration chosen at which aggregation is negligible.

Only two laboratory methods for separation of human X and Y sperm appear to be valid, reproducible and clinically applicable: albumin separation, which yields 75–80% Y sperm; and Sephadex filtration, which yields 70–75% X sperm. The separation of X and Y sperm is based on the following:

(1) Differences in the weight, density or size of the X and Y chromosomes as a result of differences in the size of different components of the sperm.

(2) Differences in haploid expression of X and Y chromosomes as a result of differences in the nature of sperm components: defective allocation (non-disjunction) of sex chromosomes, to either the gametes or, after fertilization, to early cleavage products, will result in individuals with somatic cells containing only a single X chromosome (XO; YO is lethal) or an extra X or Y chromosome (XXX, XXY or XYY) (Table 13.4).

Layered separation over albumin columns

When semen is layered over columns of serum albumin, increased numbers of Y sperm are recovered from the albumin layers. Semen aliquots of 0.5 ml (diluted 1 : 1 with Tyrode's solution) are layered for 1 h over a 7.5% solution of serum albumin in a glass column (8×75 mm). The initial sperm layer is then removed by pipette, the albumin centrifuged at 2800–3200 rpm for 10 min, and the sperm disc is resuspended in Tyrode's solution. The resuspended sperm is then layered over a two-layer serum albumin column. At 1 h, the sperm layer is removed, and after another 30 min, the 13% layer is removed. The 20% serum albumin is then centrifuged for 10 min, and the sperm disc is resuspended in 0.25 ml of Tyrode's solution, which is then inseminated into the uterus.

Flow cytometry and sorting

With flow cytometry, high-speed measurements of components and properties of individual cells are made in a liquid suspension. Laser light is used for monochromatic illumination of cells stained with fluorescent dyes. Light detectors sample the fluorescence produced by the interaction of light with dye and produce electrical signals proportionate to the intensity of fluorescent light from each object. This technique is useful in the evaluation of the degree of separation needed to produce populations enriched in X or Y sperm.

Table 13.4 Techniques to separate X- and Y-chromosome bearing sperm

Technique	*Results*
Sedimentation of immobilized sperm on media	Insemination with sperm that had sedimented the greatest distance produced 70% females
Skim-milk powder, glycine, sodium citrate, glycerol	Increase in number of male offspring when sperm from the top layers was used
Albumin column	Successful results with frozen sperm preselected on albumin column before cryopreservation
Velocity sedimentation	Sedimentation rates depend on size, density and shape of sperm
	Cell size difference is predominant factor in separation of types; shape is usually the least important factor Sperm heads have extremely aspherical shapes
Centrifugation through density gradients	Sperm separated according to their sedimentation rates by centrifugation through density gradients, provided the density of the gradient material is less than that of the sperm. The advantage is that the time required for separation is much shorter. Shorter time does not improve theoretical resolution of separation, because diffusion is insignificant
Motility and electrophoretic separation	Immotile sperm electrophoretically attracted to the anode at neutral pH. When electrophoretic separation is under conditions consistent with sperm motility, sperm migrate to the cathode. Sperm are oriented by electric field and swim in direction the head is facing. If negatively charged, sperm can be oriented so that the tail is facing the anode by virtue of its greater negative charge density and their intrinsic motility is greater than the electrophoretic mobility
Isoelectric focusing	Separation performed in columns with the fluid stabilized using density gradients Sperm layered on, or suspended in, this solution migrate electrophoretically until reaching an isoelectric point
HY antigens	Sperm treated with HY antisera. Insemination with mouse sperm treated with antisera to a Y-linked histocompatibility antigen produced 45% males compared with 53% for controls
Flow sorting by DNA content	Y-sorting is 72–80% successful. Disadvantages: low sorting rate and lack of sperm viability after sorting
Sephadex column	Some 70% of X sperm found in certain fractions of the filtrate when sperm were placed on top of a column of Sephadex 65–85% X sperm found in certain fractions of filtrate

GENETIC ENGINEERING (FIGURES 13.8 AND 13.9)

Innovative technologies to enhance the efficiency of experimental gene transfer in different species are desperately needed. Such techniques would not only reduce the cost of individual projects, but would also increase the likelihood of new innovations in many disciplines. It is envisaged that procedures will be modified and enhanced as new advances are reported. There are several specific achievements that would significantly enhance experimental productivity:

(1) Development of alternative DNA delivery systems (e.g. liposome-mediated gene transfer or targeted somatic cell techniques);

(2) Identification of optimal conditions for a given gene transfer procedure and identification of breeds best suited to the specific technologies;

(3) Complete animal genome mapping and identification of homologies to human genes;

(4) Establishment of routine and efficient germplasm culture and preservation systems (from preservation of gonadal tissue to culture and cryostorage of gametes).

Recent advances in genetic engineering have enabled scientists to uncover, rearrange and make copies, or clones, of genes. For example, each animal cell contains some 100 000 genes. At least 22 000 of these genes have been isolated, and some of their specific functions have been identified. Primary considerations for genetic manipulations and gene transfer are not only limited to management (including surgical manipulations and embryo handling), but also to

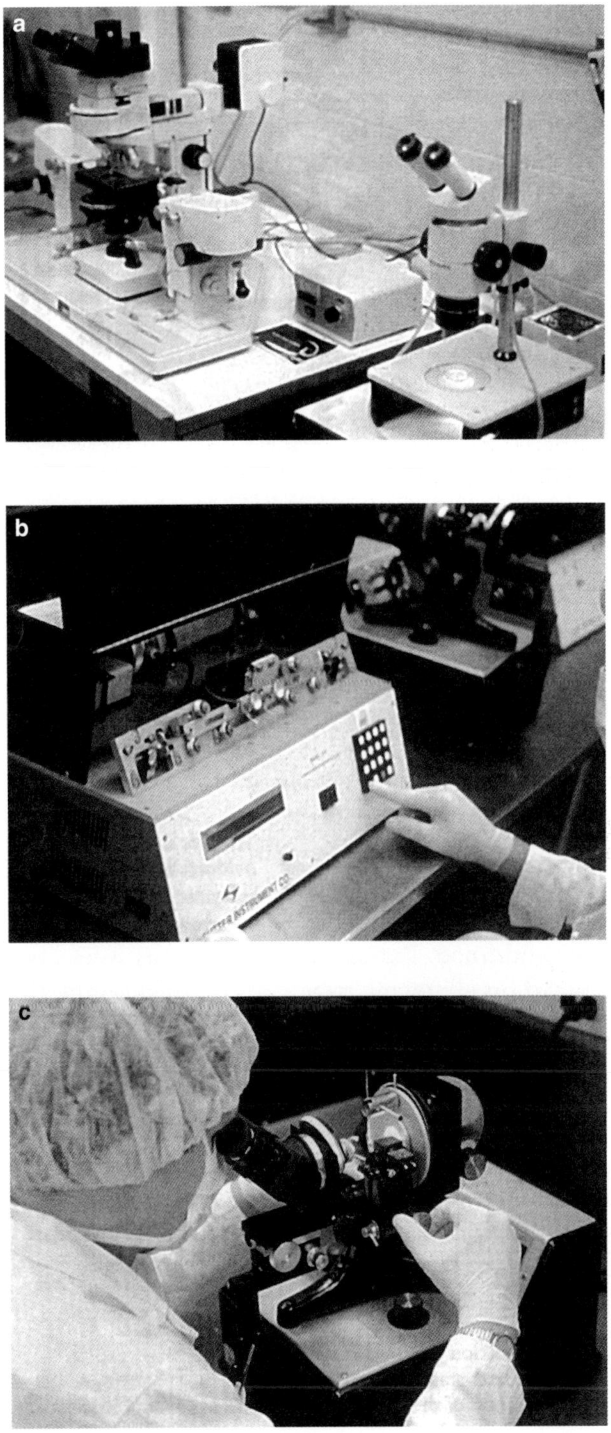

Figure 13.8 (**a**) Microinjection station includes a dissecting microscope (right) used for batch preparation of embryos and cells (and embryo transfer in mice) and microinjection microscope (left). Flanking the microinjection microscope, micromanipulators aid in precise manipulations with embryos, cells and buffers. (**b**) Pipette puller. Microneedles can be prepared with uniform tapers and shapes using an electronic or gravity-driven pipette puller. (**c**) Microforge. Needles may be fire-polished or bent to desired specifications using the microforge assembly that includes a microscope assembly for visualization of the finished product

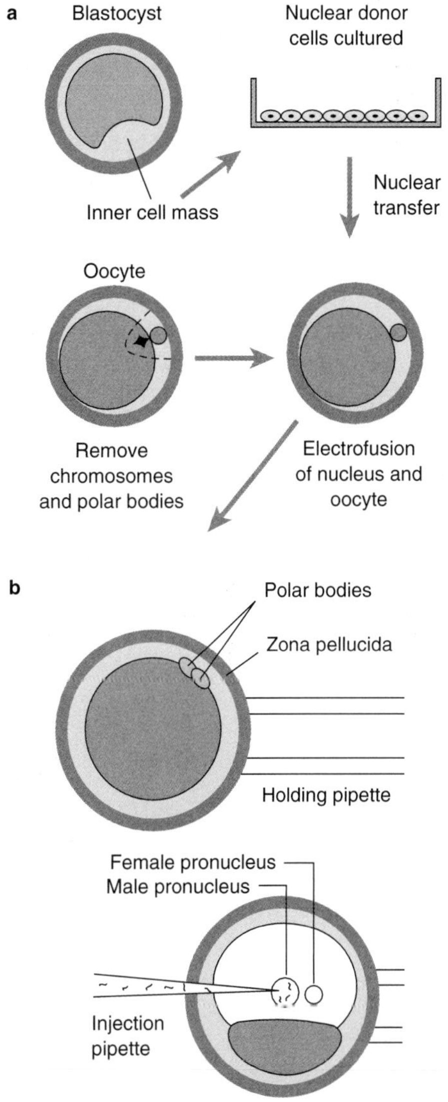

Figure 13.9 Nuclear transfer and microinjection. (**a**) Nuclear transfer and cloning. Cells from blastocysts (e.g. inner cell mass cells) or other somatic tissues are obtained and grown in culture. These cells are used as nucleus donors for transfer into enucleated oocytes. In contrast to DNA microinjection, this genetic-engineering process includes an electrofusion step to fuse the transferred nuclei and enucleated oocytes. The fused 'couplets' (transferred nucleus plus oocyte) are transferred to recipients and live-born offspring are then evaluated for the genetic modification. (**b**) Microinjection of a zygote. Most zygotes are lipid-rich and relatively opaque

expertise in tissue/cell culture, molecular biology techniques and sperm analysis/quantitation.

Maternal-to-zygote transmission

Maternal-to-zygotic transmission has at least three functions that are required for continued development:

Table 13.5 Definitions, basic principles and types of human embryonic stem cells. Adapted from Amit *et al.*, 2003 and Revelli *et al.*, 2003

Cell type/principle	*Definition*
Embryonic stem (ES) cells	Derived from the preimplantation embryo Pluripotent, capable of differentiating into representative cells of all three germ layers of the embryo Immortal, with long-term proliferation at the undifferentiated stage (self-maintenance) Maintain normal karyotype after prolonged culture Capable, after injection into blastocysts, of contributing to all three embryonic germ layers, including the germ line, and into mature chimeric animals Express unique markers, such as transcription factor Oct-4 or cell-surface markers like stage-specific embryonic antigen
Embryoid bodies (EBs)	Tumor-derived cell lines able to differentiate *in vitro* into a variety of cell types, including muscle and nerve cells, to aggregate into cell clusters in which part of the cells differentiate spontaneously, to form teratocarcinomas after their injection into recipient
Cloning	Development of a colony of cells from one cell by repeated mitosis: all cells have the same genetic constitution Transplantation of a somatic cell nucleus into an ovum for the purpose of developing an embryo through asexual reproduction

(1) Destruction of oocyte-specific transcripts, such as the RNA-binding protein MSY2 and histone $H1_{00}$, that are not subsequently expressed. The destruction of these mRNAs restricts the period of time during which the genes can function.

(2) Replacing of maternal transcripts that are also degraded during oocyte maturation and following fertilization, and that are common to the oocyte and the early embryo (e.g. actin) with zygotic transcripts. If these maternal transcripts are not replenished, development will shortly arrest owing to the embryo's inability to execute basic cellular functions. Expression of these genes does not result in reprogramming of gene expression in the classical sense; nonetheless, their expression is essential.

(3) Promoting of the dramatic reprogramming in the pattern of gene expression that is coupled with the generation of novel transcripts not expressed in the oocyte. This reprogramming of gene expression is likely to be the molecular basis for the transformation of the differentiated oocyte into totipotent 2-cell-stage blastomeres.

Stem cells

The definitions, basic principles and types of human embryonic cells are summarized in Table 13.5. The body contains several self-renewing systems, including hematopoietic tissue, intestinal epithelium and epidermis. Spermatogenesis originates from spermatogonial stem cells, and the continuous production of progenitor cells supports male reproduction throughout adulthood. Extensive investigations were conducted on allergenic stem cell transplantation, the hematopoietic system and transplantation of allergenic hematopoietic stem cells for therapy of several hematological malignancies, metabolic disorders and solid tumors. Future research is needed to evaluate the immunological response to transplantation of other types of allergenic stem cells, particularly how they are affected by histoincompatibility. A technique was developed to transfer spermatogonial stem, in which the stem cells are transplanted into the seminiferous tubules of infertile recipient animals. The transplanted stem cells proliferate on the basement membrane and establish colonies of spermatogenesis. Spermatogonial stem cells are unique among the many types of stem cells in that they reside in an immunologically privileged environment.

Several methods have been used for gene transfer. The advantages and disadvantages of DNA microinjection and retrovirus-mediated gene transfer are described in Table 13.6.

Transgenic animal models have been applied in the fields of embryology, endocrinology, genetics, immunology, neurology, oncology, pathology, physiology, toxicology and virology (Table 13.7).

Table 13.6 Advantages and disadvantages of different methods of gene transfer. Adapted from Pinkert (2000) (personal communication)

Technique	*Advantages*	*Disadvantages*
DNA micro-injection	Relatively high frequency of generating transgenic animals (20–30% of live-born offspring)	Random and potentially significant influence that the site of integration may exert on transgene expression (positional effects)
	High probability of germ-line transmission of the transgene	Potential for undesired insertional mutagenesis
	Relative lack of constraints on the size or type of DNA construct used	Occasional production of mosaic founders
	Relative stability of the transgene as it is transmitted from generation to generation	Occasional lack of germ-line incorporation
	Low frequency of mosaicism or double integrations (combined estimate of 10–30% of founders)	Time and expense required to obtain micromanipulation and microinjection skills
Retrovirus-mediated gene transfer	Uncertain	Low copy number integration
		Additional steps required to produce retroviruses
		Limitations on the size of the foreign DNA insert (usually 9–15 kb) transferred
		Potential for undesired genetic recombination that may alter the retrovirus
		High frequency of mosaicism
		Possible interference by integrated retroviral sequences on transgene expression

Genetic manipulation of embryonic stem cells

Genetic manipulation can be performed in human embryonic stem (ES) cells. Extensive investigations have been conducted on differentiation of human ES cells in both spontaneous- and directed-differentiation models. For example, human ES cells have been spontaneously differentiated into cardiomyocytes with their characteristic features: typical myofibril organization consistent with early stage cardiomyocytes, positive staining with specific cardiomyocytic markers including anticardiac myosin heavy chain, anti-α-actinin, antidesmin, expressed specific cardiac genes and physiological features of cardiac cells. At present there are more than 70 human ES cell lines in several laboratories around the world (National Institutes of Health, NIH; index.htm). Derivation of human ES cells can reproduced with reasonable success. The most common procedure used to isolate the inner cell mass (ICM) is immunosurgery, with the aim of selectively isolating the ICM of the blastocyst from the outer layer of the trophoectoderm. The zona pellucida is removed using Tyrode's solution, and the embryo is exposed to antihuman whole antiserum.

Interspecies somatic cell nuclear transfer

Securing human blastocysts is a prerequisite factor for developing novel medical biotechnologies, such as cell replacement therapy using ES cells. However, an inevitable increase in the use of human embryos is anticipated with continuing technical improvements and their subsequent clinical application. Recent development of somatic cell cloning makes it possible to obtain human blastocysts without the use of human embryos; however, this raises concerns about human cloning and provokes ethical concerns. To date, strict regulation has prohibited human cloning and several countries have even limited the production of human cloned embryos.

To obtain human blastocysts, an interspecies somatic cell nuclear transfer (iSCNT) technique using human somatic cells and animal enucleated oocytes was suggested. Although disputes and serious concerns

Table 13.7 Use of transgenic animal models and gene transfer techniques

Uses
Genetic bases of human disease and the design and testing of therapeutic strategies
Gene therapy
Disease resistance in man
Drug and product efficacy testing and screening, toxicological screening protocols can now incorporate transgenic technology
Novel or improved products
Models range from enhancing production traits of interest to 'foreign' protein production and human organ replacement (xenotransplantation)
Techniques
Blastomere/embryo aggregation
Teratocarcinoma cell transfer
Retroviral infection
Microinjection
Electrofusion
Nuclear transplantation
Embryonic stem cell transfer
Sperm-mediated transfer and spermatogonial cell-mediated transfer
Particle bombardment and jet injection

about interspecies cloning have been provoked, iSCNT is the only alternative to avoid the abuse of human embryos and even oocytes. The feasibility of interspecies cloning has been demonstrated in previous studies; blastocyst formation was possible after the transfer of mouse, bovine, porcine or rabbit somatic cells into bovine enucleated oocytes. It has now been applied to various animal research models. In terms of accessibility and ethics, human cord fibroblasts and enucleated bovine oocytes were selected as somatic cell donors and recipient cytoplasts.

DNA microinjection

Several experimental studies have been conducted on DNA microinjection, egg cytoplasm/gene control in development, translation of globin mRNA transgenic technology and altering the genome by homologous recombination. However, all these experiments were conducted on farm animals, using the mouse model (Brinster *et al.*, 1980; Cappechi, 1989; Gurdon, 1977; Hogan *et al.*, 1994; Houdebine, 1997; Monastersky and Robi, 1995; Pinkert, 1994a; Pinkert, 1994b; Pinkert, *et al.*, 1997; Pinkert and Murray, 1998). Very little is known about the possible application to human reproduction.

DNA microinjection techniques

DNA microinjection generally involves the use of micromanipulators and air- or oil-driven microinjection apparatus physically to inject the DNA construct solution into the ova. Almost any cloned DNA construct can be used. With few exceptions, microinjected gene constructs integrate randomly throughout the host's genome, but usually only at a single chromosomal location (the integration site). This fact can be exploited to co-inject simultaneously more than one DNA construct into a zygote. The constructs will then co-integrate together at a single, randomly located, integration site. During integration, a single copy of multiple copies of a transgene (actually as many as a few hundred copies of the particular sequence) are incorporated into the genomic DNA, predominantly as a number of copies in head-to-tail concatemers. Because DNA microinjection is usually accomplished in ova at the one-cell stage, transgene incorporation occurs in essentially every cell that contributes to the developing embryo. Incorporation of the transgene into cells that will eventually contribute to development of germ cells (sperm or ova) is a common occurrence with this method.

Host DNA near the site of integration frequently undergoes various forms of sequence duplication, deletion or rearrangement as a result of transgene incorporation.

Advantages of the DNA microinjection method are:

(1) Relatively high frequency of generating transgenic animals (20–30% of liveborn offspring);

(2) High probability of germ-line transmission of the transgene;

(3) Relative lack of constraints on the size or type of DNA construct used;

(4) Relative stability of the transgene as it is transmitted from generation to generation;

(5) Low frequency of mosaicism or double integrations (combined estimate of 10–30% of founders) (Rosnina *et al.*, 2000).

In contrast, disadvantages of this method include:

(1) Random and potentially significant influence that the site of integration may exert on transgene expression (positional effects);
(2) Potential for undesired insertional mutagenesis;
(3) Occasional production of mosaic founders;
(4) Occasional lack of germ-line incorporation;
(5) Time and expense required to obtain micromanipulation and microinjection skills.

Transgene-encoded mRNA expression

While absence of mRNA expression is probable for loss-of-function models and may only represent a confirmatory step of minor significance, the analysis of expression of the transgene is absolutely essential in determining the usefulness of a particular transgenic animal. Technically, the most critical step in analyzing transgene expression is the isolation of RNA. Care must be taken to avoid contamination of RNA preparations with ribonucleases (enzymes that degrade RNA). The presence of a specific mRNA is usually determined by RNA slot blot or Northern blot hybridization. Northern blotting is more informative as it confirms not only the presence but also the size of the mRNA transcript of interest (Rosnina *et al.*, 2000).

Transgene-encoded protein expression

Various techniques are often employed to identify the unique protein or perhaps a specific enzyme activity. The immunoblotting technique, in which proteins are resolved on a polyacrylamide gel, transferred to a membrane and detected with a labeled antibody, is useful in verifying the appropriate molecular weight of the protein product of interest. To identify which cells within a tissue contain the protein product of the transgene, immunohistochemical staining of tissue sections with a labeled antibody can also be employed. Additionally, the use of 'reporter genes' (e.g. an oncogene, or a growth hormone or fluorescent protein gene) can often simplify determination of expression levels by producing a protein that is easily and unequivocally determined.

CLINICAL PARAMETERS

Preimplantation genetic diagnosis

Preimplantation genetic diagnosis (PGD) involves the assessment of the chromosomal status of an embryo *in vitro*, before its transfer to the uterus. Biopsy of one or two blastomeres is performed on day 3 of development, when the embryo is at the 6- to 10-cell stage. Each isolated cell is fixed and screened for chromosomal content using fluorescence *in situ* hybridization (FISH) with chromosome-specific DNA probes. PGD is applied to determine the sex of embryos from patients with X-linked disease and to identify chromosomally abnormal embryos from patients with an altered karyotype. Although blastomere culture may increase the number of cells available for chromosomal analysis, the high frequency of nuclear defects and the occurrence of polyploidy and mosaicism among cultured cells discourage the use of blastomere isolation and proliferation strategy for use in preimplantation genetic diagnosis.

Extensive investigations are needed in the areas of male sex determination, prenatal differentiation, postnatal development, cellular organization, paracrine regulation, male germ apoptosis, gonadotropin receptors, septo-optic dysphasia, related malformations, magnetic resonance imaging of hypothalamic–pituitary region in non-tumoral hypopituitarism; clinical aspects of interest include cancer of the male reproductive organs, blood–testis barrier, testicular descent and the prevention of male infertility after gonadotoxic cancer treatment in prepubertal boys.

Such information will be valuable for scientists, general pediatricians, endocrinologists and andrologists.

Identical twins

Identical twins have identical genes, as do a clone and its progenitor. Identical twins do look alike and even teachers mix them up. Identical twins are strikingly similar in many ways, but research shows that they are not completely alike. Identical twins are more identical than clones will ever be. As a group, identical twins are more similar to each other in personality than ordinary siblings or fraternal twins, who develop from two separate eggs; this is true even when the identical twins are apart.

Even identical twins are influenced by non-genetic factors, beginning *in utero* and extending to parents, friends, opportunities in life and chance occurrences. Since a clone and its progenitor would be born into different families at different times, these non-genetic factors could be expected to be more powerful. In the case of identical twins, there are also some genetic differences that are surprising.

Schizophrenia is clearly influenced by genes, for example. However, if one identical twin has schizophrenia, the chance that the other also has it is only 40–50%. Not even physical traits like height and weight are perfectly duplicated between pairs of identical twins. Height is among the traits most heavily influenced by genes, but identical twins may differ by as much as 4 inches. The correlation between identical twins is strong for height, strong for IQ, weaker for weight and weaker still for personality. Sexual and religious attitudes exhibit the same level of genetic influence as does personality, while attitudes on taxes and politics appear to be less influenced by genes. These findings are only population averages and cannot be used to predict anything about similarities between individual clones and their progeny. The degree of similarity for various traits roughly follows this pattern in identical twins. There is no perfect replica.

Cloned food/federal agencies

According to the FDA, 400–500 cows and bulls have been produced by cloning. The FDA's Veterinary Medicine Advisory Committee stated that there are no biological reasons, based on either underlying scientific assumptions or empirical studies, to indicate that consumption of edible products from clones of cattle, pigs, sheep or goats poses a greater risk than consumption of those products from their non-clone counterparts. The National Academy of Sciences declared that while food from such clones posed a 'low level of food safety concern', more data were needed.

FUTURE RESEARCH

Additional research is needed in the following areas:

(1) Sperm motility: sperm isolate themselves based on different progressive motility.

(2) Sperm dimensions or density: cells sorted through a device sensitive enough to detect minute differences.

(3) Sperm cytogenetics: chemical or immunological reaction capable of selecting on sex chromosome content.

(4) Sperm environment: hormone or chemical condition resulting in penetration of the egg by an X or Y sperm.

(5) Search for Robertsonian chromosome rearrangements that include a sex chromosome: the availability of such chromosomes could facilitate specific breeding schemes suitable for sex selection.

(6) Cytogenetic sexing of cells isolated from an embryo and transfer of the selected embryo after short *in vitro* culture.

14

Molecular reproduction in men

Extensive investigations have been conducted on the genes expressed in various reproductive processes (Abdel-Rahman *et al.*, 1995; Agulnik *et al.*, 1994; Ariel *et al.*, 1994; Bathgate *et al.*, 1996; Branford *et al.*, 1997; Cao *et al.*, 1995; Check *et al.*, 1996; Cornwall and Hann, 1995; Domashenko *et al.*, 1997; Furuya *et al.*, 1995; Gerwin *et al.*, 1995; Juneja and Koide, 2000; Nayernia *et al.*, 1996; Sarge *et al.*, 1994; Vani and Rao, 1997; Worrad and Schultz, 1997; Xu *et al.*, 1995). Many genes coding for important factors and receptors are expressed during the development of the testes (Figures 14.1 and 14.2; Table 14.1). The relaxin-like factor (RLF) gene is highly expressed in the testes.

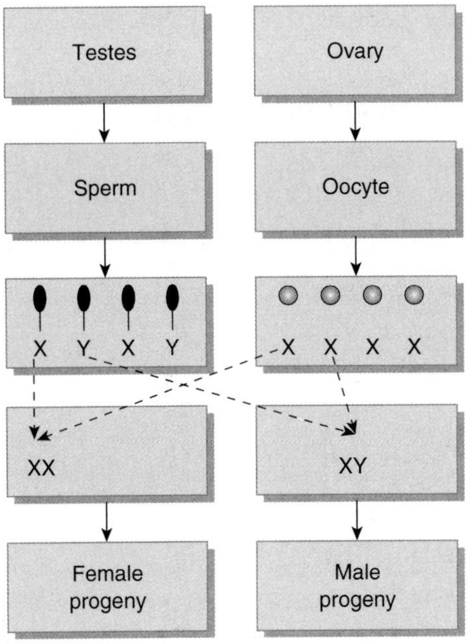

Figure 14.1 Schematic representation of the generation of two different progenies by fertilization between two distinct populations of sperm and eggs

MOLECULAR PARAMETERS OF CHROMOSOMES/GENES

Deoxyribonucleic acid

Deoxyribonucleic acid (DNA) is the molecule that contains and transfers genetic information from one generation to the next. DNA molecules, in association with histones and various proteins, are organized to form complex intracellular structures called

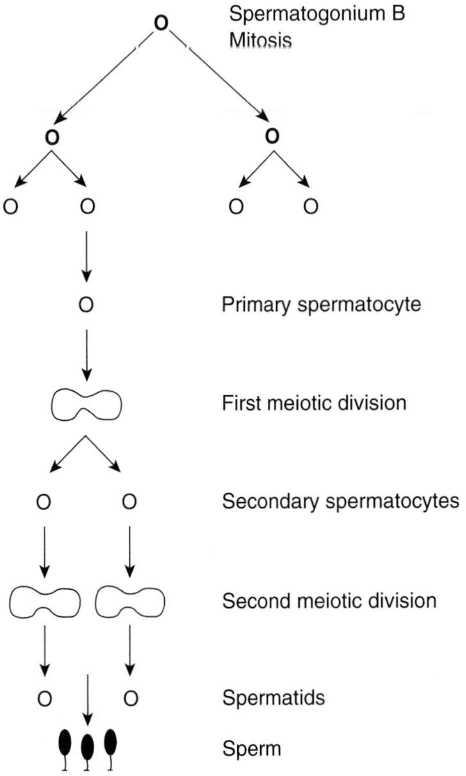

Figure 14.2 Series of events occurring during spermatogenesis

Table 14.1 Genetic control of testes determination

Gene	*Role during testes development*
Tdy (testes determining factor in mice)	Act on supporting cell lineage and inducing differentiation of supporting cells to Sertoli cells
Sry (Y-chromosome specific gene)	Different homologs of Sry have a common open reading frame which has 41% homology to a DNA-binding motif HMG-box; Sry-encoded protein might have DNA binding activity
Sox6 (Sry-related gene), Sox5	Overlapping functions in the regulation of gene expression during spermatogenesis in the adult mouse
Sox9	Critical Sertoli cell differentiation factor
TAZ83	Coding at early to midpachytene germ cell stage
TAZ4	Testes specific gene located on chromosome 11
TNZ1	Expressed in neonatal Leydig cells

'chromosomes'. Mammalian gametes are the direct products of the reductive division of chromosomes, termed meiosis, and thus contain the haploid number (abbreviated n) of hereditary determinants. Both gametes contribute equally to the genetic make-up of new progeny by transmitting the haploid number (n) of chromosomes to the newly formed diploid zygote ($2n$) of the next generation. The general mechanisms and genes expressed during spermatogenesis, fertilization and implantation are shown in Table 14.1. DNA contains hereditary information within its helical structure, and also provides the basis for the evolutionary process.

DNA directs cellular growth and proliferation, and also regulates the differentiation of the fertilized egg to form the multitude of specialized cells required for organogenesis and proper functioning of mature animals. The majority of DNA is located within the nucleus in the form of coiled rods and is an integral part of chromosomes. Each species of farm animal has a fixed number of chromosomes, and each chromosome occurs as duplicates (homologous chromosomes). During the formation of gametes, reductive division, designated as meiosis, occurs, whereby the number of chromosomes in the cells is reduced to a haploid number (n), or half the diploid number ($2n$), found in somatic or non-sex cells. Men are the heterogametic sex, since one pair of sex chromosomes consists of an X and a Y type. This produces two distinct populations of spermatozoa, one bearing an X and the other a Y chromosome (Figure 14.1). The male gametes determine the sex of the new progeny. Following advances in genetics and techniques for separating chromosomes, X- or Y-bearing sperm can be selected and used to fertilize an egg and obtain progeny having the desired sex. However, there are no known inherent advantages of fertilizability between X- and Y-bearing gametes.

CELLULAR PROTEINS

Tyrosine phosphorylation plays an important role in cell growth, differentiation and apoptosis. Src family tyrosine kinases (SFKs) are key signaling molecules regulating the tyrosine phosphorylation of a number of cellular proteins.

Recombinant proteins

Synthetic human proteins are useful therapeutic agents. Polypeptides are simple to make: a gene is transcribed, the message translated, and the resulting protein may not even require post-translational modification. In other words, little intermediary metabolism is needed to produce most proteins; such products can be secreted directly into the milk of transgenic animals. Advantages of recombinant protein production over purification from source (e.g. from animals or human cadavers) include greater consistency of product quality, higher efficiency of production, lower immunogenicity than animal proteins, reduced infectivity compared to tissue-derived products, and genetic engineering of 'super proteins' with high activity. The only disadvantage of recombinant technology is that such proteins are difficult to detect when used for illicit purposes – the abuse of erythropoietin and growth hormone by athletes (Tseng, 1980).

MOLECULAR PARAMETERS OF SPERMATOGENESIS

Extensive investigations have been conducted on the genetic control of testes determination, genes involved in testicular development and function, Y-linked genes, spermatogenesis, T-type Ca^{2+} channels and alpha1E expression in spermatogenic cells, and their possible relevance to the sperm acrosome reaction (Chandley and Cooke, 1994; Harley, 1993; Hutchinson, 1993; Johnson and Barry, 1995; Lamb, 1995; Lievano *et al.*, 1996).

The two compartments of the testes, seminiferous tubules and interstitium, are under the hormonal control of gonadotropins, acting on either Sertoli cells or Leydig cells. During spermatogenesis, these different cell types, and in particular germ cells, express four specific sets of genes, which are regulated at either the transcriptional or transductional level. Some are detected exclusively in haploid cells, whereas others are initially expressed before or during meiosis and continue to be expressed in spermatids:

(1) Male germ cell-specific gene homologs (e.g. glyceraldehyde-3-phosphate dehydrogenase);

(2) Unique genes expressed exclusively during spermatogenesis;

(3) Germ cell-specific alternate transcripts leading to specific isoforms;

(4) Genes developmentally regulated during germ cell differentiation (e.g. c-Abl protooncogene).

Mitosis

Germ cells present in immature testes are reactivated at puberty and undergo mitosis, while situated in the basal compartment of the tubule. These generated spermatogonial stem cells give rise to cells with distinct morphological characteristics, classified as A1 spermatogonia. The emergence of these cells marks the beginning of spermatogenesis. Each spermatogonium undergoes a defined number of mitotic divisions unique to the species, giving rise to a 'clone' of cells which differ morphologically from their parents. The nuclear division during mitosis (karyokinesis) is complete, whereas the cytoplasmic division (cytokinesis) is incomplete, resulting in primary spermatocytes connected by thin cytoplasmic bridges. This interconnecting syncytial state of germ cells exists throughout the entire process of spermatogenesis.

Meiosis

During meiosis, a number of genes present on autosomes are expressed; however, genes located on sex-chromosomes remain inactive. Later during spermatid formation, the autosomes cease RNA production and their DNA becomes highly condensed or heterochromatic.

Postmeiotic phases

Spermiogenesis involves major remodeling of the structure of spermatids to form spermatozoa, which are composed of three distinct parts: head, middle piece and tail. The nucleus, which is present in the head region, contains compact packaged haploid chromosomes. On completion of spermatogenesis, the spermatozoa are released into the lumen of the seminiferous tubules by spermiation. Different species have varying periodicity in the spermatogenesis cycle. Nonetheless, within a given species the rate of progression of germ cell differentiation through the various stages of spermatogenesis is remarkably constant.

Spermatogenesis provides an interesting system for examining the regulation of gene expression during development and differentiation. The genes expressed during spermatogenesis can be divided into two main groups: diploid-expressed genes, e.g. the proacrosin gene, and haploid-expressed genes, e.g. the gene encoding the transition protein 2, a novel gene from the rat protamine gene cluster (Prm3), and a spermatid-located calpastatin gene. A number of novel genes that play a role during spermatogenesis have been identified (Tables 14.2 and 14.3).

MOLECULAR ASPECTS OF FERTILIZATION

Immotile and immature spermatozoa undergo a series of changes during their transit through the rete testes, ductuli efferentia and epididymis to become motile and mature. Expression of the BE-20 epididymal protein gene is detected in the cauda epididymis and the proximal segment of the ductus deferens, suggesting a role in sperm maturation and its capacity to fertilize ova.

Sperm–egg interactions

Sperm–egg binding between the outer membrane of the sperm and the outermost glycoprotein covering (zona pellucida 3, ZP3) of the egg occurs initially as a species-specific interaction. The sperm receptor present on the surface of the unfertilized egg involved in sperm–egg binding has been identified as ZP3. Sperm–egg binding triggers the acrosome reaction in the sperm head, which involves fusion of the outer acrosomal membrane with the overlying sperm plasma membrane. The net result of the acrosome reaction is the release of hydrolytic enzymes and exposure of the inner acrosomal membrane. Together with increased motility (hyperactivation), and the liberated hydrolytic enzymes, the acrosome-reacted sperm has the potential to penetrate its way through the zona pellucida and enter the perivitelline space. The sperm head next sinks into the oocyte, triggering the second meiotic division, which leads to the formation and extrusion of the second polar body.

Table 14.2 Genes expressed during reproduction

Reproductive process	*Gene*
Spermatogenesis	Proacrosin gene
	Smcy, Hya, Sdma, CRES
	Spx1, MSH2, HSF2
	Pgk2, ApoA1, Oct3/4
Oogenesis	RLF gene, oxytocin gene
Fertilization	BE-20
Preimplantation and	Cytokines, Sry
implantation	Myc, Sp1
	Oct4, Oct6, PIBF
	EGF

MOLECULAR ASPECTS OF INFERTILITY

Translocation and preimplantation genetic diagnosis

Translocation carriers have a high risk of infertility, recurrent spontaneous abortion and conception of a chromosomally abnormal pregnancy. Unbalanced embryos are as likely as normal embryos to develop to the blastocyst stage, thus implanting and resulting in spontaneous abortion and/or affected offspring at the same rate (Escudero *et al.*, 2003). Preimplantation genetic diagnosis (PGD) is offered to carriers of translocations as an alternative to prenatal diagnosis and pregnancy termination of unbalanced fetuses. PGD for translocation is performed using several techniques of fluorescence *in situ* hybridization (FISH). Patients undergoing PGD of translocations obtain a pregnancy rate comparable with routine *in vitro* fertilization (IVF) patients and a very significant reduction in the frequency of spontaneous abortions. Patients with ≤65% chromosomally abnormal sperm have a good chance of conceiving; patients with higher rates would need to produce ten or more good-quality embryos to have a reasonable chance of conceiving (Escudero *et al.*, 2003).

Table 14.3 Genes involved in spermatogenesis and their function

Gene	*Role during spermatogenesis*
Smcy	Y-chromosome gene; isolated from the region encoding spermatogenesis gene Spy
Hya, Sdma	Regulatory role in the expression of the male-specific minor histocompatibility antigen HY
CRES (cystatin-related epididymal and spermatogenic) gene	Specialized role during sperm development and maturation
YRRM (Y-located RNA recognition motif) gene	Candidate for azoospermia factor
Spx1 (X-linked homeobox gene), MSH2 (mismatch repair gene), HSF2 (heat shock factor 2)	Regulatory role during spermatogenesis
Pgk2, ApoA1, Oct3/4	Role in sperm maturation process
Gene encoding T-type Ca^{2+} channel	Voltage-sensitive calcium-channel sensitive to blocking agents dihydropyridine and nifedipine

Growth factors

Interleukin-10 (IL-10) is an apheliotropic cytokine secreted by leukocytes and somatic cells with well characterized anti-inflammatory and immune-deviating properties. IL-10 inhibits proliferation and cytokine synthesis in type-1 T lymphocytes, and does not induce responsiveness or energy. Conversely, IL-10 favors differentiation and function of lymphocyte subsets with pivotal roles in immune tolerance, namely the newly discovered T regulatory (Tr1) cells and T helper cells. The ability of IL-10 to skew immune outcomes is indirect and is mediated through programming antigen-presenting cells preferentially to support expansion of alternative types of T cells. Moreover, IL-10 terminates inflammatory responses and limits inflammation-induced tissue pathology by inhibiting synthesis of tumor necrosis factor-α (TNF-α), interleukin-1, and a large array of other proinflammatory cytokines and chemokines in monocytes and macrophages.

Cell transfection

'Stable transfectants' are cells that permanently express a recombinant DNA sequence, or construct cells. In these cells the target DNA is stably integrated into the genome. Genomic integration may be achieved using a selectable marker linked to the gene of interest. Such integration may take place during genetic recombination; DNA modified by such incorporation is known as 'recombinant'. Alternatively, cells may express the inserted gene for only a few days (typically 12–72 h) before ejecting the plasmid DNA. These transient transfectants are used for short-term experiments that demand gene expression without accurate simulation. Gene expression can be observed by intracellular microinjection of specific mRNA transcripts – either 'sense' or 'anti-sense'. This technique is limited to short-term experimental analysis of small cell numbers.

15

Sperm processing

Ejaculated semen is processed to separate viable from non-viable sperm for artificial insemination (AI), intrauterine insemination (IUI), or for assisted reproductive technology (ART). Sperm concentration is one of the major semen parameters to be evaluated before semen processing. The clinical diagnosis of male partner fertility relies primarily on the outcome of standard semen analysis. It is therefore imperative that the concentration of sperm be determined accurately and reliably. Although the initial sperm concentration of a semen sample has been shown to have a relatively low value postpreparation, concentrations are routinely used for the accurate insemination of oocytes *in vitro*. The parameter can be measured manually or by a computer-assisted semen analyzer system (CASA). Several reusable and disposable chambers are available for both manual and computerized evaluation. Before a chamber can be used for the routine evaluation of sperm concentration, its accuracy and precision has to be evaluated by comparison to a hemocytometer (Neubauer, Germany), Makler chamber (Sefi Medical Instruments, Israel) or disposal Leja chamber (Leja, Nieuw-Vennep, The Netherlands) (Figures 15.1–15.4).

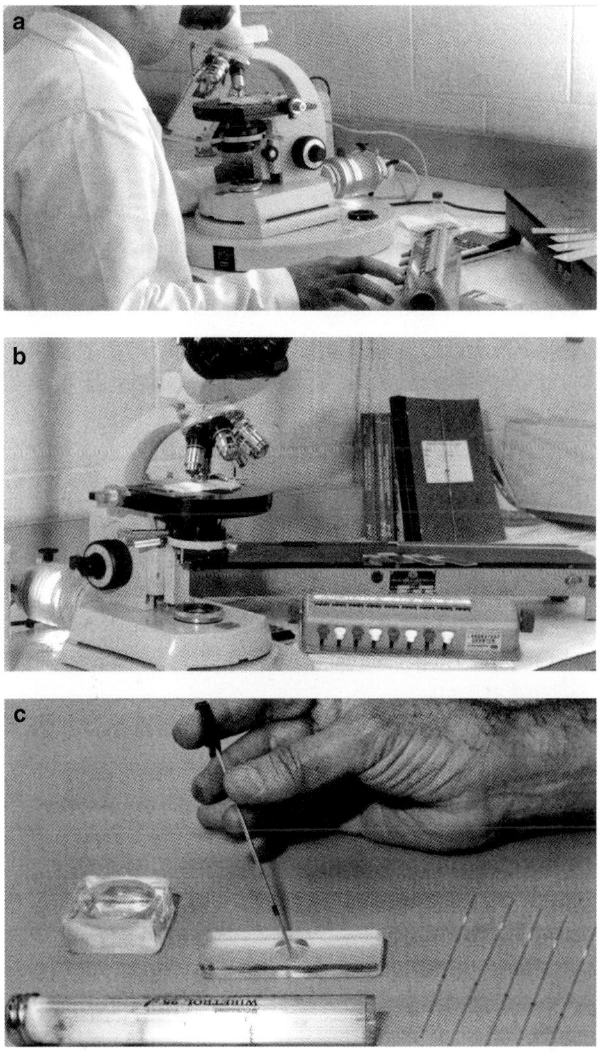

Figure 15.1 Microscopic examination using hemocytometer to count sperm in the ejaculate (**a**) and (**b**). Note an automatic counter at the bottom of (**b**) to count simultaneously viable and non-viable sperm, leukocytes, debris and other cell contaminants. (**c**) Micropipetting for evaluation, counting and storage in cryopreservation straws for sperm and eggs

SPERM SEPARATION METHODS (TABLES 15.1 AND 15.2)

Separation of viable from non-viable sperm

The semen of both human and animal ejaculates contains a mixture of viable and non-viable spermatozoa; the non-viable cells can exceed 80% of the total, consisting of dead, immotile or abnormal cells. In cases where the proportion of viable cells is low,

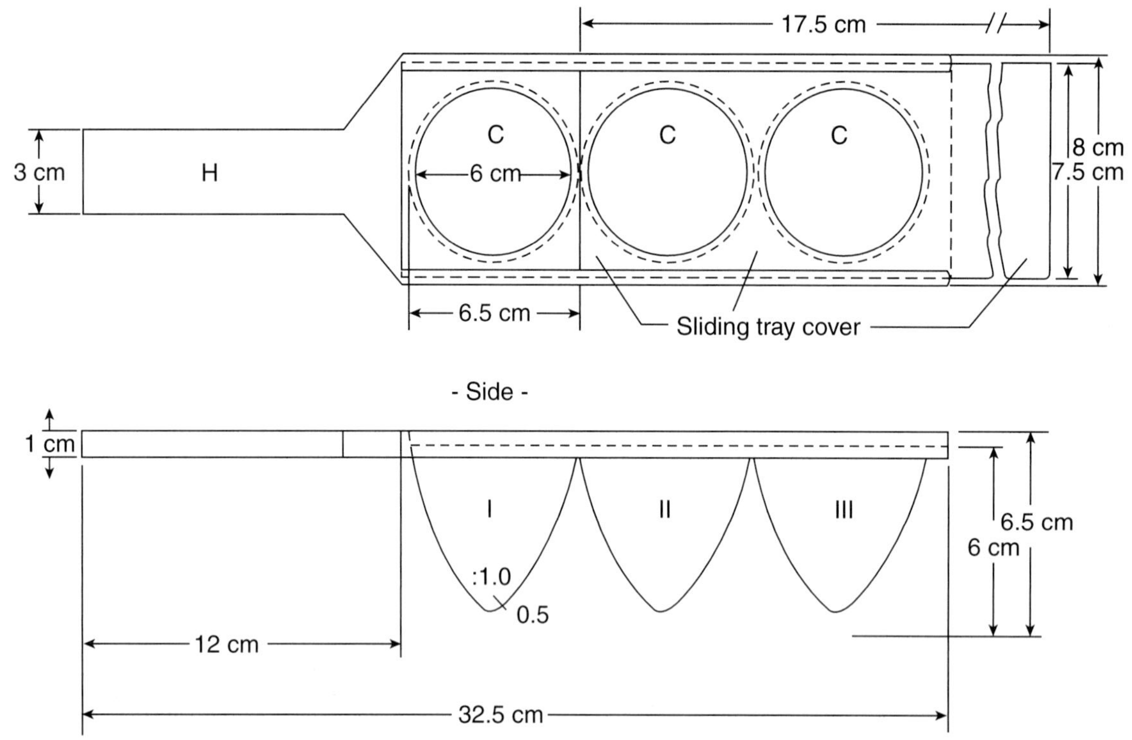

Figure 15.2 Model tray for the collection of a split ejaculate. The tray consists of three cups (C) which are attached to each other, a handle (H) and a tray cover. Each cup is oval and rounded with a cross-sectional diameter of 6 cm to allow entry of the glans penis. Approximately 1 cm from the bottom of the tray the cup comes to a point. The depth at the point of each cup is 6 cm. Volume markings are present at the bottom of each cup for easy volume measurement. Each cup is numbered to indicate the ejaculate fraction (I, II or III). The tray is made from clear plastic with no spermicidal properties. The handle is 12 cm long and rounded, with a diameter of 3 cm, so that it fits easily into the hand. The cups are covered with coverslips after ejaculation so that spillage is avoided (designed by Hafez, Zaneveld and Polakoski)

problems regarding the fertility of the subject arise, using both natural and AI. Therefore, it is necessary to develop methods of enchancing the proportion of viable cells present when AI is to be attempted using a donor semen.

Separation of human sperm

Sbracia *et al.* (1996) applied the following technique to separate human sperm:

(1) Nycodenz isotonic solution (27.6% w/v Nycodenz) is supplemented with 1 mg/ml human serum albumin.

(2) Ham's F-10 medium containing 1 mmol/l calcium lactate, 20 mmol/l $NaHCO_3$, 5 mmol/l $KHCO_3$, 0.5 mmol/l $MgSO_4$, 50 mg penicillin G, 50 mg/ml streptomycin and 1 mg/ml human serum albumin is prepared.

(3) Four aliquots of Nycodenz solution are prepared by dilution of the stock solution with the F-10 medium.

(4) The aliquots are carefully layered into 12-ml centrifuge tubes (under-layering will preserve the interface between the layers more efficiently).

(5) Liquified semen is diluted with 1–2 volumes of medium, loaded on top of the gradient and centrifuged at 350 *g* for 10 min.

(6) After centrifugation the seminal fluid is removed together with the 9.7% and 13.8% layers and any cells that had settled on the 13.8/17.9% interface; these aliquots are discarded.

(7) The 17.5% layer is collected, diluted with medium and mixed gently by inversion.

(8) After centrifugation at 350 *g* for 10 min, the supernatants are discarded and the pellets containing the motile cell fraction are gently resuspended in fresh medium.

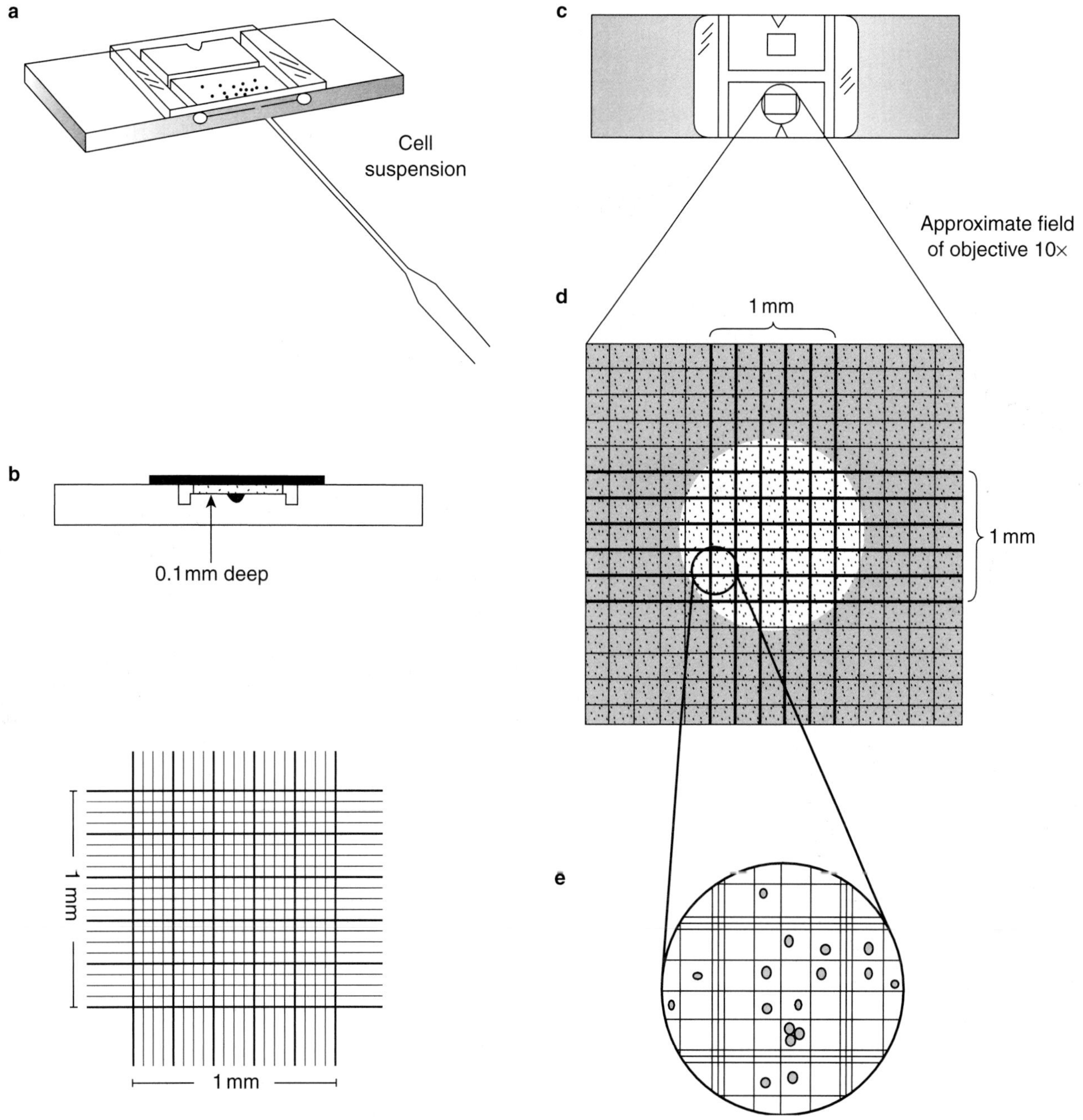

Calculation of sperm cell concentration

Establish average sperm count from two chambers.

Dimensions of the large central area of the Neubauer counting chamber are 1 mm (width) ×1 mm (height) ×0.1 mm (depth) for a volume of 0.1 mm^3. Since sperm cell concentration is normally reported in sperm number per milliliter (ml), the sperm count must be multiplied by a factor of 10 000. Since the semen is diluted at a 1 : 100 ratio prior to the sperm count, the final sperm count must be multiplied by an additional factor of 100.

Example

Sperm count of diluted semen in chamber 1 = 240
Sperm count of diluted semen in chamber 2 = 250
Average sperm count = 245
Sperm cell concentration = $245 \times 10^4 \times 10^2$/ml or 245×10^6/ml

Figure 15.3 Measurement of sperm concentration using a hemocytometer (**a**), and (**b**), the semen suspension is placed under the coverslip of the hemocytometer, (**c**) the sperm count is conducted under approximately 10× magnification, (**d**) and (**e**) sperm are counted in squares. CELL-VU® (not shown) is a disposable hemocytometer that can be used for all manual cell counting needs, from blood (full blood count) and sperm to body fluids, such as cerebral spinal fluid

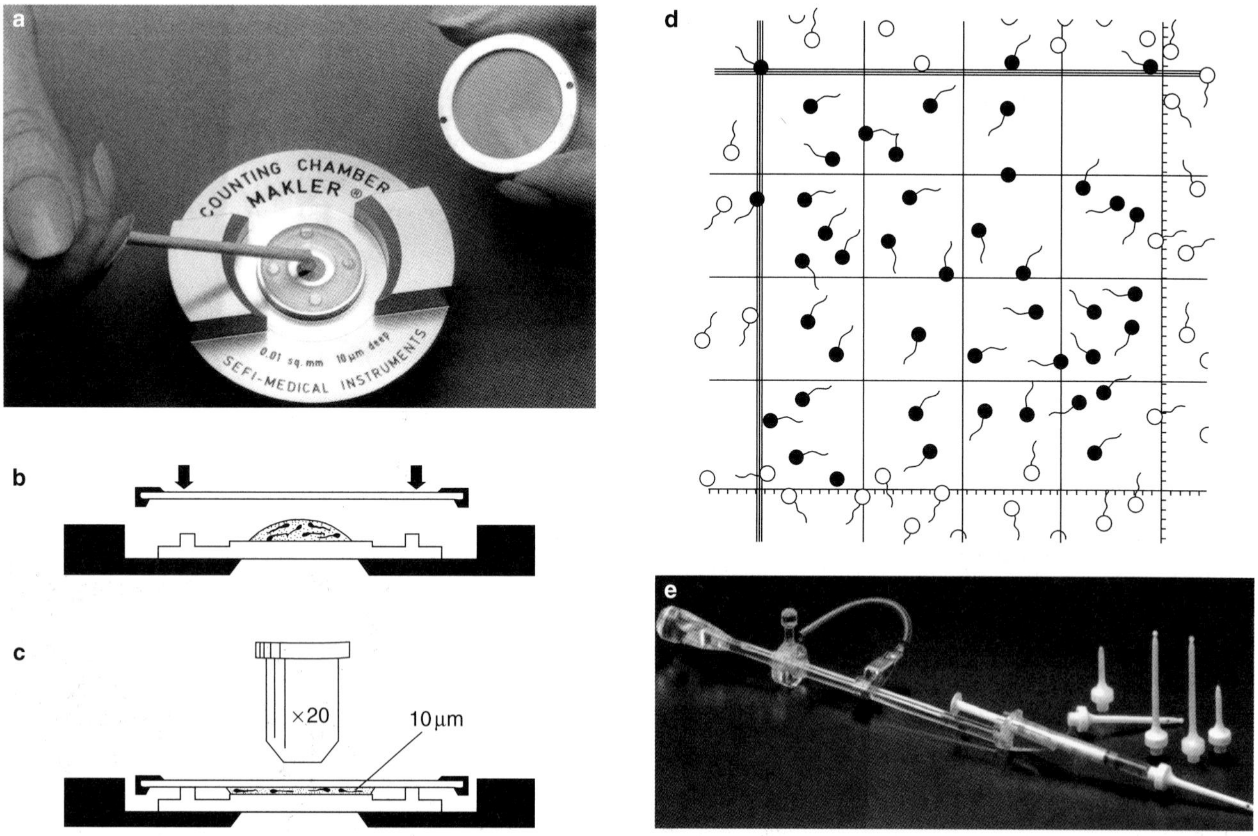

Figure 15.4 (**a**) Makler® counting chamber used for rapid semen analysis from undiluted specimens. For rapid results the number of spermatozoa counted in ten squares of the grid indicates their concentration in million/ml. The grid is built into the cover glass. There is no need to insert a grid into the microscope eyepiece. The optimal depth of 10 µm eliminates blurring and enables free sperm movement for easy motility evaluation. Sperm count, motility evaluation and morphology determination can all be undertaken in one chamber, which is economical, reusable and easily cleaned with disinfectant solution. Calibration is unnecessary and repeated use does not alter the accuracy. (**b**) Cross-section of the Makler chamber with a drop of semen placed on the center of the lower part; (**c**) when covered with the coverslip which is placed upon the four slightly elevated pins the drop becomes 10-µm thick. Sperm cells are spread in one focal plane where they can move. (**d**) One of the 0.2 × 0.2 mm squares, bounded by double lines and subdivided into 16 small squares in which sperm are counted, the sperm with white heads are ignored. (**e**) Makler insemination device designed to seal the cervix preventing the leakage of injecting semen (courtesy Sefi Medical Instruments Ltd., Haifa, Israel)

Sperm filtration

Human periovulatory mucus is an effective barrier against seminal fluid containing decapacitating factors, non-motile or dead sperm, leukocytes, prostaglandin and various infective agents. Cervical mucus is particularly selective in allowing only progressively motile sperm of normal shape and size to penetrate and migrate through the cervix.

Sperm processing methods that mimic this periovulatory-mucus selectivity may therefore favorably influence the outcome of oocyte fertilization. The simplest sperm washing techniques are those which merely concentrate the most favorable sperm and remove seminal plasma; however, these may not be adequate owing to their imprecise nature. Other sperm preparations have been developed that more closely mimic cervical mucus selectivity. Such procedures specifically recover a select population of normal motile sperm from the raw ejaculate.

Psychosocial parameters of infertile couples

Infertile couples are characterized by various psychosocial parameters, including anger, grief, guilt, frustration, depression, feelings of isolation and

Table 15.1 Sperm processing methods (Acosta and Kruger, 1996; Jeyendran, 2003; Keel and Webster, 1990; Lipschultz and Howard, 1997; Speroff *et al.*, 1999; Trounson and Gardner, 2000; WHO, 1999)

Density gradient centrifugation

Utilizing either a continuous or discontinuous density gradient in conjunction with centrifugation to separate sperm selectively based on their size, motility or density differential
Density gradient should have no or minimal osmotic effect when added to media. Gradient should also have very low viscosity to have a minimal effect on sperm sedimentation rate
Two substances are used

- colloidal silica-based density gradient
- iodixanol-based density gradient

Silica-based density gradient

'Percoll' colloidal coated with polyvinylpyrrolidone, withdrawn by manufacturer, many similar products marketed to replace Percoll: 'PureSperm' and 'PureCeption', 'Sperm Grad' and 'Enhances Plus'

Although continuous density gradients are used with normozoospermic ejaculates, they are not as effective as discontinuous density gradients. Discontinuous density gradients are prepared with either two layers consisting of 40% and 80%, or three layers consisting of 45%, 70% and 90%, respectively

Gradient centrifugation

- Preferred method for normozoospermia
  - gently layer 1.5–2.0 ml fresh liquefied semen on top of 1.0 ml 90% gradient in centrifuge tube using transfer pipette or two tubes of semen if volume is more than 2.0 ml
  - centrifugation at 600 *g* for 20 min or 30–40 min for viscous samples
  - gradient and seminal fluid removed without disturbing sperm pellet, leaving a small amount of density gradient over the pellet
  - note: if no sperm pellet is clearly visible, remove all but 0.4 ml of density gradient layer. This will allow for collection of sperm suspended in density gradient
  - using syringe, add 3–5 ml fresh medium and resuspend pellet by gently flicking tube with fingers
  - centrifugation at 600 *g* for 5 min to wash away residual silica
  - sperm pellet resuspended in 0.4 ml of media
  - sperm quality evaluated before insemination

Iodixanol

Iodixanol is currently available under trade names 'Opti Prep' and 'Accudenz'
Iodixanol, a non-toxic inert and iodinated acyclic hydrocarbon, is used for *in vitro* isolation of organelles
Sperm selected according to density differential between various ejaculate components
Motile sperm with normal morphology band together at interface between two density gradients, and thereby do not accrue into dense pellet form
Density gradient prepared by layering 1 ml 1.09 g/ml iodixanol over 1 ml
Semen placed over top of density gradient and centrifuged at 600 *g* for 20 min; upper layers containing abnormal sperm discarded
Motile sperm harvested from 1097 to 1165 interface, washed and centrifuged for 10 min at 200–400 *g*; supernatant washed sperm pellet resuspended in 0.4 ml media, sperm quality evaluated before use

Silanized colloidal silica

Used when sperm counts or motility are suboptimal
Density gradient prepared by layering 2 ml 40% silanized colloidal silica over 2 ml 80% silanized colloidal silica in centrifuge tube with lid
Semen placed up to 1.5 ml over top of density gradient
Centrifugation at 200–400 *g* for up to 30 min depending on the quality of pellet formation
2 ml 40% silanized colloidal silica/semen supernatant discarded without disturbing sperm pellet
Sperm pellet aspirated/mix with 10 ml of media in different centrifuge tube
Centrifugation for 10 min at 200–400 *g*
Supernatant discarded; sperm pellet resuspended in 0.4 ml of media

(Continued)

Table 15.1 (Continued)

Sephadex column filtration

A column made of hydrated Sephadex G15, an inert polysaccharide, in conjunction with a glass wool barrier support, separates motile and functionally intact sperm within an ejaculate; non-functional sperm adhere to the column, effectively inhibiting their migration, thereby filtering motile sperm capable of passing through the filter; glass wool could be replaced by cotton wool or any other synthetic fibers
Two types of filtration columns were developed for functional sperm separation within an ejaculate
Semen is washed using media and placed over adherence column for filtration by gravitational force using Sephadex column filtration procedure or glass column filtration procedure

Sephadex column filtration procedure

- 20% (w/v) Sephadex suspension and allowed to hydrate for a few hours at room temperature, or overnight at 5°C
- 3 ml suspension into a 3-ml disposable syringe with glass wool at the bottom, to allow media to drain by gravity, sperm are washed
- sperm concentrated in an ejaculate placed over hydrated Sephadex column and allowed to filter by gravity, column rinsed with 3 ml of media to complete filtration
- filtrate centrifuged at 200–400 *g* for 10 min, supernatant discarded, sperm pellet resuspended in 0.4 ml media
- Sephadex column is commercially available as Sperm Prep I and II

Glass wool column filter

- procedure developed to decrease semen viscosity/increase percentage sperm motility
  - tightly packed soda lime glass wool
  - filtration yielded a particularly high recovery of motile sperm, but increased number of sperm with short or broken tails;
  - filtration efficacy depends on type of glass wool: glass wool microfiber code number 112 appeared optimal (efficacy is also influenced by density of filter column) (too tightly packed vs. too loosely compressed)
- filter column prepared by inserting glass wool into a 3-ml disposable syringe to a depth of 2–3 mm
- repeated rinsing of glass wool column until no fibers observed in filtrate under microscope
- sperm washed, concentrated sperm extended to a volume of 0.4 ml
- glass wool column filter is commercially available as Cook sperm filter

powerlessness, depression, marital problems, separation and divorce. However, sporadic conception is noted in infertile couples after or during romantic holidays, after adoption, or after abandoning infertility-clinic treatment. Spontaneous pregnancy occurs in 10% of untreated infertile couples with oligozoospermic men, in patients who have been on a waiting list for *in vitro* fertilization (IVF) or intracytoplasmic sperm injection (ICSI) for 2 years. 'Psychogenic infertility' is associated with chronic and acute stress with transitory azoospermia or oligospermia.

SPERM PREPARATION FOR ASSISTED REPRODUCTIVE TECHNOLOGY

Various procedures have been applied to maximize the use of naturally ejaculated fresh semen and stored, cryopreserved semen (Tables 15.3–15.5):

(1) *In vitro* fertilization (IVF);

(2) Gamete intrafallopian transfer (GIFT);

(3) Intracytoplasmic sperm injection (ICSI);

(4) Intrauterine insemination (IUI);

(5) Epididymal sperm aspiration/testicular biopsy sperm extraction;

(6) Testicular/epididymal sperm cryopreservation;

(7) Cryopreservation of specimens with extremely low sperm count or motility.

The female reproductive tract naturally induces sperm capacitation. Thus IVF and GIFT procedures, although requiring fewer viable sperm than IUI, nonetheless require *in vitro* means of capacitation.

The various techniques of sperm preparation for assisted reproduction are directed to the separation of sperm from seminal fluid and from other cellular components of the semen as well as to the concentration of the motile sperm population. The most frequently used techniques are: sperm 'washing' in various media; 'swim-up' or 'swim-down' preparations, in which

Table 15.2 Sperm collection methods (Acosta and Kruger, 1996; Jeyendran, 2003; Keel and Webster, 1990; Lipschultz and Howard, 1997; Speroff *et al.*, 1999; Trounson and Gardner, 2000; WHO, 1999)

Testicular epididymal sperm extraction (TESE) procedure

Patient, in supine position, shaved minimally and under anesthesia, testis grasped between cupped hands to make a 2–3-cm transverse incision in scrotum; incision deepened through dartos and tunica vaginalis layers to expose testis

Hemostasis is induced by monopolar electrocautery

Testes palpated to diagnose any pathological blood supplies to testes medially/posterior, then squeezed forcing some tubules to extrude through the opening in tunica albuginea; tubules are removed with curved tenotomy scissors, curved upwards

Epididymovasostomy

Recommended surgical procedure when epididymal obstruction is evident, or in cases where an initial vasovasostomy does not result in patency, only after scrotal exploration to decide which procedures are most appropriate in patients with suspected primary vasal obstruction, a thorough medical examination/evaluation should be undertaken before any procedures

Several decisive factors can facilitate accurate diagnosis

Epididymal fullness accompanied by mild tenderness suggests secondary epidermal rupture or hydraulic 'blowout'

Definitive epididymal blockage diagnosis is typically impossible without epididymal exploratory surgery

Complete fertility evaluation should be performed prior to surgery

Testicular fine-needle aspiration (TFNA)

Outpatient procedure effective for obstructive zoospermia patients, with high sperm recovery rates

Main limitations include lack of visual confirmation and increased likelihood of missing entire spermatogenesis areas in non-obstructive azoospermia

0.5% lidocaine used to perform spermatic cord/scrotal skin block

Testicle immobilized to hold skin taut over testes, 23-gauge, sharp, beveled fine needle inserted 2.5 cm, attached to 10-ml syringe, into anterior portion of midpole testes

Needle advanced back/forth with gentle back-pressure on plunger until aspirate enters tubing (aspirate is off-white or opaque)

When adequate fluid is collected in tubing, needle is withdrawn with maintenance of suction during withdrawal

Tubing flushed with modified human tubal fluid supplemented with 0.3% bovine serum albumin, then transferred into test-tube for further processing or cryopreservation

TFNA mapping

Employed to locate heterogeneous sperm production in non-obstructed azoospermia

Used to diagnose sperm presence/determine sperm production location for subsequent site-directed TESE retrievals

Presence of sperm confirmed microscopically: slides fixed with Papanicolaou, stained with undiluted olivine blue for 15 s; bright-field microscopy indicates the presence of sperm with tails, systematic findings from TFNA at different sites of testes to construct testes map

Testicular micro-dissection (TMD)

Procedure performed to maximize sperm retrieval from azoospermic patients by microdissection to locate seminiferous tubules which appear to be engorged, a visual sign of ongoing spermatogenesis

In presence of spermatogenesis, large quantities of testicular tissue are easily harvested

In presence of sperm, procedure is repeated and sperm collected for cryopreservation for ART

Tunica albuginea opened for 3–4 cm using micro knife along axis direction of testicle, tubules gently teased with blunt forceps to identify areas of engorged tubules to be removed with curved tenotomy scissors

Postmortem sperm retrieval

Postmortem sperm retrieval is relatively straightforward but the legal ramifications are complex

Different procedures are employed: transpelvic seminal-vesiculectomy, simple vasectomy, TFNA, PESA, orchiectomy and electroejaculation (morally acceptable/ethically sound, practical/highly effective)

ART, artificial reproductive technologies; PESA, percutaneous epididymal sperm aspiration

Table 15.3 Sperm processing procedures for intrauterine insemination (IUI) (Acosta and Kruger; 1996; Hafez *et al.*, 2003; Hafez and Hafez, 2003; Jeyendran, 2003)

Sperm migration

This procedure is similar to the concept of sperm migration through ovulatory cervical mucus

Motile healthy sperm swim from one medium to another, whereas non-motile sperm and sperm with morphological anomalies have greater difficulty to swim through

Sufficient population of viable sperm are filtered for use in IUI and *in vitro* fertilization (IVF)

Swim-down

Semen samples or washed sperm are layered over a heavier, more viscous media. Sperm migrate into/towards gravitational force, 'swimming down', thereby separating motile sperm from the remaining sample, which is left above

Sperm washed and concentrated

4.0 ml media with either 7.5% bovine serum albumin or 20% human serum albumin is prepared

2.0 ml prepared media placed into each of two centrifuge tubes, 0.5 ml washed sperm layered on top of prepared media

Incubation vertically for 30 min based on initial sperm concentration/motility

Aspiration to discard upper overlay

Centrifugation at 300 *g* for 10 min, pellet resuspended in 0.4 ml final volume for insemination

Swim-up

Without centrifugation

- light, low-viscosity media layered over the semen
- sperm naturally migrate up against gravity leaving behind non-dynamic contaminants within the sample
- semen sample dispensed in 2 round-bottom tubes with lid or screw-cap
- supernatant carefully decanted without disturbing sperm pellet, 0.5–1.0 ml of media gently added over pellet
- incubation for 30–50 min (high concentrated sperm requires a shorter incubation period), with tubes at 45° angle
- upper supernatant gently aspirated into sterile centrifuge tube
- sperm pellet resuspended in proportional volume of media
- sperm exposed to antigravitational relative centrifugal fold

With centrifugation

- 0.5–1.0 ml semen gently placed under 1 ml of media in tube
- tube placed at 45° angle incubated at 37°C for 10–30 min or until medium appears cloudy
- upper supernatant aspirated into sterile centrifuge tube which is centrifuged at 300 *g* for 10 min
- sperm pellet resuspended in 0.4 ml of medium for insemination
- two commercially available products come as complete kits, which incorporate all necessary items for insemination
    (1) sperm select system employs a high-purity preparation of 3000 kDa sodium hyaluronate, a naturally occurring polysaccharide in ovulatory cervical mucus. Semen placed below a layer of hyaluronate solution incubated at 37° for 45 min, fine-mesh structure of hyaluronate system allows migration of motile sperm and filtering out cellular debris and immotile defective sperm
    (2) ZSC II combines the swim-up/swim-down techniques to yield a greater number of high-quality, morphologically normal, motile sperm; medium is layered over the semen, and sperm are allowed to migrate for 45 min to 1 h

the motile sperm population migrates away from the non-motile elements of semen; and centrifugation of sperm through various density gradients exploiting the higher density of mature sperm that completed cytoplasm extrusion during spermatogenesis (Figures 15.5 and 15.6).

Concerns about the adverse 'iatrogenic' effects of sperm preparation techniques have focused on three issues regarding the choice of sperm preparation media, the mechanical damage owing to centrifugation/resuspension, and the propagation of lipid peroxidation during sperm pelleting owing

Table 15.4 Assisted reproductive technology procedures (Acosta and Kruger, 1996; Hafez *et al.*, 2003; Hafez and Hafez, 2003; Jeyendran, 2003)

In vitro sperm capacitation
Once decapacitation factor(s) present in seminal plasma have been removed from the sperm, they may be artificially induced to undergo capacitation
Capacitation incubation time might actually be hastened by using the correct type of media with *in vitro* fertilization (IVF) and gamete intrafallopian transfer (GIFT)
Several commercially available media have been used
10 medium
human tubal fluid medium and modified human tubal fluid (MHTF) medium
preimplantation stage one (P-1) medium
Protein supplements are commercially available
Synthetic serum substitute (SSS)
Human serum albumin
When standard sperm sources are impractical, visible viable sperm can be extracted directly from the male reproductive tract
In certain cases sperm cannot undergo capacitation due to idiopathic infertility or unexplained intrinsic sperm factor(s)
Thus sperm can be treated with TEST yolk media
IVF
Sperm processed as for intrauterine insemination (IUI)
Prepared sample is suspended in IVF media
Sperm concentration is evaluated since some merely 50 000–100 000 sperm are needed
Sample volume sufficient to deliver these numbers can then be calculated
Motile sperm are then added to the oocyte
Testicular biopsy sperm extraction
Tissue placed in large, sterile Petri dish with 2–3 ml MHTF containing 5% SSS, on warming stage under a dissection microscope
Seminiferous tubules are gently squeezed with sterile, watch-maker forceps to isolate tubular content
Aliquots are periodically examined for motile sperm until at least 0.1 million total sperm are found
Optimal recovery is > 1–2 million motile sperm
Tubular contents are collected into centrifuge tube for cryopreservation
Remainder of biopsy is placed into sterile glass tissue grinder with 2 ml MHTF containing 5% SSS, with gentle grinding with pestle with large clearance to avoid cell shearing
Epididymal sperm aspiration
Equipment required: phase-contrast microscope, Makler sperm counting chamber, 20 ml MHTF containing 5% SSS (prewarmed to 37°C), sterile, disposable transfer pipettes, individually wrapped 5-ml tissue culture tubes
Medium preloaded into a syringe aspirated into tissue culture tube
Counting chamber loaded with aspirated aliquot and examined microscopically
Sperm motility/concentration evaluated and data given to surgical staff
Specimen transported to IVF lab maintaining temperature close to 37°C until processed for cryopreservation
Cryopreservation of testicular epididymal sperm
Specimens pooled in centrifuge tube, centrifuge at 350 *g* for 5 min
Supernatant decanted/resuspended pellet in MHTF containing 5% SSS

(Continued)

Table 15.4 (Continued)

Sperm concentration/motility evaluated
Aliquot 0.1–1.0 million motile sperm into each 0.8-ml vial
MHTF added supplemented with SSS to bring final volume
Mixing with equal volume of freezing medium
Cryopreserve specimen with glycerol
Sperm stored in liquid nitrogen at −196°C
GIFT
Processing similar to that for sperm IVF
Whereas sperm number is fixed for IVF, sample volume is fixed for GIFT
Final adjusted concentration should allow the minimal requisite of 100 000 motile sperm to be loaded into catheter
Intracytoplasmic sperm injection (ICSI)
Sperm processing similar to that as for IVF
If insufficient sperm result, sperm resuspended within minimal media volume
Small drop of sperm suspension placed under minimal oil in a culture dish, incubation at 37°C for 5–10 min
Motile sperm removed from edge of drop and transferred to another dish in preparation for ICSI
In cases of azoospermia or severe oligozoospermia sperm are aspirated or extracted directly from male reproductive tract

Table 15.5 Physiological action and clinical applications of products (courtesy Nidacon International AB, Goteborg, Sweden)

Product	*Physiological action*	*Clinical application*
Sperm CryoProtect™	Cryopreserving human sperm	Freezing solutions containing egg yolk, high concentrations of glycerol can be toxic to sperm; thus, it is free from egg yolk and contains a reduced concentration of glycerol. It is an optimized solution for protecting human sperm from damaging freezing/thawing effects. The solution contains osmotically active ingredients to reduce intracellular water, and cryoprotectants to reduce injury caused by ice crystal formation. Human serum albumin is added to serve as a cryoprotectant, counteract the detrimental effects of reactive oxygen species (ROS), and prevent sperm aggregation/adherence to laboratory equipment It can be also used as a cryoprotectant for untreated ejaculates. However, when untreated ejaculates are used, the number of motile sperm post-thawing will be reduced Seminal plasma, a source of prostaglandins, ROS and pathogens, should be removed from the sperm suspension before intrauterine insemination (IUI)
PureSperm®100	Improved stock suspension	Improved formulation so the gradient works even more efficiently and cleanly than before PureSperm® stock suspension should be diluted with PureSperm® Buffer to provide layers of different densities required for the gradient Sperm pellets are washed in PureSperm® Wash. These three products, PureSperm 100 diluted with PureSperm Buffer, and PureSperm Wash, form an optimized system to prepare sperm for assisted reproductive technologies (ART)
Ready Swim™	Solution for optimized swim-up	Balanced salt solution that maximizes sperm survival during 'swim-up' *In vivo*, motile sperm quickly migrate from liquefying semen into the cervix, thereby removing themselves from the presence of both seminal plasma and ROS arising from cell debris. *In vitro*, this process is imitated by allowing sperm to swim into a layer of medium, thereby separating them from remainder of ejaculate

(Continued)

Table 15.5 (Continued)

Product	*Physiological action*	*Clinical application*
		Ionically balanced solution to avoid premature hyperactivation. Sudden pH and osmolatity changes during the sperm movement from semen sample to the fertilization medium are minimized. Avoiding premature hyperactivation conserves energy resources and improves fertilization potential
		During swim-up, motile sperm move away from extraneous cells and damaging factors in the ejaculate: ROS/seminal plasma. Damage to sperm DNA and structural molecules caused by ROS is minimized by removal of immature sperm/lymphocytes, key sources of ROS
		Motile sperm separated from immotile sperm, epithelial cells/cell debris. When unopened can be stored for 1 year at room temperature. The use of borosilicate Type I glass bottles ensures that Na^+ ions do not leach into the preparation. This prevents any changes in Na^+ levels and osmolality which can impair sperm survival and function, and cause premature hyperactivation
PureSperm® Wash	Washing sperm pellet	A balanced salt solution containing EDTA/human serum albumin. Designed specifically for washing sperm pellet obtained from a PureSperm gradient
	Rapid method to prepare human sperm	'Swim-up' does not remove sperm with abnormal morphology or damaged DNA, and does not separate out bacteria and viruses from the sperm preparation. There is commercially available 'Speedkit', a kit containing sufficient sperm preparation material for five patients, together with glass centrifuge tubes, five semen collection tubes, one for each patient, and empty tubes to balance the centrifuge rotor
		PureSperm is a single layer of colloid, ready-to-use in the centrifuge tube: medium added to 1.5 ml of patient semen and centrifuged. The sperm pellet is then transferred to the centrifuge tube containing SpermAssist™ which is a washing solution and maintenance medium. After centrifugation, most of the supernatant is removed. The sperm pellet is then resuspended in the last 0.5 ml of the washing solution, creating a sperm preparation ready to transfer directly to the patient. Instructions included in pack insert
Sperm Catch™	Used for ICSI	A natural alternative to polyvinyl plastic for slowing sperm ICSI
		The only products available for slowing sperm motility contained polyvinylpyrrolidone; injecting this artificial product into the oocyte along with the sperm may cause damage to acrosomal, mitochondria plasma membranes and chromosomal DNA
		It contains only substances normally found in mammalian reproductive tract, it slows sperm, and mimics the naturally occurring sequence of events during IVF
NidOil™	Selected for its purity and suitability for use with embryos	Some procedures for IVF and ICSI use an oil overlay to protect small volumes of culture medium from evaporation in the incubator and to help dampen the effects of sudden changes in temperature, gas saturation and pH. Likewise, gamete manipulation under the microscope requires the gametes to be held in small drops of medium under oil, to maintain a constant environment within the culture medium
		NidOil, a paraffin oil product designed for gametes/embryos is neither sticky nor too viscous, to facilitate pipetting, but is sufficiently viscous to prevent movement of drops of media around culture dish
Sperm Assist™	For IUI	HEPES-buffered salt solution formulated specifically to resuspend sperm for IUI; with ionic balance to meet sperm requirements avoiding premature hyperactivation
		Sperm survival/fertilizing ability and pregnancy rates improved, avoiding media which cause premature hyperactivation
		Does not contain any coloring or preservatives, which can be toxic to sperm
		Used to suspend sperm prepared on a PureSperm® gradient, (made from either PureSperm® Buffer or ready-to-use PureSperm® 40 + PureSperm® 80) and washed with PureSperm® Wash gives optimal results. Yield of motile sperm is maximized, sperm survival is increased

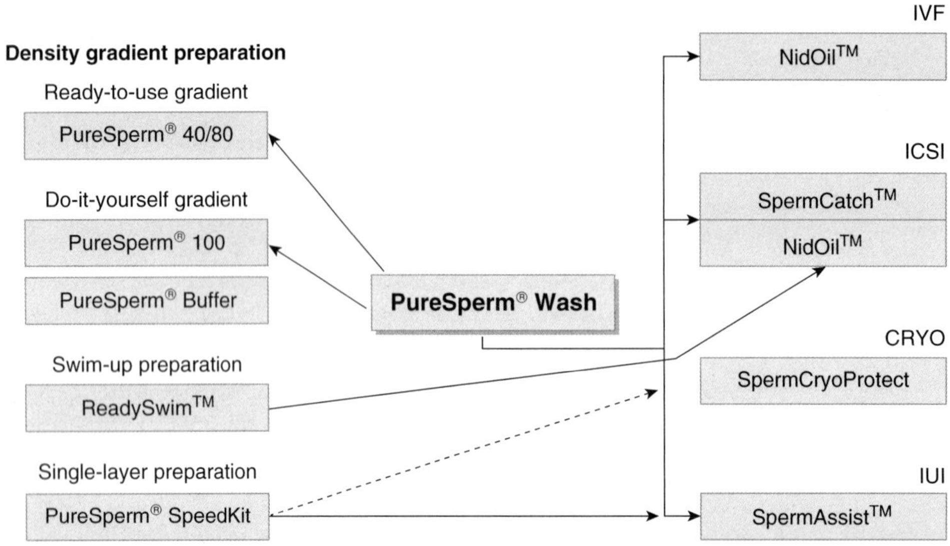

Figure 15.5 PureSperm® product range that uses integrated and optimized sperm preparation for assisted reproductive technology (Nidacon International AB, Goteborg, Sweden). IVF, *in vitro* fertilization; ICSI, intracytoplasmic sperm injection; CRYO, cryoprotectant; IUI, intrauterine insemination

to the close vicinity of already-damaged leukocytes and spermatozoa that may generate reactive oxygen species.

Sperm processing for intrauterine insemination

Several methods have been applied to separate and eliminate decapacitation factor(s) and contaminants from the seminal plasma. These may be in the form of cellular debris (gelatinous pieces, epithelial cells), bacteria, mycoplasmas, chlamydia, trichomonads and various blood components (leukocytes/erythrocytes). This is accomplished through filtering the motile sperm, and recovery of the most viable sperm. The three methods that are reliable, repeatable and simple to perform are sperm migration, column adherence and density gradient centrifugation (swim-up and swim-down).

Gamete interaction and intracytoplasmic sperm injection

Extensive investigations have been conducted on the micromanipulation techniques used to enhance fertilization and successful pregnancy in sheep and goats with specific emphasis on direct sperm injection into oocytes. Exogenous oocyte activation was not mandatory for fertilization, and subsequent normal fetal development. Several techniques have been applied for domestic and exotic mammalian species.

Gamete interaction involves recognition between a sperm receptor located in the plasma membrane and an oocyte receptor located in the zona pellucida (ZP3). ZP3 induces the acrosome reaction. Closer interaction occurs between ZP2 and an inner acrosomal membrane receptor. Certain acrosomal proteins are necessary for this process. The acrosome is necessary for the sorting and correct organization of plasma membrane proteins. Immotile sperm used for ICSI give results comparable to those of motile sperm if the initial ejaculate contained $\geq$20% viable sperm and specific criteria were used to select the immotile sperm.

Testicular sperm processing method

Little is known about processing testicular sperm in men. Figure 15.7 shows the cystoscopic view after transurethral resection of the ejaculatory ducts, the appearance of vasal anastomosis after inner-layer suturing, the epididymis after epididymal tunic aperture creation, and the longitudinally or transversely incised scrotum.

SEMEN PROCESSING PRODUCTS (TABLE 15.5)

Several commercially available products are optimized for purification of human sperm for assisted reproductive technology. All batches are strictly tested to assure high levels of sterility, low endotoxin levels

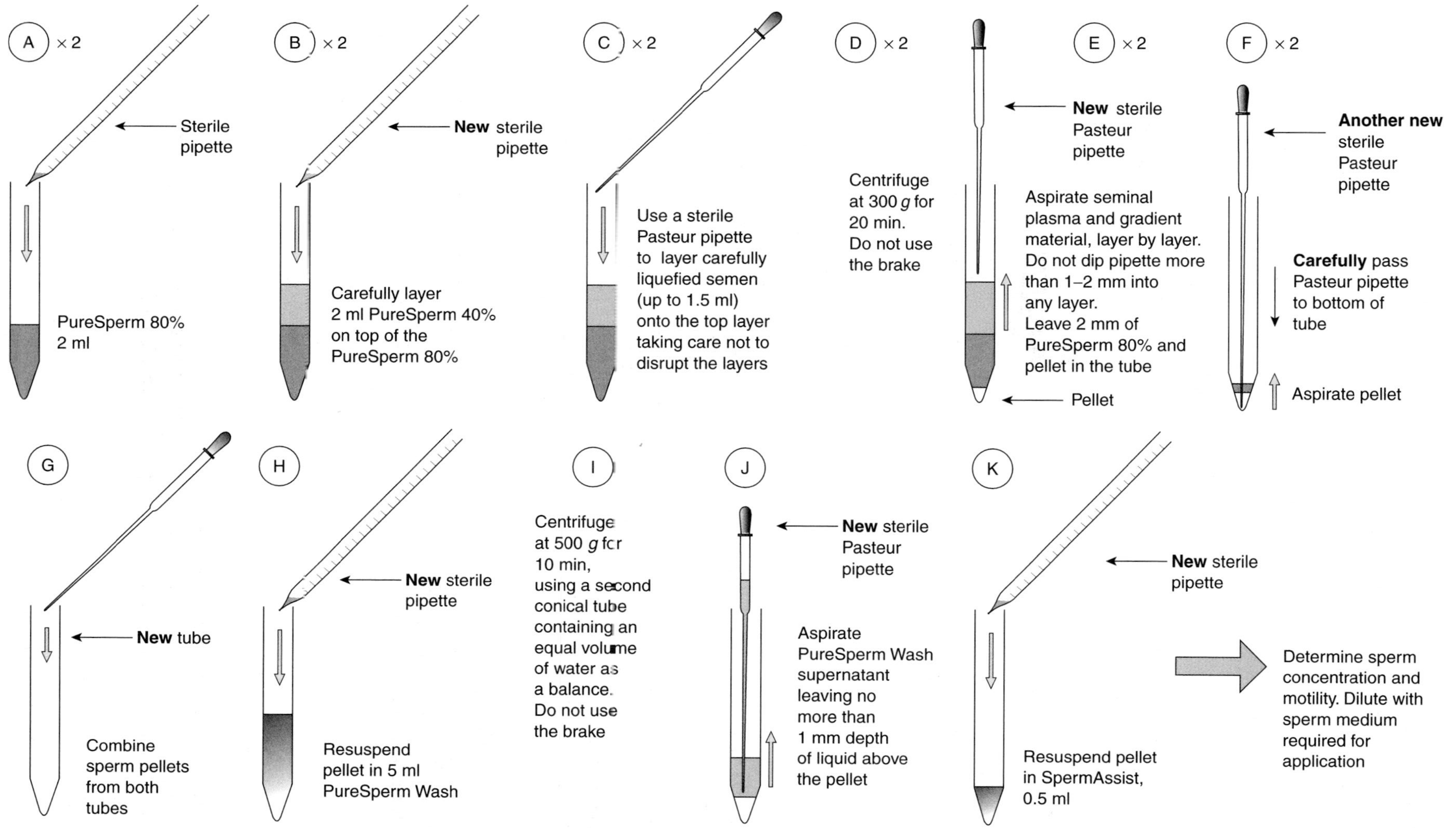

Figure 15.6 Preparation of PureSperm® density gradients for human sperm. It is recommended to prepare two gradients for each ejaculate in steps A–F (Nidacon International AB, Goteborg, Sweden)

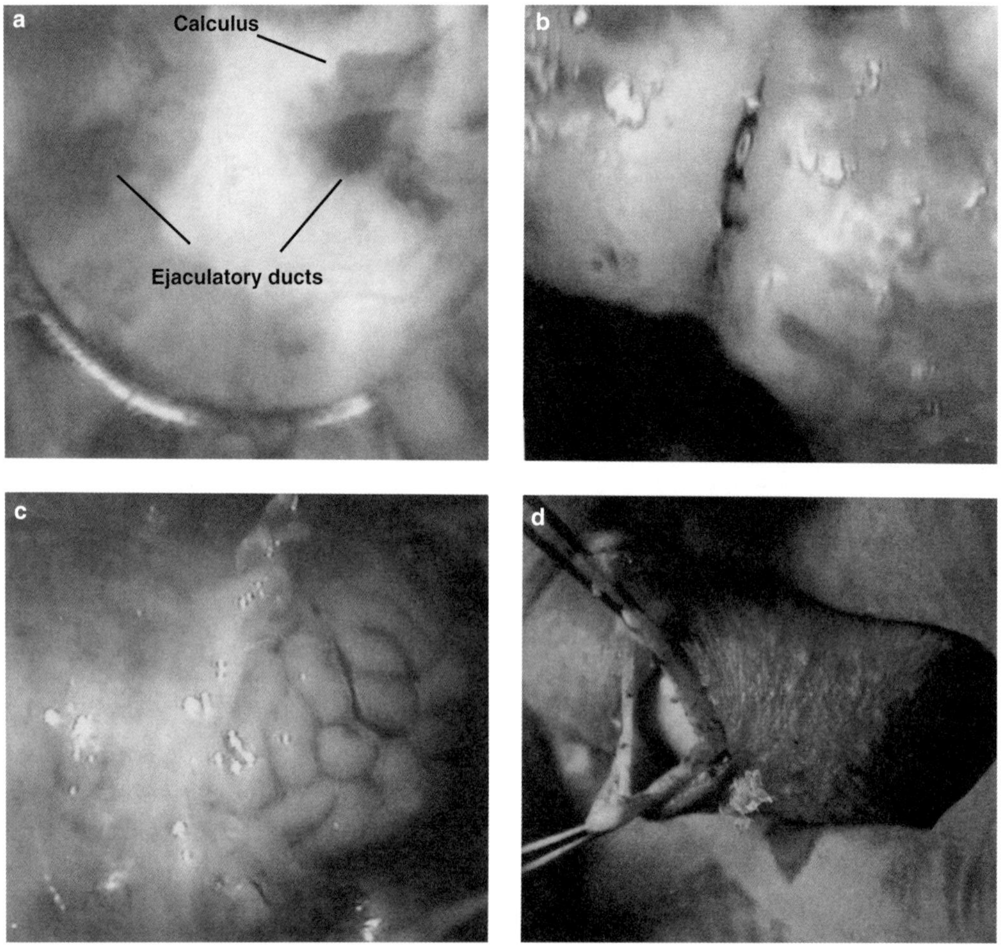

Figure 15.7 Testicular sperm processing methods. (**a**) Cystoscopic view after transurethral resection of the ejaculatory ducts, showing obstructing ductal calculi within lumens, bilaterally. (**b**) Appearance of the same vasal anastomosis after inner-layer 10-0 nylon sutures have been tied and cut. The inner layer has been completed, and the anastomosis is watertight. (**c**) View of the epididymis after epididymal tunic aperture creation. Note pearly white and dilated tubule appearance. (**d**) Scrotum longitudinally or transversely incised. Tunica vaginalis longitudinally deepened. Tunica albuginea is exposed surface. From Brannigan *et al.*, 2003, with permission

and optimal performance. Ready-to-use products, such as 40% and 80% dilutions (PureSperm® 40 and PureSperm® 80, respectively), save preparation time in the laboratory. PureSperm 40 and PureSperm 80 are formulated to minimize sudden pH and osmolality changes during the transition of sperm from the semen sample to the fertilization medium. This helps to avoid premature hyperactivation and improves the fertilization potential. They maintain a pH between 7.4 and 7.8 at room temperature and at 37°C, thus providing suitable conditions for good sperm motility, survival time and fertilization potential. The preparation contains glucose as a usable energy substrate for normal cell metabolism and sperm function.

Nicotine (systematic name, 5-(*N*-2,3-dihydroxypropylacetamido)-2,4,6-tri-iodo-*N*,*N'*bis(2,3-dihydroxypropyl)isophthalamide) is a non-ionic iodinated gradient medium which readily dissolves in water to produce non-toxic autoclavable solutions. To separate viable cells in a morphologically intact state by isopycnic centrifugation, it is necessary to use a gradient medium that provides gradients of an appropriate density/tonicity. It is important to maintain isotonic conditions throughout the gradient; otherwise, the cells will change in volume and, therefore, density, and large changes in tonicity across the gradient can damage the cells irreversibly. The properties of iodinated gradient media make them suitable for separating cells and sperm (Ford and Rockwood, 1982).

'Accudenz' facilitates a higher rate of recovery of sperm and motile sperm. Sperm motility is lower in Accudenz compared to Percoll pellets; however, the long-term retention of sperm motility is substantially improved in Accudenz at 24 h. Sperm activation status monitored by chlortetracycline fluorescence indicated that after 4 h of incubation the incidence of fully acrosome-reacted spermatozoa in the Accudenz versus Percoll pellets was $6.2 \pm 0.3\%$ versus $13.1 \pm 1.0\%$, a 100% increase in Percoll.

Accudenz yields a higher concentration of motile sperm with improved retention of motility, velocity and acrosomal integrity and without an increase of sperm with diminished cellular maturity.

TEST yolk treatment

TEST (TES and Tris buffer) yolk treatment enhances sperm quality by increasing the ability of sperm to penetrate zona-free hamster oocytes. Such treatments also enhance the ability of sperm to bind to the human zona pellucida, further improving IVF outcome. These sperm enhancement functions have been substantiated (and with no apparent deleterious effects on sperm). To enhance fertilization potential further, the treated sperm sample can be additionally processed using column adherence methods.

SPERM PREPARATION EQUIPMENT

Table 15.6 shows the equipment, separation media and techniques for sperm preparation and IVF.

Table 15.6 Equipment, supplies, media and techniques for sperm preparation and *in vitro* fertilization (IVF)

Routine basic equipment for IVF	
Dissecting, inverted and light microscopes	
Incubator with accurately regulated temperature and CO_2	
Centrifuge for sperm preparation	
Warmed stages or surfaces for culture manipulations	
Refrigerator/freezer	
Dry heat oven for drying and sterilizing	
Disposable general supplies	
Non-toxic tissue culture	
Culture vessels	
Needles, catheters, oocyte aspiration/embryo	
Glass pipettes (soaked/rinsed with tissue culture media)	
Equipment for sperm preparation	
Semen sterile collection 60-ml pot	
Counting chamber (Makler, Sefi Medical Instruments or Horwell hemocytometer	
Centrifuge with swing-out rotation	
Microscope slides/coverslips	
Disposable test tubes: 4 ml, 10 ml	
Culture media: MediCult Percoll Medium, Sil-Select (MICROM)	
Glass Pasteur pipettes	
Disposable pipettes: 1, 5, 10 ml	
Spirit burner plus methanol or gas Bunsen burner	
Supply of liquid nitrogen/storage Dewars	
Sperm preparation	
Overlay and swim-up, multiple overlay	
Discontinuous buoyant density gradients	
mini	95/70/50%
two-step	40/80, 45/90, 47.5/5/95%
one-step	95%
High-speed centrifugation and washing sedimentation under oil, 'fishing' with micromanipulator swim-out under oil	
Manufacturing companies for IVF media	
Scandinavian IVF Science AB, Molndalsvagen 30A, P.O. Box 1410, Gothenburg, Sweden	
Menezo B2: Bio-Merieux, France	
Ham's F-10, EBSS: Flow Laboratories, UK	
HTF: Irvine Scientific, USA	
Bio-Care International, San Diego, CA 92121, USA	

Real-time sperm separation Wang tubes (Figures 15.8 and 15.9)

This system encompasses the application of newly designed separation tubes and innovative methods. Several biological and biophysical phenomena, and basic and theoretical principles, have been applied in the real-time sperm separation system:

(1) Non-pathological spermatozoa do not transfer microorganisms.

(2) The motility pattern and swim-up capacity of infected sperm or pathological sperm are limited or disturbed.

(3) The faster the sperm migrate and the greater distance they cover, the more normal are the sperm.

(4) Spermatozoa that are different from what is expected for their stage of development and sperm with morphological or physiological disorders can be identified by characteristics such as different migration velocities and distances.

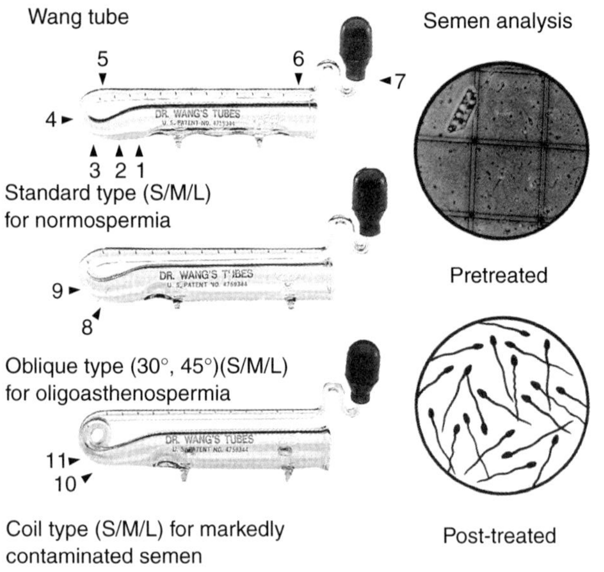

Figure 15.8 Wang tube system is the most effective method of obtaining a high-degree of sperm isolation and purification, which separates motile sperm from microorganisms, highly motile cells from less-motile or non-motile cells in a mixed sample, and double-stranded (normal) from single-stranded (abnormal) DNA sperm, while retaining an adequate volume of tissue culture medium, with an absence of cell debris, seminal plasma or other impurities in semen

(5) Highly motile sperm can be easily separated from other live cells such as leukocytes, red blood cells, lymphocytes and cellular debris.

(6) Tissue culture medium has a low viscosity, which does not favor the adhesion of the microorganisms to highly motile sperm.

(7) The specific gravity of a sperm pellet is greater than that of the tissue culture medium, so that the pellet will fall steadily to the bottom of a Wang tube, allowing the motile sperm to migrate.

(8) The velocity and direction of sperm migration are quite different from the random active or passive movement of microorganisms.

(9) The Wang tube system is a multidirectional challenge/migration (MCM) technique. It is not just a simple swim-up technique. The spermatozoa are allowed to migrate along multiple directions and pass through carefully designed, computerized curvatures of critical angles. The challenge facilitates the selection of high-quality sperm.

(10) These formulae are based on the theories of Bernoulli's equation and application of hydrodynamics.

GENETIC PARAMETERS

Gender selection

An Egyptian myth relates how the goddess Isis was once compelled by the fertility god Osiris to make all her progeny male by sorcery. This idea has not been entirely discarded and has recently re-emerged as advances have been made in separating X from Y spermatozoa. With increasing success, sex preselection has become a matter of general concern. Khatame *et al.* (1999) evaluated the success of gender selection using semen samples separated by a modified swim-up technique. They retrospectively compared the gender outcome of two treatments (A and B) for either male or female offspring with those who conceived spontaneously. The treatment groups consisted of 52 pregnancies for couples who conceived with the separation technique. Of these 52 participants, 15 desired female offspring and were placed into treatment group A and 37 desired male offspring and were placed into treatment group B. The control groups consisted of 162 women who presented with initial consultation for gender selection and conceived spontaneously. Control group A consisted of 80 women who initially chose female offspring, and control group B consisted of 82 participants who initially chose male offspring. In treatment group A, one timed IUI was performed using the bottom 0.5 ml of the separated semen on cycle days 12–14, when the follicle was 18–22 mm. Patients in this group were also administered clomiphene citrate and human chorionic gonadotropin. In treatment group B, one timed IUI was performed with the top 0.5 ml of the separated semen, when the follicle was 18–22 mm. The gender outcome of the pregnancies in the treatment and control groups was evaluated based on the known desired gender. The success rate for conceiving a female child after intervention (treatment group A) was 86.7% effective ($p=0.0002$) as compared to control group A. Couples seeking a male child (treatment group B) were 89.2% effective ($p=0.0002$) as compared to control group B. It would appear that the modified swim-up method with additional monitoring results in statistically significant gender preselection.

Chromosomal anomalies and genetic deletions

Genetic infertility includes chromosomal anomalies, genetic deletions such as Y deletion and cystic fibrosis.

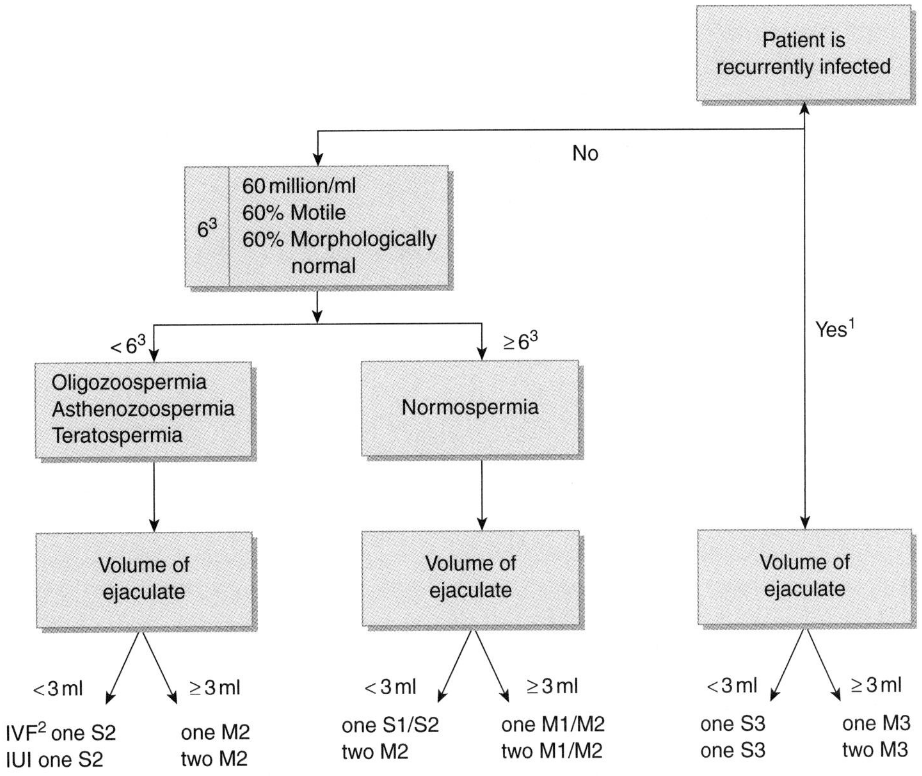

Figure 15.9 Flow chart for selection of correct Wang tube. (1) More than six white blood cells in raw semen under high-power field; (2) selection of Wang tube for gamete intrafallopian transfer, zygote intrafallopian transfer or tubal embryo transfer is identical to that for *in vitro* fertilization (IVF); (3) more Wang tubes are suggested for more sperm preparations. IUI, intrauterine insemination

Oligozoospermic men have a high risk (5%) of sex chromosome and autosome anomalies. There are some 250 genes pertinent to spermatogenesis on the autosomal chromosomes. Most miscarriage/pregnancy failure in older women is a result of chromosome anomalies arising in the embryo. Most common genetic disorders associated with primary infertility in females are chromosome anomalies, e.g. Turner's syndrome (monosomy X) and Stein–Leventhal syndrome (polycystic ovarian disease). Causes of genetic male infertility include Klinefelter's syndrome, X-autosome reciprocal translocation, Y-chromosome microdeletion, congenital absence of the vas deferens, cystic fibrosis and obstructive azoospermia in Young's syndrome. Successful pregnancy can be initiated in most of these syndromes by oocyte donation, ICSI or related assisted reproductive technologies. Disorders associated with specific potential dysgenic outcome of ICSI include sex chromosome numerical anomalies (45X, 47XXY), Y-chromosome microdeletion and cystic fibrosis.

16

Micromanipulation and assisted conception

MICROMANIPULATION OF OVA AND BLASTOCYSTS (TABLES 16.1 AND 16.2)

Various methods have been employed for embryo sexing, such as separation on the basis of sexual dimorphism, detection of sex chromatin mass, fluorescence *in situ* hybridization, detection of the HY antigen and use of a Y-specific DNA probe. Several processes are involved in nuclear transfer including use of a particle gun, sperm-mediated gene transfer, injection of the pronuclei, retroviral-mediated gene transfer, injection of the oocyte cytoplasm and germinal vesicle gene injection.

Zona pellucida

The zona pellucida, an extracellular lipoprotein matrix, serves several functions during the induction of the sperm acrosome reaction, which is stimulated by exposure of sperm to intact or digested zonae, during cleavage, and hatching of the blastocyst. Release (hatching) of the blastocyst from the zona pellucida occurs in the uterus 6 days postovulation (Figure 16.1). Several techniques have been used for embryo micromanipulation (Figure 16.2). The success of the techniques depends on the use of agar gel to seal incisions made in the zona pellucida during micromanipulation. The agar protects the blastomeres from damage by uterine secretions and leukocytes until the embryo has developed sufficiently to survive *in utero* without a zona.

Zona drilling/cracking

Zona drilling may be complete or partial zona drilling (PZD) (Figure 16.3). Zona drilling is accomplished mechanically or by local application of a zona solvent such as acid Tyrode's or alpha-chymotrypsin solution using a microneedle. In the case of PZD the zona is mechanically torn with a glass needle or cracked by piercing it with a glass holding pipette. PZD is usually followed by microinsemination (Figure 16.4). For 'cracking' of the blastocyst, two fine glass hooks are controlled by a micromanipulator. In blastomere transfer, part of the cell, specifically the nuclei, or whole cells are transferred. Fusion of cytoblast/karyoplasms with host cells is inhibited by electrofusion. For blastocyst biopsy one or two blastomeres are removed (for preimplantation diagnosis of sex or genetic anomalies) allowing the remaining embryos to develop.

Bisection of blastocysts

Six microinstruments are placed in the optical field of an inverted microscope. Two micropipettes controlled by type-B micromanipulators hold the blastocyst and the empty zona pellucida by negative pressure. Instruments with a sharp tip positioned in front of the blastocyst are controlled by a type-A micromanipulator. The micropipette on the left and the microscalpel on the right are controlled by a type-B micromanipulator. Two sharp microneedles cut the zona pellucida over as short a distance as possible along the middle. The blastocyst is subsequently rotated through 90° with the two microneedles to show the slit. The micropipette is introduced through the slit inside the zona, while a small volume of medium is injected to expel the embryo. Bisection of the blastocyst is achieved using the microscalpel along the sagittal plane. Using the suction of the micropipette, each 'half' embryo is put back into an empty

Table 16.1 Effect of sperm–oocyte interaction on the binding and penetration of sperm to the zona pellucida

Sperm binding/penetration
Oocyte maturity affects the number of sperm bound to the zona
Number of sperm bound to mature oocyte = 51 ± 50
Number of sperm bound to immature oocyte = 7 ± 12
Number of sperm bound to atretic oocyte = 10 ± 18
Fertilized mature oocytes have a higher number of sperm bound to the zonae 81 ± 53, compared to unfertilized oocytes 42 ± 47
Sperm motility/the number of motile sperm used to inseminate oocytes correlates with the number of sperm bound to the zona, whereas sperm morphology and concentration do not correlate
Second insemination
Second insemination is performed if fertilization does not occur within 18 h after first insemination
The oocyte does not fertilize due to either its own maturity or difficulty in sperm penetration of the zona pellucida
Secondary insemination leads to fertilization since blastomeres are seen 18 h after this secondary insemination
This activity in the oocyte is delayed following the first insemination and is not related to the second one
Secondary insemination yields 5–7% fertilization, similar to that of immature oocytes
Secondary insemination is performed only in cases of unfertilized oocytes that were immature when first insemination was performed
Polyspermy
Despite exposure of eggs to supernumerary sperm, the incidence of polypoid fertilization is 2–10%
This incidence maybe related to the functional ability of the polyspermic block of the oocyte rather than to the high number of sperm in the dish
Polypronuclear fertilization is more frequent in cycles with high fertilization or improved pregnancy rates
This emphasizes the important role of the oocyte in polyspermy

zona pellucida. 'Half' (demi) embryos are then incubated at 37°C for 2 h. They reconstitute the blastocele, and it is possible to distinguish again the inner cell mass in each 'half' blastocyst. The cells destroyed during the bisection adhere to the outer surface of the 'half' blastocyst.

CRYOPRESERVATION OF GAMETES AND EMBRYOS (FIGURE 16.5)

The main advantage of cryopreservation of embryos, instead of just the sperm or oocytes, is that the embryo contains the complete genome, i.e. the full quota of chromosomes for the individual, and it can be transferred to a foster mother of known or unknown genetic background without the risk of genetic change. Since the pioneering efforts of Audrey Smith in 1952 concerning the effect of low temperature on further development of mammalian ova, much progress in embryo cryopreservation has been made. Cryopreservation of embryos of different mammalian species has been attempted with variable degrees of success.

Principles of cryobiology

The biophysical principles that apply to cryopreservation of living cells and tissues also apply to cryopreservation of embryos. Embryos may be damaged during cryopreservation and/or thawing by either the formation of large intracellular ice crystals or the increased intracellular concentration of solutes and the accompanying changes that result from dehydration of the cells during cryopreservation (solution effects). Whereas fast freezing minimizes damage from solution effects, it leads to the formation of large ice crystals that cause severe mechanical damage. On the other hand, while slow freezing prevents large ice crystal formation, it leads to increased damage from solution effects. Therefore, the optimal freezing rate for a given tissue depends on its relative tolerance to damage from ice crystals and toxicity from solution effects.

Table 16.2 Assisted fertilization and assisted blastocyst hatching

Indications for assisted fertilization by ICSI	
Necrozoospermia	
Extreme oligozoospermia	
Extreme asthenozoospermia	
Extreme mixed teratozoospermia	
Uniform teratozoospermia	
Antibodies to sperm	
Duct obstruction or absence	
Aneuploidy	
Pronuclear/syngamy disorder	
Female infertility	
Unexplained fertilization failure	
Indications for assisted blastocyst/fragment removal	
Elevated zona thickness	
Elevated maternal age	
Unexplained failure of implantation	
Reduced embryonic development rate	
Elevated basal FSH level	
Fragmentation above 15%	
ICSI	
Advantages of assisted hatching	
Technically simple	
Not labor intensive	
Normal rate of congenital malformation	
Elevates implantation	
Promotes earlier implantation	
Disadvantages of assisted hatching	
Possible risk of conjoint twinning	
High rate of embryo loss with standard embryo transfer	
Low success rate with standard transfer techniques	

ICSI, intracytoplasmic sperm injection; FSH, follicle stimulating hormone

The critical range of temperatures at which slow rates are necessary for optimal survival during cooling are from –70°C to –20°C. Human embryos can be preserved for prolonged periods in a state of suspended animation if they are able to withstand cryopreservation to temperatures at which no further biological activity occurs. Liquid nitrogen at –196°C satisfies this condition.

Cryopreservation of embryos (Tables 16.3–16.5)

Various techniques have been used for cryopreservation and thawing. Embryos selected for cryopreservation should be of the highest quality and at the correct stage of cleavage. They are handled with sterile techniques using a dissecting microscope. Embryos are transferred to sterile, freshly prepared culture media for microscopic classification and storage until use. If embryos are stored for longer than 2 h before transfer, they should be transferred into fresh medium every 2 h. The embryos are aspirated into micropipettes with a small volume of medium (less than 0.2 ml) to prevent contamination of the fresh medium. The embryos are handled gently to avoid any physical damage. Manipulation and evaluation are accomplished as quickly as possible to enable the embryos to be returned to a stable culture environment. To gain experience with handling embryos, operators are trained to use commercially available micropipettes to pick up Sephadix® particles with a diameter similar to that of mammalian eggs. Pieces of debris, unfertilized ova or degenerating ova can also be used for practice.

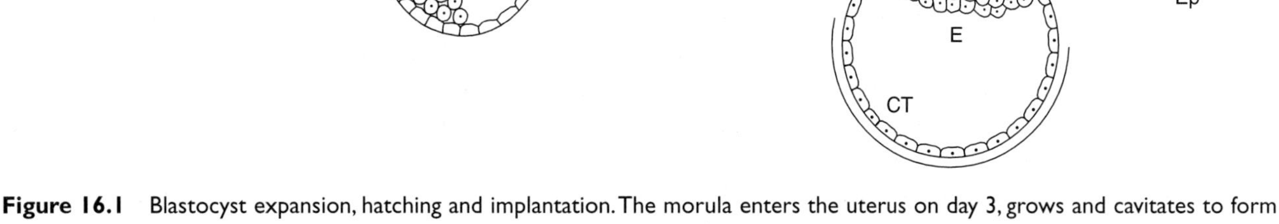

Figure 16.1 Blastocyst expansion, hatching and implantation. The morula enters the uterus on day 3, grows and cavitates to form a blastocyst. (**a**) Blastocyst, hollow ball of cells surrounded by zona pellucida (ZP). (**b**) Blastocyst hatching: blastocyst expands and ruptures ZP, emerging as a dumb-bell shape. (**c**) Early implantation in the endometrium. BV, blood vessel; C, cytotrophoblast; E, embryoblast; Ep, epithelium; En, endometrium; ST, syncytiotrophoblast; T, trophoblast; UG, uterine gland

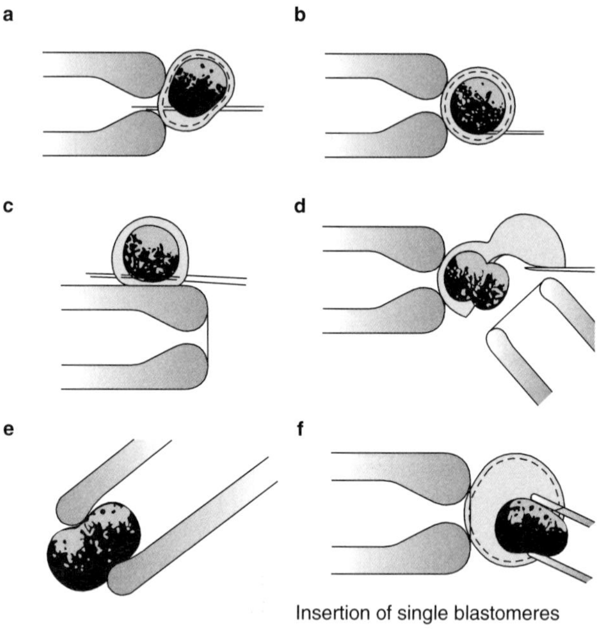

Figure 16.2 (**a**)–(**d**) Micromanipulation of the ovum to remove the zona pellucida to be used for biological assay. (**e**) and (**f**) Insertion of single blastomere into the zona pellucida

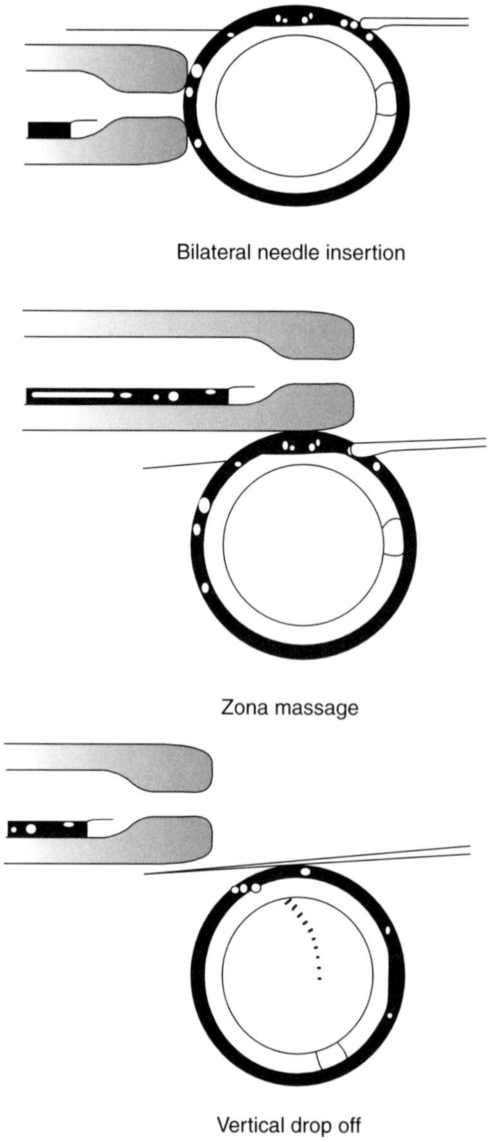

Figure 16.3 Partial dissection of zona pellucida

Post-thaw embryo survival

Several maternal, technical and operational factors influence the survival rate of embryos:

(1) Physiological and biophysical characteristics and developmental stage of embryos;

(2) Time interval and *in vitro* treatment from embryo collection to initiation of cryopreservation;

(3) Type of computerized freezers and program of cryopreservation;

(4) Osmotic shock during various stages of cryopreservation;

(5) Exposure of embryos to excessive light during microscopic examination;

(6) Osmotic and colloid osmotic pressures of fluids, prepared media and cryoprotectants;

(7) Nature and extent of 'seeding' and 'plunging';

(8) Microbiological contaminants in glassware, freezer and storage.

Semen cryopreservation

Cryopreservation is a useful and often necessary process for semen storage. During cryopreservation, sperm are kept in a state of suspended animation within a deep-frozen medium (liquid nitrogen). Azoospermic patients have extremely abnormal sperm quality, and may be infected with a sexually transmissible disease (STD), such as acquired immune deficiency syndrome (AIDS). Donor (homologous semen) sperm is required for procreation and must be cryopreserved and quarantined for at least 6 months before use to prevent STD infections. If the husband is unable to provide a semen sample on demand, or is unable to provide a semen sample in the future (as in cases of chemotherapy), the husband's ejaculate (autologous semen) has to be cryopreserved at the time of insemination; the cryopreserved sample is then thawed and processed for use.

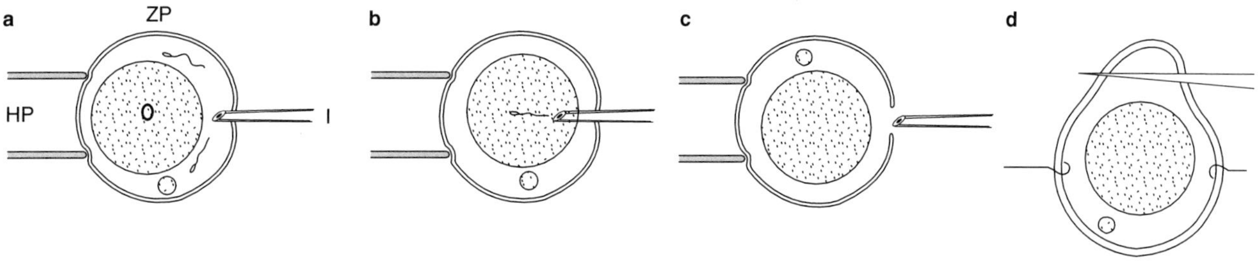

Figure 16.4 Sperm microinjection/microinsemination. (**a**) Microinsemination sperm transfer (MIST): egg held by holding pipette (HP), while sperm are injected into perivitelline space (PVS) beneath zona pellucida (ZP) using fine injecting needle (I). (**b**) Sperm microinjection directly into cytoplasm of oocyte. One sperm is injected directly in ooplasm. (**c**) Zona drilling: hole in zona drilled using acid Tyrode's medium, through which sperm introduced into PVS. (**d**) Microinsemination: zona opening or zona cutting using hooked needles and partial zona dissection (PZD) where opening is made with microneedle insemination of oocyte

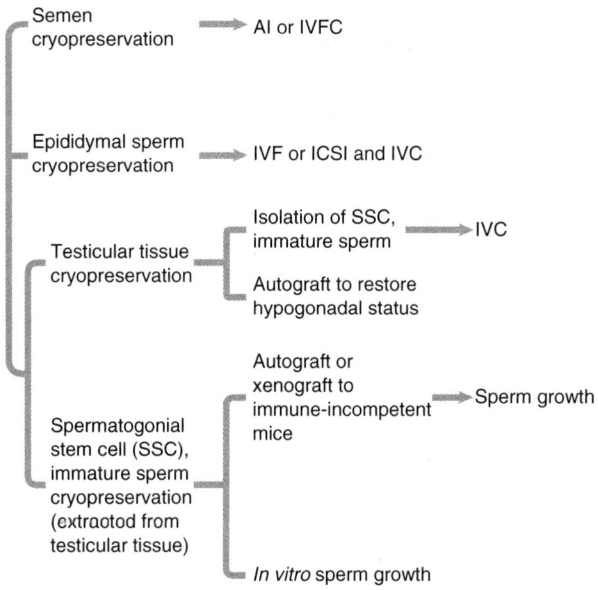

Figure 16.5 Possible options for restoring fertility using cryopreserved immature and mature male germ lines. AI, artificial insemination; IVF, *in vitro* fertilization; IVFC, *in vitro* fertilization and culture; IVC, *in vitro* culture; ICSI, intracytoplasmic sperm injection

Several extending media are used for semen cryopreservation and perform different functions, including providing nutrients as a source of energy, protecting against the harmful effect of rapid cooling, providing a buffer to prevent harmful shifts in pH as lactic acid is formed, maintaining the proper osmotic pressure and electrolyte balance, inhibiting bacterial growth and protecting the sperm cells during freezing. A simple carbohydrate, such as glucose, usually is added as a source of energy for the sperm. Both egg yolk and milk are use to protect against cold shock of the sperm cells as they are cooled from body temperature to 5°C. These substances also contain nutrients that can be used by sperm. A variety of buffers may be used to maintain a nearly neutral pH and an osmotic pressure of approximately 300 mmol/l, which is equivalent to that of semen and blood plasma.

Sperm after cryopreservation

The sperm plasma membrane contains high levels of unsaturated fatty acids and is therefore particularly susceptible to peroxidative damage with subsequent loss of membrane integrity and impaired cell function of sperm. After storage of the frozen semen for 1 month and 2 years the percentage of damaged sperm is almost the same. There is no significant difference in the fertilizability of semen. In bull sperm after thawing, selenium and vitamin E stimulate sperm motility and viability. In medium containing 0.5 mg vitamin E/ml diluted semen, the fertility of thawed sperm is 5% higher. The addition of different antioxidants to diluents at storage/cryopreservation is recommended to improve the quality of semen used for artificial insemination (AI).

Programmable freezers

Electronically programmed machines are used to monitor the temperature over the critical phase of the cooling curve before the vials containing embryos are plunged into liquid nitrogen. Several types are completely self-contained and capable of obtaining controlled rates of cryopreservation with or without liquid nitrogen and without mechanical refrigeration devices or the use of conventional refrigerants. The three major systems are freezers with a cylindrical chamber with circulating air cooled by microprocessor controlled thermoelectric cells, freezers operated with liquid nitrogen and freezers operated with alcohol or other agents.

Table 16.3 Precooling, cooling, seeding, plunging and storage and thawing of embryos

Process	*Techniques employed*
Collection of embryos	Selection and superovulation of donor, insemination during estrus
	Collection of embryos from female reproductive tract or ovaries (surgical, non-surgical or postmortem)
	Washing of embryos in sterile culture media
	Microscopic evaluation and classification of embryos
Cryoprotectant solutions	Gradual step-wise concentration of cryoprotectant (DMSO, glycerol or ready-made commercially available cryoprotectant)
	Small volume is freshly prepared
	Solutions to which serum is added are not stored more than 3–5 days, because protein denaturation occurs even at optimal temperatures
	Solutions are deep refrigerated or frozen until use
Precooling preparation	Embryos transferred in serial concentrations of cryoprotectant
	Straws attached to syringe using rubber adapter to aspirate medium or air bubbles and embryo
	Straws and cane labeled for future identification
	Straws heated or filled with phosphate-buffered saline
	Straws dipped in blue or red PVC at both ends
Cooling procedures	Slow cooling rate ranges from 0.5 to 1.6°C/min
	Rapid cooling rate ranges from 17 to 30°C/min
	Cooling rate 1°C/min from ambient temperature to –7°C
	Cooling rate 0.3°C/min to –35°C
	Cooling rate 0.1°C/min to –38°C
Freezing, seeding and plunging	Straws placed in freezer at –6°C and maintained for 10 min
	Forceps cooled in liquid nitrogen
	Straws grasped near embryos with cooled forceps until ice crystals form
	Seeded straw placed into programmable freezer and cooling regimen applied
	Thermos flask filled with liquid nitrogen
	Cane containing frozen embryos removed from freezer and plunged into liquid nitrogen
	Straws loaded in aluminum canes and stored in liquid nitrogen container at –196°C
Thawing	Thawing ranges from 20°C/min in slow warming to 360–500°C/min for the rapid thawing; optimal temperature for cryopreservant thawing ranges between 20 and 37°C
	Temperature of water bath adjusted to 37°C
	Color-marked canes identified and straws removed from cane to small canister containing liquid nitrogen; labels are checked before removing from liquid nitrogen
	Straws are held by neck, placed in 37°C water bath and removed when ice melts
	Embryos remain on bottom of vial and are observed under a microscope, counted and removed with a micropipette to avoid the occasional loss of embryos experienced by washing embryos out of the straw
	Straws are thawed for 4 s in a 37°C water bath and removed when ice melts
	Water is wiped from straws
Cryoprotectant removal	Heat seal or PVC plug cut from tips of straws
	Embryos washed through drops of serial dilutions of cryoprotectant mixture in sterile Petri dish (35 mm diameter)
	Embryos examined using a stereoscope to evaluate their quality

DMSO, dimethyl sulfoxide; PVC, polyvinyl chloride

Table 16.4 Morphological classification of embryos before and after cryopreservation and thawing

Parameter	*Classification*	
Stage of embryonic development	Unfertilized (UFO)	
	2–12-cell	
	Early morula	
	Morula	
	Early blastocyst	
	Blastocyst	
	Expanded blastocyst	
	Hatched blastocyst	
	Expanding hatched blastocyst	
Criteria for classification of embryos	Compactness of blastomeres	
	Regularity in shape of embryo	
	Variation in cell size	
	Color and texture of the cytoplasm	
	Presence of vesicles	
	Presence of extruded cells	
	Diameter	
	Regularity of the zona pellucida	
	Presence of cellular debris	
Quality of embryo	Excellent:	perfect embryo for its stage. Blastomeres are of similar size with even color and texture; they are neither very light nor very dark. Cytoplasm is not granular or unevenly distributed and contains some moderate-sized vesicles. Perivitelline space empty and of regular diameter; zona pellucida even and neither wrinkled nor collapsed
	Good:	trivial imperfections such as an oval zona, a few small excluded blastomeres and slight asymmetry
	Fair:	definite but not severe problems such as moderate numbers of excluded blastomeres, small size and small amounts of degeneration
	Poor:	partly degenerated, vesiculated cells, greatly varying cell size, very small, and/or similar problems
	Very poor:	severely degenerated, probably not worth transferring, unfertilized, zona only, ghost-like, 3-cell, debris, bacteriological contamination
Artifacts	Air bubble, debris, empty zona pellucida, denuded oviductal epithelium	

ASSISTED REPRODUCTIVE TECHNOLOGY (TABLES 16.6 AND 16.7; FIGURE 16.6)

During the recent past there have been dramatic changes in the field of male infertility. The introduction of intracytoplasmic sperm injection (ICSI) and specialized sperm retrieval procedures has made it possible to circumvent some of the most severe forms of male infertility. If at least one viable sperm cell is available, the pregnancy rate with ICSI depends on the age of the woman and the number of oocytes

Table 16.5 Freezing of human testicular biopsies (Schulze, 2001)

Freezing of human testicular biopsies
SpermFreeze (MediCult, Denmark) as ready-to-use medium: Earle's balanced salt solution plus 15% glycerol as cryoprotectant, HEPES-buffered (18 mmol/l)
Submerge biopsies into 0.5 ml SpermFreeze within Nunc Vials, equilibrate for a maximum of 15 min
In Nicoolbag 10 System (Air Liquide, Germany): cool to –60°C within 5 min
Submerge samples into liquid nitrogen until use
Enzymatic sperm extraction from frozen testicular tissue
Thaw sample in 37°C water bath for approximately 3 min
Transfer to 1 ml culture medium (MediCult) and dissect gently
Incubate sample for 30 min (37°C; 5% CO_2)
Add collagenase (sigma) at a final concentration of 400 U/ml
Incubate for 30 min, dissect further without squeezing the tubules
Incubate for another 60 min with collagenase (total incubation time can be modified according to the previous finding in the test-TESE, in severe cases overnight)
Squeeze remaining tubules, remove debris mechanically
Suspend the sediment, transfer to test-tube and centrifuge (500–800 *g* for 10 min)
Remove collagenase supernatant, resuspend pellet in small volume of culture medium
Transfer suspension into medium droplets under oil and incubate for at least 30 min
Collect sperm from the edges of the droplets
Perform ICSI as usual
Indications for testicular biopsy with cryo-TESE option
During surgery for post-testicular obstruction
Inoperable post-testicular obstruction
Bilateral aplasia of the vasa deferentia
Idiopathic normogonadotropic azoospermia
Hypergonadotropic azoospermia
Anejaculation (resistant to treatment)
Cryptozoospermia
Necrozoospermia

TESE, testicular epididymal sperm extraction; ICSI, intracytoplasmic sperm injection

retrieved. Wood and associates (1993) at the Liverpool Women's Hospital, UK, reported that motile epididymal sperm retain their fertilizing capacity after cryopreservation. The data on testicular sperm suggest that, although cryopreservation may reduce the fertilizing capacity of testicular sperm, there is no decrease in pregnancy rate.

Table 16.6 Embryo sexing, nuclear transfer, maturation media and cloning in mammals

Embryo sexing techniques
Separation on basis of sexual dimorphism
Detection of the sex chromatin mass
Fluorescence *in situ* hybridization
Detection of the HY antigen
Use of Y-specific DNA probes
Chromosome analysis
Factors involved in nuclear transfer
Use of particle gun
Sperm-mediated gene transfer
Injection of the pronuclei
Retroviral-mediated gene transfer
Injection of the oocyte cytoplasm
Germinal vesicle gene injection
Methods of gene transfer (cloning)
Quality of the cytoplast
Quantity of cytoplasm in the recipient oocyte
Age of cytoplast
Source of donor blastomeres
Cell stage of the cytoplast
Cell stage of donor blastomeres
Types of bovine serum for maturation media
Fetal calf serum
Pro-estrous serum
Steer serum
Estrous cow serum
Serum substitutes
Superovulated cow serum

Embryo donation

The American Society for Reproductive Medicine (ASRM) provides recommendations for the evaluation of potential sperm, oocyte and embryo donors, incorporating recent information about optimal screening

Table 16.7 Assisted reproductive technology/andrology (ARTA) and *in vitro* semen manipulation

Method	*Techniques*	
Assisted reproductive technology/ andrology (ARTA)	IVFET	(*in vitro* fertilization/embryo transfer)
	GIFT	(gamete intrafallopian transfer)
	PROST	(pronuclear-stage tubal transfer)
	ZIFT	(zygote intrafallopian transfer)
	TEST	(tubal embryo-stage transfer (embryos in premorula cleavage stages))
	Embryo bank	(cryopreservation of oocytes/morulae)
Zona drilling	Mechanical or by local application of a zona solvent such as acid Tyrode's or alpha-chymotrypsin solution using a microneedle	
Partial zona drilling (PZD)	Zona is mechanically torn with a glass needle or cracked by piercing on a glass holding pipette	
Subzonal injection (SUZI)	Injection of one or more sperm into perivitelline space	
Intracytoplasmic sperm injection (ICSI)	Injection of immotile live sperm directly into vitellus	
Semen manipulation *in vitro*	Swim-up/swim-down	
	Use of semen additives	
	In vitro capacitation	
	In vitro hyperactivation	
	Separation of X and Y sperm	
	Cryopreservation/semen banks	

and testing for sexually transmitted infections (STIs), genetic diseases and psychological assessments. This represents an effort to make the screening guidelines for embryos and gametes more consistent and incorporates recent information from the Centers for Disease Control (CDC), Food and Drug Administration (FDA) and American Association for Tissue Banks (AATB). The term 'screening' refers to specific historical factors that place an individual at high risk for a given disease such as human immunodeficiency virus (HIV) and transmissible spongiform encephalopathy (TSE) or Creutzfeldt–Jakob disease (CJD). 'Testing' refers to specific laboratory studies such as serological tests.

ASRM also established guidelines for assisted reproductive technology (ART) clinics wishing to offer embryo donation, guidelines for couples who wish to donate an embryo, guidelines for potential recipients, record keeping and protection of confidentiality. Genetic screening is established for various ethnic groups including Ashkenazi Jews (for Tay–Sachs disease, Canovan disease), African-Americans (for sickle cell anemia); Mediterranean people (for β-thalassemia); south-east Asians and Chinese (for α-thalassemia) and Caucasians with European descent (for cystic fibrosis).

Intrauterine insemination versus *in vitro* fertilization/intracytoplasmic sperm injection

A variety of cases of infertility are treated with intrauterine insemination (IUI), with or without controlled ovarian hyperstimulation (COH), rather than with ICSI and *in vitro* fertilization (IVF). IUI is efficient and cost-effective for the treatment of unexplained and not severe male factor infertility. IUI is also applied to specific types of female infertility such as oligo-inoculators, cervical factor and corrected minimal tubal obstruction. The IUI outcome, in terms of clinical pregnancy rate, is influenced by various factors including the results of COH, timing/number of insemination(s), duration/cause of infertility, age of the woman, number of follicles, endometrial thickness or organization at the time of ovulation. Of parameters related to the male partner, the most important determinant of pregnancy outcome is sperm progressive motility.

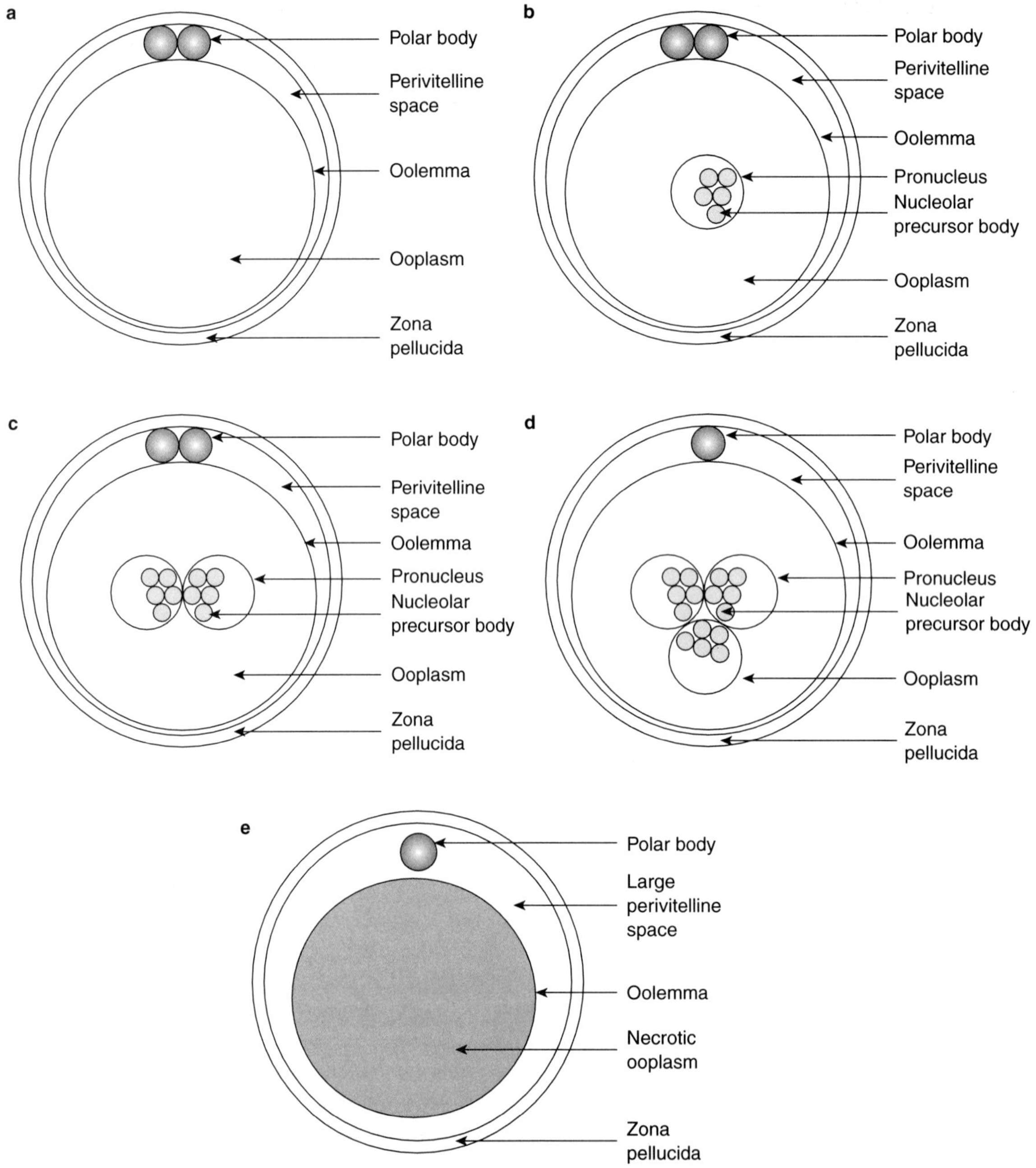

Figure 16.6 At the time of fertilization, the morning following the day of injection of oocytes they typically appear: (**a**) unfertilized, (**b**) monopronucleate, (**c**) fertilized, (**d**) triploid, (**e**) degenerate. From Fleming and King (2003), with permission

However, samples with an acceptable number of motile sperm can be processed efficiently.

Smoking and IVF/ICSI

Cigarette smoking by men and/or their female partners reduces fecundity and the success rate of IVF and ICSI, owing to the harmful effect of benzopyrene and nicotine, noxious metabolites of cigarette smoke. This is associated with a reduction in sperm motility and/or morphology as well as alteration in sperm membrane function, with a subsequent decrease in the ability to undergo capacitation and oocyte penetration. Apart from putative adverse effects during fertilization, altered DNA in sperm might hamper development of the embryo (Zitzmann *et al.*, 2003).

ICSI and calcium ionophore oocyte activation

Severe oligoasthenoteratozoospermia is usually treated with ICSI, since such patients have no or very low fertilization rates using conventional IVF. Couples with unexplained infertility after superovulation and IUI undergoing IVF have an 11–23% chance of fertilization failure that can be easily overcome by using ICSI. The fertilization rate after ICSI is some 70%. Total fertilization failure after ICSI can be due to various mechanisms related to the oocytes or qualitative or quantitative low semen characteristics, such as total immotile or rounded-head sperm. Calcium ionophore oocyte activation seems to be a useful method in cases of repeated failed fertilization after ICSI (Eldar-Geva *et al.*, 2003).

Anabolic steroid–induced azoospermia

Power lifters, body-builders and other related professional athletes are known for anabolic steroid abuse. Anabolic steroids increase lean muscle mass while suppressing the hypothalamic–pituitary–gonadal axis. This is associated with hypogonadotropic hypogonadism and oligospermia or azoospermia. Menon (2003) was able to treat this condition with the combined administration of human chorionic gonadotropin (hCG) and human menopausal gonadotropin (hMG).

UROLOGICAL SURGERY

Care must be taken during andrological surgery, including use of aseptic techniques, meticulous hemostasis, counting of sponges before wound closure and follow-up care.

Pathophysiology, risk factors, complications and related management of urological surgery

Damage to the urinary sphincter during transurethral resection of the prostate can cause incontinence which may also be due to underlying neuro-urological problems undiagnosed before the procedure. A thorough history and physical examination is imperative before assuming that lower urinary symptoms are owing solely to bladder outlet obstruction as opposed to bladder dysfunction. If bladder outlet obstruction necessitates surgical intervention, resection of prostatic tissues is limited to tissue proximal to the verumontanum, using video-cystoscopy/photography of the external urinary sphincter. The introduction of α-blockers has radically changed the management of benign prostatic hyperplasia (BPH). Patients who fail medical therapy require transurethral resection of the prostate.

Scrotal pain in the prepubertal male is testicular torsion until 'proven otherwise'. Testicular torsion occurs at any age, and must be included in the differential diagnosis of any male with acute onset of scrotal discomfort. If misdiagnosised as epididymitis the patient is given a prescription for antibiotics and anti-inflammatories and sent home. An anterior lie of the epididymis and absence of the cremasteric reflex on the symptomatic side can be signs of testicular torsion. The diagnosis of acute testicular pain is aided by either Doppler ultrasonography or nuclear scrotal scintigraphy.

Hematoma formation, the most common surgical complication after vasectomy, occurs as a result of vasospasm during the procedure with delayed bleeding after wound closure, or suture material or surgical clips which fall off. A hematoma can become infected resulting in loss of the testis. No-scalpel vasectomy can reduce the incidence of complications.

Epididymitis/orchitis can occur even with antibiotic prophylaxis. Patients should be informed that the effectiveness of the procedure must be demonstrated by semen analysis before the cessation of contraception.

Both radical and partial nephrectomy for renal cell cancer are performed laparoscopically. Benefits to patients are shorter hospital stay, less pain and faster recovery to baseline. Patient candidates for nephrectomy are given the option of having the procedure performed laparoscopically. Furthermore, informed consent should consider all possible treatment options, including open/laparoscopic radical nephrectomy, partial nephrectomy or cryosurgical ablation of the lesion. Patients should be informed of potential injury to the bowel, blood vessels and other adjacent structures during these procedures. A second additional procedure (repair of bowel injury) may be necessary if patients are willing to undergo such a procedure if needed. Symptoms of hyponatremia can start as mental confusion, or muscle cramps, and progress to convulsions, then coma or death.

The syndrome can be avoided by limiting resection time to less than 1.5 h, since the volume of glycine irrigant absorbed is proportional to the length of the procedure. Transurethral resection syndrome must be suspected in a patient who experiences hemodynamic changes, including hypertension and bradycardia. These may be the only signs of hyponatremia in the anesthetized patient. In more severely affected patients, seizures can occur. The anesthesiologist must note these changes and communicate with the surgeon. Awareness of the symptoms of hyponatremia and aggressive therapy once diagnosis is suspected are critical to optimal management.

Radical prostatectomy, the 'gold standard' for treatment of localized prostate cancer, is associated with significant intra-/postoperative morbidity. Large-volume blood loss occurring in the perioperative period requires blood transfusion. Injury to the rectum is one of most feared complications during radical prostatectomy. While it is possible to perform primary repair of an injury to the rectum, some patients may require a temporary colostomy. Appropriate preoperative bowel preparation (mechanical and antibiotic) allows for primary repair of a rectal injury, thereby avoiding colostomy.

Long-term complications associated with radical prostatectomy include incontinence, stricture formation at the bladder neck and impotence. These complications can be managed medically or may require surgery. Insertion of radioactive seeds within the prostatic tissue (brachytherapy) has gained significant popularity. Improvements in imaging technology have enabled mapping of the prostate and precise radioactive seed placement. This procedure is performed on an ambulatory basis and does not require prolonged catheterization, unlike radical prostatectomy. Brachytherapy is efficacious for appropriately selected patients. Morbidity following brachytherapy includes urinary incontinence, urethral stricture, impotence and recto-prostatic fistula formation.

Cryosurgery is performed for both primary and recurrent disease. With the routine use of urethral warming devices and rigorous temperature monitoring within the prostate and at the Denonvilliers' fascia, the extent of the tissue freezing can be precisely controlled. Technical advances in cryosurgery are of significant potential for both short- and long-term morbidity, including urethral sloughing, irrigative voiding symptoms and recto-prostatic fistula formation.

Prostate-specific antigen (PSA) testing, digital rectal examination and improvements in biopsy techniques have enabled prostate cancer to be diagnosed in more males at an earlier and, therefore, presumably curable stage. All men over 50 years of age should be screened for prostate cancer. Screening should be performed annually using PSA and digital rectal examination. For African-American males or those with a family history of prostate cancer, screening should begin even earlier (40 years). Screening should also be undertaken when various complications occur, including urethral tears, creation of false passages into the urethra, urinary tract infections, bleeding, undermining of the bladder neck/bladder perforation during manipulation of the penis or urethra or when the site of urethral perforation is the bulbar urethra, because of the curvaceous course of the urethra at this point. In bladder neck perforation of the urethra at the bulb, use of internal, self-retaining ureteral stents improves patient comfort/reduces the likelihood of stent migration. Because of the nature of these devices, one can lose track of them until complications arise. The most common complications are bacterial or fungal urinary tract infections. Encrustation of the stent from prolonged retention, making endoscopic removal of the stent impossible, is another complication. One preventive measure is to keep a log of all stents placed, with the date of stent removal. Common causes of complications are compression or occlusion of the vasculature of the spermatic cord, causing closure of the internal inguinal ring; direct clamping or cutting, damaging the cord structures/injuring the testicular artery; painful, tender/swollen testis; herniorrhaphy causing protracted discomfort, ischemic injury or testicular dysfunction; damage as a result of the mesh used in inguinal herniorraphy of the spermatic cord, the mesh eroding into the vas deferens or causing fibrotic reaction/vasal obstruction; and vas deferens injured during dissection of the hernia sac from cord structures or during sac ligation (Meray *et al.*, 2002).

Percutaneous nephrolithotripsy is a 'minimally invasive' procedure associated with reduced morbidity, compared with open procedures. As guide wires or needles are blindly introduced via the flank into the kidney, perforation of the kidneys, arteries, veins and even bowel can occur. In the event of complications, a nephrectomy or other procedure to repair lacerated blood vessels or bowel may be necessary. The patient must be informed of potential complications despite the minimally invasive nature of this procedure and should be willing to undergo additional procedures in case of intra-operative complications.

Patients are motivated and, in the case of inflatable prosthesis placement, must possess dexterity to utilize the device effectively. Patients should be properly evaluated before surgery. Patients must have realistic expectations and understand the risks and benefit limitations of prosthetic surgery. Lack of sterile technique, poor placement with crossover of the penile cylinders or improper sizing cause penile deformity, curvature and/or erosion of the prosthesis through the penis or urethra. Penile prosthetic devices may cause postoperative infection even under the best aseptic conditions.

Priapism may result from systemic disease, such as sickle cell anemia, malignancy or pharmacological therapy for impotence. Careful dose titration of the intracorporeal agent to be administered is essential. Patient selection and education regarding the frequency of dosage, injection technique and complications are essential prior to initiation of self- injection therapy. Aggressive therapy with oral α-adrenergic or intracavernosal irrigation is indicated. Patients should be informed of risks and the potential sequela of priapism prior to initiation of intracavernosal injection therapy.

INSTRUMENTATION, WATER AND AIR FILTRATION AND CULTURE MEDIA

Ultrapure water

Distilled and bottled water leach new organics as little as 1 hour after storage. Unfortunately, storage problems are just one of the drawbacks to using distilled or bottled water. There are also problems of higher operating and maintenance costs and contaminant carryover. Laboratory water purification has undergone dramatic changes since the 1980s. Chemists, life scientists and medical technicians are now routinely concerned with impurity levels that were impossible to measure until recently. Today, deionization, reverse osmosis, carbon absorption and membrane microfiltration are in some respects superior to distillation. Various systems of water ultrafiltration are now commercially available. These systems cost less than distilled or bottled water, and there is no contaminant carryover. Unlike stills, which require regular acid cleaning, ultrafiltration cartridges can be replaced in minutes.

Air filtration

Laminar airflow is airflow in which the entire body of air within a designated space moves with uniform velocity in a single direction along parallel flow lines. Laminar-flow biological safety cabinets (hoods) are devices designed to minimize biohazards inherent in work with low- and moderate-risk biological agents. Vertical laminar-flow containment hoods not only provide product protection by using a filtered downflow of air, but also provide operator protection through a negative-pressure air barrier created along the front opening. With proper aseptic conditions and good laboratory procedures, risk levels are substantially reduced.

Microscopy

Several commercially available microscopes are easy to operate; these include inverted microscopes with a single-laser beam delivered through the objective for gamete micromanipulation, and optional three beam for sperm trapping, tail cutting and/or zona pellucida cutting.

References

Abbas AK, Lichtman AH, Pober JS. Cellular and Molecular Immunology, 3rd edn. Philadelphia: WB Saunders, 1997

Abdel-Rahman B, Fiddler M, Rappolee D, et al. Expression of transcription regulating genes in human preimplantation embryo. Hum Reprod 1995; 10: 2787–92

Acosta A, Kruger T. Human Spermatozoa in Assisted Reproduction, 2nd edn. New York: Parthenon Publishing, 1996

Agulnik AL, Mitchell MJ, Lerner JL, et al. A mouse Y chromosome gene encoded by a region essential for spermatogenesis and expression of male-specific minor histocompatibility antigens. Hum Mol Genet 1994; 3: 873–8

Aitken J. The biochemistry and physiology of human spermatozoa: consequences for fertility and sterility. In Van Blerkom J, ed. The Biological Basis of Early Human Reproductive Failure: Application to Medically-Assisted Conception and Treatment of Infertility. New York: Oxford University Press, 1994: 252–82

Aitken RJ, Clarkson JS, Fishel S. Generation of reactive oxygen species, lipid peroxidation and human sperm function. Biol Reprod 1989; 41: 183–97

Aitken RJ, Harkiss D, Knox W, et al. A novel signal transduction cascade in capacitating human spermatozoa characterized by a redox-regulated, cAMP-mediated induction of tyrosine phosphorylation. J Cell Sci 1998; 111: 645–56

Altman R. The Prostate Answer Book. New York: Warner Books, 1993

Amit M, Suss-Toby E, et al. Human embryonic stem cells and embryo cloning. In Revelli A, Tur-Kaspa I, Holte JG, Massobrio M, eds. Biotechnology of Human Reproduction. Lancaster, UK: Parthenon Publishing, 2003

Anderson DJ, Hill JA. Cell-mediated immunity in infertility. Am J Reprod Immunol 1988; 17: 2230

Araki Y, Suzuki K, Matusik RJ, et al. Immortalized epididymal cell lines from transgenic mice over-expressing temperature-sensitive simian virus 40 large T-antigen gene. J Androl 2002; 23: 854–69

Ariel M, Cedar H, McCarrey J. Developmental changes in methylation of spermatogenesis-specific genes include reprogramming in the epididymis. Nat Genet 1994; 7: 59–63

Arnoult C, Kazam IG, Visconti PE, et al. Control of the low voltage-activated calcium channel of mouse sperm by egg ZP3 and by membrane hyperpolarization during capacitation. Proc Natl Acad Sci USA 1999; 96: 6757–62

Aurech E, Chen R, Wang F, et al. Effect of antioxidants on motility and membrane integrity on chilled-stored stallion semen. Theriogeneology 1997; 48: 185–92

Aversa A, Bonifacio V, Moretti C, et al. Re-dosing of prostaglandin E1 versus prostaglandin E1 plus phen tolamine in male erectile dysfunction: a dynamic color power Doppler study. Int J Impot Res 2000; 12: 33–40

Bajpai M, Asin S, Doncel GF. Effect of tyrosine kinase inhibitors on tyrosine phosphorylation and motility parameters in human spermatozoa. Arch Androl 2003; 49: 229–46

Barboza JM, Medina H, Doria M, et al. Use of atomic force microscopy to reveal sperm ultrastructure in HIV-patients on highly active antiretroviral therapy. Arch Androl 2004; 50: 121–9

Basson R. Assessing erectile dysfunction in the primary care setting. Med Aspects Hum Sex 2001; 29: 14–18

Bastacky SE, Wojno KJ, Kuo N, et al. Pathological features of hereditary prostate. Prostate 1995; 253: 987–92

Bathgate R, Balvers M, Hunt N, et al. Relaxin-like factor gene is highly expressed in the bovine ovary of the cycle and pregnancy: sequence and ribonucleic acid analysis. Biol Reprod 1996; 55: 1452–7

Baum N, Spiefer B. Medical management of premature ejaculation. Med Aspects Hum Sex 2001; 29: 15–18, 23–25

Beernink FJ, Ericsson RJ. Male sex preselection through sperm isolation. Fertil Steril 1982; 38: 493

Beernink FJ. Factors influencing the human sex ratio. Presented at the Annual Meeting of the American Fertility Society, New Orleans, 1984

Beernink FJ. Techniques for separating X- and Y-spermatozoa In Fredericks CM, Paulson JD, Decherney AH, et al., eds. Foundations of In Vitro Fertilization. New York: Hemisphere, 1986

Benitz et al. Effect of different culture media on sperm DNA integrity. Adv Reprod 2002; 7: 100–20

Bennet D, Boyce EA. Sex ratio in progeny of mice inseminated with sperm treated with H-Y antiserum. Nature 1973; 246: 308

Ben-Yosef D, Yogev L, Hauser R, et al. Testicular sperm retrieval and cryopreservation prior to initiating ovarian stimulation as the first line approach in patients with non-obstructive zoosperm. Hum Reprod 1999; 14: 1794–801

Berry R, Schaid DJ, Smith JR, et al. Linkage analysis at the chromosome 1 loci 1q24-25 (HPC1), 1q42.2 (PCAP), and 1p36 (CAPB) in families with hereditary prostate cancer. Am J Hum Genet 2000; 66: 539

Bhasin S. The dose-dependent effects of testosterone on sexual function and on muscle mass and function. Mayo Clin Proc 2000; 75 (Suppl): 570–6

Bhattacharya BC, Bangham AD, Cro RJ, et al. An attempt to determine the sex of calves by artificial insemination with spermatozoa separated by sedimentation. Nature London 1966; 211: 863

Bischof RJ, Brandon MR, Lee CS. Studies on the distribution of immune cells in the uteri of prepubertal and cycling gilts. J Reprod Immunol 1994; 26: 111–29

Bischof RJ, Lee CS, Brandon MR, et al. Inflammatory response in the pig uterus induced by seminal plasma. J Reprod Immunol 1994; 26: 131–46

Boismenu R, Havran WL. An innate view of T cells. Curr Opin Immunol 1997; 9: 57–63

Bostwick DG, MacLennan GT, Larson TR. Prostate Cancer: What Every Man – And His Family – Needs to Know, revised edn. New York: Villard Books, 1999

Bourgeon FB, Evrard M, Brillard-Bourdet M, et al. Involvement of semenogelin-derived peptides in the antibacterial activity of human seminal plasma. Biol Reprod 2004; 70: 768–74

Branford WW, Zhao GQ, Valerius MT, et al. Spx1, a novel X-linked homeobox gene expressed during spermatogenesis. Mech Dev 1997; 65: 87–98

Brannigan RE, Schoor RA, Ross LS, et al. In Jeyendran RS, ed. Sperm Collection and Processing Methods: A Practical Guide. New York: Cambridge University Press, 2003

Brinster RL, Avarbock MR. Germline transmission of donor haplotype following spermatogonial transplantation. Proc Natl Acad Sci USA 1994; 91: 11303–7

Brinster RL, Chen HY, Trumbauer ME, et al. Translation of globin messenger RNA by the mouse ovum. Nature London 1980; 283: 499–501

Brinster RL. Stem cells and transgenic mice in the study of development. Int J Dev Biol 1992; 3: 89–99

Brow SL, Settel AD, Strohl KP, et al. Vasculogenic impotence and cavernosal oxygen tension. Int J Impot Res 2000; 12: 19–22

Calamera JC, Doncel GF, Olmedo SB, et al. Modified sperm stress test: a simple assay that predicts sperm-related abnormal in-vitro fertilization. Hum Reprod 1998; 13: 2484–8

Cao QP, Gaudette MF, Robinson DH, et al. Expression of the mouse testis-determining gene Sry in male preimplantation embryos. Mol Rep Dev 1995; 40: 196–204

Cappechi MR. Altering the genome by homologous recombination. Science 1989; 244: 1288–92

Carani C, Scuteri A, Marrama P, et al. The effects of testosterone administration and visual erotic stimulation on nocturnal penile tumescence in normal men. Horm Behav 1990; 24: 435–41

Carrell DT, Emery BR, Hamilton B. Seminal infection with *Ralstonia picketti* and cytolysosomal spermophagy in a previously fertile man. Fertil Steril 2003; 79: 1665–7

Catt JW. Intracytoplasmic sperm injection (ICSI) and related technology. Anim Reprod Sci 1996; 4: 239–50

Chandley AC, Cooke HJ. Human male fertility – Y-linked genes and spermatogenesis. Hum Mol Genet 1994; 3: 1449–52

Chang KH, Lim JM, Kang SK, et al. Karyotypes of interspecies blastocysts from human fibroblast into bovine blastocysts. Fertil Steril 2003; 80: 1380–7

Chauvin TR, Griswold MD. Characterization of the expression and regulation of genes necessary for myo-inositol biosynthesis and transport in the somniferous epithelium. Biol Reprod 2004; 70: 744–51

Check JH, Szekeres-Bartho J, O'Shaughnessy A. Progesterone induced blocking factor seen in pregnancy lymphocytes soon after implantation. Am J Reprod Immunol 1996; 35: 277–80

Chehval MJ, Doshi R, Kidd CF, et al. Antisperm autoantibody response after unilateral vas deferens ligation in rats: when does it develop? J Androl 2002; 23: 669–73

Chen Y, Cann MJ, Litvin TN, et al. Soluble adenyl cyclase as an evolutionarily conserved bicarbonate sensor. Science 2000; 289: 625–8

Chen Y, Lee NPY, Mruk DD, et al. Fer kinase/Fer T and adherens junction dynamics in the testis: an in vitro and in vivo study. Biol Reprod 2003; 69: 656–73

Chew KK, Earle CM, Stuckey BG, et al. Erectile dysfunction in general medicine practice: prevalence and clinical correlates. Int J Impot Res 2000; 12: 41–5

Choi JM, Chung P, Veeck L, et al. AZF micro deletions of the Y chromosome and in vitro fertilization outcome. Fertil Steril 2004; 81: 337–42

Christ GJ, Lerner SE, Kim DC, et al. Endothelin-1 as a putative modulator of erectile dysfunction. 1. Characteristics of contraction of isolated corporal tissue strips. J Urol 1995; 153: 1998–2003

Christ GJ. The penis as a vascular organ: the importance of corporal smooth muscle tone in the control of erection. Urol Clin North Am 1995; 22: 727–45

Cohan P, Korenman SG. Erectile dysfunction. J Clin Endocrinol Metab 2001; 86: 2391–4

Cohen OJ, Fauci AS. Current strategies in the treatment of HIV infection. Adv Intern Med 2001; 46: 207–46. Review

Colpo LM. Evaluation, treatment and management of erectile dysfunction. An overview. Urol Nurs 1988; 18: 100–6

Comhaire FH. Andropause: hormone replacement/therapy in the aging male. Eur Urol 2000; 38: 655–62

Cornwall GA, Hann SR. Transient appearance of CRES protein during spermatogenesis and caput epididymal sperm maturation. Mol Reprod Dev 1995; 41: 37–46

Corson SL, Baatzer FR, Alexander NH, et al. Sex selection by sperm separation and insemination. Fertil Steril 1984; 42: 756

Costa P, Bressolle F, Mottet N, et al. Pharmacokinetics of moxisylyte in healthy volunteers after intravenous infusion and intracavernous administration with and without a penile tourniquet. J Ther Drug Monit 1996; 18: 135–44

Cote HCF, Brumme ZL, Craib KJ, et al. Changes in mitochondria DNA as a marker of nucleoside toxicity in HIV-infected patients. N Engl J Med 2002; 346: 811–20

Craft I, Tsirigotis M, Courtauld E, et al. Testicular needle aspiration as an alternative to biopsy for the assessment of spermatogenesis. Hum Reprod 1997; 12: 1483–7

D'Amico AV, Schultz D, Loffredo M, et al. Biochemical outcome following external beam radiation therapy with or without androgen suppression therapy for clinically localized prostate cancer. JAMA 2000; 284: 1280–3

Dalzell LH, Thompson-Cree MEM, McClure N, et al. Effects of 24-hour incubation after freeze-thawing on DNA fragmentation of testicular sperm from infertile and fertile men. Fertil Steril 2003; 79: 1670–70

De Lamirande E, Leclerc P, Gagnon C. Capacitation as a regulatory event that primes spermatozoa for the acrosome reaction and fertilization. Mol Hum Reprod 1997; 3: 175–94

Dimbro MR. Griffith's 5-Minute Clinical Consul. New York: Lippincott Williams & Wilkins, 2003

Domashenko AD, Latham KE, Hatton KS. Expression of myc-family, myc-interacting, and myc-target genes during preimplantation mouse-development. Mol Reprod Dev 1997; 47: 57–65

El Garem YF, Depuydt CE, El Arini AF, et al. Relationship between seminal plasma-soluble transferrin receptor and spermatogenesis in azoospermic patients. Fertil Steril 2003; 79: 1668–9

Eldar-Geva T, Brooks B, Margalioth EJ, et al. Successful pregnancy and delivery after calcium ionophore oocyte activation in a normozoospermic patient with previous repeated failed fertilization after intracytoplasmic sperm injection. Fertil Steril 2003; 79: 1656–8

Ericsson RJ, Glass RH. Functional differences between sperm bearing the X- or Y-chromosome. In Amann RP, Seidel GE Jr, eds. Prospects for Sexing Mammalian Sperm. Boulder: Colorado University Associated Press, 1982

Escalier D. New insights into the assembly of the periaxonemal structures in mammalian spermatozoa. Biol Reprod 2003; 69: 373–8

Escudero T, Abdelhadi I, Sandalinas M, et al. Predictive value of sperm fluorescence in situ hybridization analysis on the outcome of preimplantation genetic diagnosis for translocations. Fertil Steril 2003; 79: 1528–34

Eskin BA, Troen BR. The Geripause: Medical Management during the Late Menopause. New York: Parthenon Publishing, 2003

Ezeh UI, Martin M, Dean R, et al. Correlation of testicular pathology and sperm extraction in azoospermic men with ejaculated spermatids detected by immunofluorescent localization. Hum Reprod 1998; 13: 3051–5

Fabbri A, Aversa A. Erectile dysfunction: an overview. Hum Reprod Update 1997; 3: 455–66

Fahmy WE, Bissada NK. Cryosurgery for prostate cancer. Arch Androl 2003; 49: 397–407

Fauci AS, Lane HC. The acquired immunodeficiency syndrome (AIDS). In Wilson JD, Braunwald E, Isselbacher KJ, et al., eds. Harrison's Principles of Internal Medicine, 12th edn. New York: McGraw-Hill, 1991: 1402–10

Feldman HA, Goldstein I, Hatzlchristou DG, et al. Impotence and its medical and psychosocial correlates: results of Massachusetts Male Aging Study. J Urol 1994; 151: 54–61

Fleming SD, King KS. Micromanipulation in Assisted Conception. Cambridge, UK: Cambridge University Press, 2003

Foote RH, Oltenacu EAB. Increasing fertility in artificial insemination by culling bulls or ejaculates within bulls. In Proceedings of the 8th Technical Conference on Artificial Insemination and Reproduction NAAB, British Columbia, 1980: 6–12

Foote RH. Functional differences between sperm bearing the X- or Y-chromosome. In Amann RP, Seidel GE Jr, eds. Prospects for Sexing Mammalian Sperm. Boulder: Colorado University Associated Press, 1982

Foote RH. Prospects for sexing: present status, future prospects and overall conclusions. In Amann RP, Seidel GE Jr, eds. Prospects for Sexing Mammalian Sperm. Boulder: Colorado University Associated Press, 1982

Ford TC, Rockwood D. Formation of isotonic Nycodenz gradients for cell separations. Anal Biochem 1982; 124: 293–8

Forsling ML. Pocket Examiner in Endocrinology. London: Pitman Publishing, 1984

Franken DR, Menkveld R, Kruger TF, et al. Monitoring technologist reading skills in a sperm morphology quality control program. Fertil Steril 2003; 70: 1637–43

Fujisawa M, Sawada K. Clinical application of Viagra (sildenafil citrate) for ED. Adv Reprod 2002; 6: 82–5

Furuya K, Mizumoto N, Makimura N, et al. A novel biological aspect of ovarian oxytocin: gene expression of oxytocin and oxytocin receptor in cumulus luteal cells and the effect of oxytocin on embryo genesis in fertilized oocytes. Adv Exp Med Biol 1995; 395: 523–8

Galantino-Homer HL, Visconti PE, Kopf GS. Regulation of protein tyrosine phosphorylation during bovine sperm capacitation by cyclic adenosine 3',5'-monophosphate-dependent pathway. Biol Reprod 1997; 56: 707–19

Garrido R, et al. Selection of sperm with best motility. Fertil Steril 2004; 81: 349–55

Gerwin N, Jia GQ, Kulbacki R, Gutierrez-Ramos JC. Interleukin gene expression in mouse preimplantation development. Dev Immunol 1995; 4: 169–79

Govier FE, Barr A, Yen J, et al. Experience with triple-drug therapy in a pharmacological erection program. J Urol 1997; 150: 1822–4

Gronberg H, Bergh A, Damber JE, et al. Cancer risk in families with hereditary prostate cancer. Prostate 2000; 89: 1315–21

Gronberg H, Xu J, Smith JR, et al. Early age of diagnosis in families providing evidence of linkage to hereditary prostate cancer locus (HPC1) on chromosome 1. Cancer Res 1997; 57: 4707–9

Grusby MJ, Auchincloss H, Lee R, et al. Mice lacking major histocompatibility complex class I and class II molecules. Proc Natl Acad Sci USA 1993; 90: 3913–17

Gundogan R. Effects of diluents on motility of ram sperm during storage at 5°C. Arch Androl 2003; 49: 69–75

Gurdon JB. Egg cytoplasm and gene control in development. Proc R Soc Lond B Biol Sci 1977; 198: 211–47

Habuchi T, Suzuki T, Sasaki R, et al. Association of vitamin D with receptor gene polymorphism with prostate cancer and benign prostatic hyperplasic in a Japanese population. Cancer Res 2000; 60: 305–8

Hafez B, Hafez ESE. Andropause, endocrinology, erectile dysfunction and prostate pathophysiology. Arch Androl 2004; 50: 45–68

Hafez ESE, Hafez B, eds. Reproduction in Farm Animals, 7th edn. Philadelphia, PA: Lippincott Williams & Wilkins, 2000

Hafez ESE, Hafez B, Hafez SD. Atlas of Reproductive Physiology in Men. Lancaster, UK: Parthenon Publishing, 2003

Hafs HD, Boyd LJ. Galvanic separation of X- and Y-chromosome-bearing sperm. In Kiddy CA, Hafs HD, eds. Sex Ratio at Birth: Prospects for Control. Chicago, IL: American Society for Animal Science, 1971

Hanlon AL, Watkins PR, Bruner D. Quality of life study in prostate cancer patients treated with three-dimensional conformal radiation therapy: comparing late bowel and bladder quality of life symptoms to that of the normal population. Int J Radiat Oncol Biol Phys 2001; 49: 51–63

Hansen PJ. Immunology of reproduction, In Hafez ESE, Hafez B, eds. Reproduction in Farm Animals. Philadelphia, PA: Lippincott, Williams & Wilkins, 2004

Hansen PJ. Immunology of reproduction. In Hafez ESE, Hafez B, eds. Reproduction in Farm Animals, 7th edn. Philadelphia, PA: Lippincott, Williams & Wilkins, 2000

Hansen PJ, Asbury AC. Opsonins of streptococcus in uterine flushings of mares susceptible and resistant to endometritis: control of secretion and partial characterization. Am J Vet Res 1987; 48: 646–50

Hardy DO, Scher HI, Bogenreider T, et al. Androgen receptor CAG repeat length in prostate cancer. Correlations with age or onset. J Clin Endocrinol Metab 1996; 81: 4400–5

Harley VR. Genetic control of testis determination. In d'Karester D. ed. Molecular Biology of Male Reproductive System. San Diego: Academic Press, 1993: 1–20

Heim N. Sexual behavior of castrated sex offenders. Arch Sex Behav 1981; 10: 11–19

Helmchen H, Linden M, Wernicke T. Psychiatric morbidity in the oldest old. Result of the Berlin Aging Study. Nervenarzt 1996; 67: 739–50

Hewitson L, Martinovich C, Simerly C, et al. TESA and ELSI in nonhuman primates. Fertil Steril 2002; 77: 794–801

Hoffman S, Kaynan AM, Melman A. Priapism of ambiguous classification in a sickle cell patient. Int J Impot Res 2000; 12: 59–63

Hogan B, Beddington R, Costantini F, et al. Manipulating the Mouse Embryo: A Laboratory Manual. Cold Spring Harbor, New York: Cold Spring Harbor Laboratory, 1994

Holstein AF, Roosen-Runge EC. Atlas of Human Spermatogenesis, Berlin: Grosse Verlag, 1981

Houdebine LM. Transgenic Animals: Generation and Use. Amsterdam: Harwood Academic Publishers, 1997

Hsu GL, Hsieh CH, et al. Anatomy of the human penis. The relationship of the architecture between skeletal and smooth muscles. J Androl 2004; 25: 26–31

Huszar G, Ozenci CC, Cayli S. Hyaluronic acid binding by human sperm indicates cellular maturity, viability and unreacted acrosomal status. Fertil Steril 2003; 79: 1616–24

Hutchinson JSM. Background in reproductive biology. In Hutchinson JSM, ed. Controlling Reproduction. London: Chapman and Hall, 1993

International Germ Cell Consensus Classification Group. A prognostic factor-based staging system for metastatic germ cell cancers. J Clin Oncol 1997; 15: 594–603

Irvine RA, Yu MC, Wang F. The CAG and GGC microsatellites of the androgen receptor gene are in linkage disequilibrium in men with prostate cancer. Cancer Res 1995; 57: 1937–40

Jaffe A, Chen Y, Kisch ES, et al. Erectile dysfunction in hypertensive subjects: assessment of potential determinants. Hypertension 1996; 28: 859–62

James WH. Gonadotrophin and the human secondary sex ratio. Br Med J 1980; 281: 711

Jarrow JP, Burnett AL, Geringer AM. Clinical efficacy of sildenafil citrate based on etiology response to prior treatment. J Urol 1999; 162: 722–5

Jeyendran RS. Sperm Collection and Processing Methods: A Practical Guide. New York: Cambridge University Press, 2003

Johnson L. Spermatogenesis. In Cupps PT, ed. Reproduction in Domestic Animals, 4th edn. San Diego: Academic Press, 1991

Johnson MH, Barry JE. Essential Reproduction. Oxford, UK: Blackwell Science, 1995

Joshi N, Medina, Cruz I, et al. Determination of the ultrastructural pathology of human sperm by atomic force microscopy. Fertil Steril 2001; 75: 961–5

Joshi NV, Medium H, Colasante C, et al. Ultrastructural investigation of human sperm using atomic force microscopy. Arch Androl 2000; 44: 51–7

Joshi NV, Medina H, Qsuna JA. Ultrastructural pathology of varicose spermatozoa by using atomic force microscopy (AFM). Arch Androl 2001; 47: 143–52

Juneja R, Koide SS. Molecular aspects of reproduction. In Hafez ESE, Hafez B, eds. Reproduction in Farm Animals, 7th edn. Philadelphia, PA: Lippincott, Williams & Wilkins, 2000

Kamischke A, Nieschlag E. Diagnosis and treatment of male infertility. In De Jonge CJ, Barratt CLR, eds. Assisted Reproductive Technology: Accomplishments and New Horizons, Chapter 15. New York: Cambridge University Press, 2002

Kapranos N, Petrakou E, Anastasiadou C, et al. Detection of herpes simplex virus, cytomegalovirus, and Epstein-Barr virus in the semen of men attending an infertility clinic. Fertil Steril 2003; 79: 1566–70

Keel BA, Webster BW, eds. The Handbook of Laboratory Diagnosis and Treatment of Infertility. Boca Raton, FL: CRC Press, 1990

Khatame MA, Horn SR, Wesley A, et al. A controlled study for gender selection using swim-up separation. Gynecol Obstet Invest 1999; 48: 7–13

Kolettis PN. The evaluation and management of the azoospermic patient. J Androl 2002; 23: 293–305

Korenman SG, Morley J, Mooradian AD, et al. Secondary hypogonadism in older men: its relation to impotence. J Clin Endocrinol Metab 1990; 71: 963–9

Kunej T, Zorn B, Peterlin B. Y chromosome microdeletions in infertile men with cryptorchidism. Fertil Steril 2003; 79: 1559–65

Kurup RK, Kurup PA. Isoprenoid pathway dysfunction inhuman male infertility. Arch Androl 2003; 49: 117–27

Lamb DJ. Genes involved in testicular development and function. World J Urol 1995; 13: 277–84

Lasserre A, Gonzalez-Echeverria F, Moules C, et al. Identification of human sperm proteins involved in the interaction with homologous zona pellucida. Fertil Steril 1991; 70: 1606–15

Leclerc P, de Lamirande E, Gagnon C. Interaction between Ca^{2+}, cyclic 3',5' adenosine monophosphate, the super oxide anion, and tyrosine phosphorylation pathways in the regulation of human sperm capacitation. J Androl 1998; 19: 434–43

Ledbetter DH, Engel E. Uniparental disomy in humans: development of an imprinting map and its implications for prenatal diagnosis. Hum Mol Genet 1995; 4 Sec No 1757–64

Lee EC, Tenniswood M. Programmed cell death and survival pathways in prostate cancer cells. Arch Androl 2004; 91: 662–70

Lee JC, Surridge D, Morales A, Heaton JP. The prevalence and influence of significant psychiatric abnormalities in men undergoing comprehensive management of organic erectile dysfunction. Int J Impot Res 2000; 12: 47–51

Lee NPY, Cheng CY. Nitric oxide/nitric oxide synthase, spermatogenesis, and tight junction dynamics. Biol Reprod 2004; 70: 267–76

Lievano A, Santi CM, Serrano CJ, et al. T-type Ca^{2+}, channels and alpha 1E expression in spermatogenesis cells, and their possible relevance to the sperm acrosome reaction. FEBS Lett 1996; 388: 150–4

Lin TP. Microinjection of mouse eggs. Science 1966; 151: 333–7

Linet OI, Ogrinc FG. Efficacy and safety of intracavernosal alprostadil in men with erectile dysfunction. The Alprostadil Study Group. N Engl J Med 1996; 334: 873–7

Lipshultz LI, Howard SS. Infertility in the Male, 3rd edn. St Louis, MO: Mosby-Year Book, 1997

Lue TF. Physiology of erection and pathophysiology of impotence. In Walsh PC, ed. Campbell's Urology, 6th edn. Philadelphia, PA: WB Saunders, 1992

Lue Y-H, Lasley BL, Laughlin LS, et al. Mild testicular hyperthermia induces profound transitional spermatogenic suppression through increased germ cell apoptosis in adult cynomolgus monkeys (Macaca fascicularis). J Androl 2002; 23: 799–805

Lund A, Juvonen V, Lahdetie J, et al. A novel sequence variation in the transactivation regulating domain of the androgen receptor in two infertile Finnish men. Fertil Steril 2003; 79: 1647–51

Maduro MR, Lamb DJ. Understanding new genetics of male infertility. J Urol 2002 Nov; 168: 2197–205

Maduro MR, Lo KC, Chuang WW, et al. Genetics and male infertility: what can go wrong? J Androl 2003; 24: 485–93

Mari SI, Rawe V, Biancotti, JC, et al. Biochemical and molecular studies of the proacrosin/acrosin system in patients with unexplained infertility. Fertil Steril 2003; 79: 1676–8

Marks S. Prostate and Cancer, A Family Guide to Diagnosis, Treatment and Survival. Tucson, AZ: Fisher Books, 1999

Martin RH, Greene C, Rademaker AW. Sperm chromosome aneuploidy analysis in a man with globozoospermia. Fertil Steril 2003; 79: 1662–4

Matsui Y, Zsebo K, Hogan BL. Derivation of pluripotential embryonic stem cells from murine primordial germ cells in culture. Cell 1992; 70: 841–7

McLaren A. Implantation. In Hafez ESE, ed. Reproduction in Farm Animals, 4th edn. Philadelphia, PA: Lea & Febiger, 1980

McMahon CG, Samali R, Johnson H. Efficacy, safety and patient acceptance of sildenafil citrate as treatment for erectile dysfunction. J Urol 2000; 164: 1192–6

Meistrich ML. Potential and limitations of physical methods for separation of sperm bearing an X- and Y-chromosome. In Amann RP, Seidel GE Jr, eds. Prospects for Sexing Mammalian Sperm. Boulder, CO: Colorado University Associated Press, 1982

Menon DK. Successful treatment of anabolic steroid-induced azoospermia with human chorionic gonadotropin and human menopausal gonadotropin. Fertil Steril 2003; 79: 1659–61

Meray S, Luntz H, Nagler M, et al. In Sanfilippo JS, Robinson SL, eds. The Risk Management Handbook for Healthcare Professionals. Lancaster: Parthenon Publishing, 2002

Meucci E, Milardi D, Mordente A, et al. Total antioxidant capacity in patients with varicoceles. Fertil Steril 2003; 79: 1577–83

Meyer S, Nash SC. Prostate Cancer: Making Survival Decisions, Chicago, IL: University of Chicago Press, 1994

Miller B. State Bite: Prostate cancer incidence and mortality. Source: NCI Surveillance, Epidemiology and End Results (SEER). J Natl Cancer Inst 1993; 85: 1023–30

Monastersky GM, Robi JM. Strategies in Transgenic Animal Science. Washington, DC: American Society for Microbiology Press, 1995

Monga M, Kostelec M, Kamarei M. Patient satisfaction with testosterone supplementation for the treatment of erectile dysfunction. Arch Androl 2002; 48: 433–42

Montag VV. Use of a 1.48 µm diode laser in assisted reproduction. In Kumar A, Mukhopadhyay AK, eds. Follicular Growth, Ovulation and Fertilization: Molecular and Clinical Basis. New Delhi, India: Narosa Publishing, 2001

Montie JE, Pienta KJ. A review of the role of androgenic hormones in the pathogenesis of benign prostatic hypertrophy and prostate cancer. Urology 1994; 43: 892–9

Moore HDM, Hibbitt KG. Isoelectric focusing of boar spermatozoa. J Reprod Fertil 1975; 44: 329–32

Morales A, Heaton JP, Carson CC III. Andropause: a misnomer for true clinical entity. J Urol 2000; 163: 705–12

Morrell MJ, Flynn K. Women with Epilepsy: A Handbook of Health and Treatment Issues. New York: Cambridge University Press, 2003

Morshedi M, Duran HE, Taylor S, et al. Efficacy and pregnancy outcome of two methods of semen preparation for intrauterine insemination: a prospective randomized study. Fertil Steril 2003; 79: 1625–32

Mukherjee M, Datta M, Biswas S, et al. Immotilin, a novel sperm immobilizing protein. Fertil Steril 2003; 79: 1673–5

Munell F, Suarez-Qulan CA, Selva DM, et al. Androgen-binding protein and reproduction: where do we stand? J Androl 2002; 23: 598–609

Nayernia K, Adham I, Kremling H, et al. Stage and development-specific gene expression during mammalian spermatogenesis. Int J Dev Biol 1996; 40: 379–83

Negro-Vilar A. Selective androgen receptor modulators (SARMs): a novel approach to androgen therapy for the new millennium. J Clin Endocrinol Metab 1999; 84: 3459–62

Nehra A, Goldstein I, Pabby A, et al. Mechanisms of venous leakage: a prospective clinicopathological correlation of corporeal function and structure. J Urol 1996; 156: 1320–9

Neuhausen SL, Farnham, Kort E, et al. Prostate cancer susceptibility locus HKPC1 in Utah high-risk pedigrees. Hum Mol Genet 1999; 8: 2437–43

Olson RE. Pathophysiology of osteoporotic fractures. Am J. Clin Nutr 2000; 71: 1021–32

O'Toole CM, Arnoult C, Darszon A, et al. Ca^{2+} entry through store-operated channels in mouse sperm is initiated by egg ZP3 and drives the acrosome reaction. Mol Biol Cell 2000; 11: 1571–84

Palmiter RD, Brinster L, Hammer RE, et al. Dramatic growth of mice that develop from eggs microinjected with metallothionein-growth hormone fusion genes. Nature London 1982; 300: 611–15

Panser LA, Rhodes T, Girman CJ, et al. Sexual function of men ages 40–79 years: the Olmsted County Study of urinary symptoms and health status among men. J Am Geriatr Soc 1995; 43: 1107–11

Parinaud J, Milhet P. Progesterone induced Ca^{2+} dependent 3',5'-cyclic adenosine monophosphate increase in human sperm. J Clin Endocrinol Metab 1996; 81: 1357–60

Pask AJ, Whitworth DJ, Mao CA, et al. Marsupial anti-Mullerian hormone gene structure, regulatory elements and expression. Biol Reprod 2004; 70: 160–7

Paz G, Gamzu R, Yavetz H. Diagnosis of non-obstructive azoospermic. The laboratory perspective. J Androl 2003; 24: 167–70

Pilepich MV, Krall JM, al-Sarraf M, et al. Androgen deprivation with radiation therapy compared with radiation therapy alone for locally advanced prostatic carcinoma: a randomized comparative trial of the radiation therapy oncology group. Urology 1995; 45: 616–23

Pinkel D, Gledhill BL. Sex preselection in mammals: separation of sperm bearing Y and "O" chromosomes in the vole (Microtus oregoni). Science 1982; 218: 904

Pinkert CA. Transgenic Animal Technology: A Laboratory Handbook. San Diego: Academic Press, 1994

Pinkert CA. Transgenic swine models for xenotransplantation. Xenobiotics 1994; 2: 10–15

Pinkert CA. The history and theory of transgenic animals. Lab Anim 1997; 26: 29–34

Pinkert CA. Genetic engineering in farm animals. In Hafez ESE, Hafez B, eds. Reproduction in Farm Animals, 7th edn. Philadelphia, PA: Lippincott Williams & Wilkins, 2000: 318–30

Pinkert CA, Irwin MH, Moffatt RJ. Transgenic animal modeling. In Meyers RA, ed. Encyclopedia of Molecular Biology and Molecular Medicine. New York: VCH, 1997; 6: 63–74

Pinkert CA, Murray JD. Transgenic farm animals. In Murray JD, Anderson GB, McGloughlin MM, Oberbauer AM, eds. Transgenic Animals in Agriculture. Wallingford, UK: CAB International, 1998

Pollack A, Zagars G. External beam radiotherapy dose response of prostate cancer. Int J Radiat Oncol Biol Phys 1997; 329: 1011–18

Pursel VG, Rexroad CE Jr. Status of research with transgenic farm animals. J Anim Sci 1993; 71(Suppl 3): 10–19

Ramos CE, Park JS, Ritchey ML, et al. High-flow priapism associated with sickle cell disease. J Urol 1995; 153: 1619–21

Rao CV. An Introduction to Immunology. Boca Raton, FL: CRC Press, 2002

Ravhon A. The use of recombinant FSH. Adv Reprod 2002; 6: 107–12

Rendell MS, Rajfer J, Wicker PA, et al. Sildenafil for treatment of erectile dysfunction in men with diabetes. JAMA 1999; 281: 421–6

Revelli A, Poso F, Tur-Kaspa I. New insights into gamesomeness, sperm migration, fertilization and implantation in humans. In Revelli A, Tur-Kaspa I, Holte JG, Massobrio M, eds. Biotechnology of Human Reproduction. Lancaster, UK: Parthenon Publishing, 2003: 19–42

Rexroad CE Jr, Hawk HW. Production of transgenic ruminants. In Pinkert CA, ed. Transgenic Animal Technology: A Laboratory Handbook. San Diego: Academic Press, 1994: 339–55

Rivlin J, Mendel J, Rubinstein S, et al. Role of hydrogen peroxide in sperm capacitation and acrosome reaction. Biol Reprod 2004; 70: 518–22

Roach M, Pikett B, Weil M, et al. The critical volume tolerance method for estimating the limits of dose escalation during three dimensional conformal radiotherapy for prostate cancer. Int J Radiat Oncol Biol Phys 1996; 35: 1019–25

Robaire B. Aging of the epididymis. In Robaire B, Hinton BT, eds. The Epididymis from Molecules to Clinical Practice. A comprehensive survey of the efferent ducts, the epididymis and the vas deferens. New York, Boston: Kluwer Academic Publishers/Plenum Publishers, 2002

Rodin DM, Larone D, Goldstein M. Relationship between semen cultures, leukospermia, and semen analysis in men undergoing fertility evaluation. Fertil Steril 2003; 70: 1555–9

Rosnina Y, Jainudeen MR. Genetic reproductive failure. In Hafez ESE, Hafez B, eds. Reproduction in Farm Animals, 7th edn. Philadelphia, PA: Lippincott Williams & Wilkins, 2000

Saacke RG, White JM. Presented at the 4th Technical Conference on Artificial Insemination/Reproduction, Trento, Italy, 1972

Saleh RA, Agarwal A, Nada EA, et al. Negative effects of increased sperm DNA damage in relation to seminal oxidative stress in men with idiopathic and male factor infertility. Fertil Steril 2003; 79: 1597–605

Sanz E, Olivares R. Sperm recovering efficiency, a math matical model, is designed to objectively evaluate semen processing techniques and methods. Fertil Steril 2003; 79: 1633–6

Sarapura V, Schlaff WD. Recent advances in the understanding of the pathophysiology and treatment of hyperprolactinemia. Curr Opin Obstet Gynecol 1993; 5: 360–7

Saremi A, et al. The first successful pregnancy following injection of testicular round spermatid in Iran. Arch Androl 2002; 48: 315–19

Sarge KD, Parke-Sarge OK, Kirby JD, et al. Expression of heat shock factor 2 in mouse testis: potential role as a regulator of heat-shock protein gene expression during spermatogenesis. Biol Reprod 1994; 50: 1334–43

Sarteschi LM, et al. Cavernous arterial and arteriolar circulation in patients with erectile dysfunction: a power Doppler study. J Urol 1998; 159: 428–32

Sbracia M, Sayme N, Grasso J, et al. Sperm function and choice of preparation media: comparison of Percoll and Accudenz discontinuous density gradients. J Androl 1996; 17: 61–7

Shafik A, Olfat S. Aligamentous testicle. New clinicopathologic entity in genesis of male infertility and its treatment by orchiopexy. Urology. 1979; 13: 54–7

Schiavi RC, Rehman J. Sexuality and aging. Urol Clin North Am 1995; 22: 711–26

Schultze W. The new importance of testicular biopsy in the era of assisted reproduction. In Kumar A, Mukopadyay AK, eds. Follicular Growth, Ovulation and Fertilization: Molecular and Clinical Basis. New Dehli, India: Narosa Publishing, 2001

Seftel AD, Haas CA, Brown SL, et al. High-flow priapism complicating veno-occlusive priapism: pathophysiology of recurrent idiopathic priapism? J Urol 1998; 159: 1300–1

Sherbet GV, Lakshmi MS, Rao KV. Characterization of inorganic groups and estimation of the net negative electric charge on the surface of cells using natural pH gradients. Exp Cell Res 1972; 70: 113–23

Sliwa L. Effect of heparin on human spermatozoa migration in vitro. Arch Androl 1993; 30: 177–81

Sliwa L. Heparin as a chemoattractant for mouse spermatozoa. Arch Androl 1993; 31: 149–52

Sliwa L. Chemotactic effect of hormones in mouse spermatozoa. Arch Androl 1994; 32: 83–8

Sliwa L. Chemotaction of mouse spermatozoa induced by certain hormones. Arch Androl 1995; 35: 105–10

Sliwa L. Effect of some sex steroid hormones on human spermatozoa migration in vitro. Eur J Obstet Gynecol Reprod Biol 1995; 58: 173–5

Sliwa L. Substance P and beta-endorphin act as possible chemoattractants of mouse sperm. Arch Androl 2001; 46: 135–40

Sobrinho LG. The psychogenic effects of prolactin. Acta Endocrinol 1993; 129 (Suppl 1): 38–40

Soloway MS, Sharifi R, Wajsman Z, et al. Randomized prospective study comparing radical prostectomy alone versus radical prostectomy proceeded by androgen blockage in clinical stage B2 (T2bNxMo) prostate cancer: The Lupron Depot Neoadjuvant Prostate Cancer Group. J Urol 1995; 164: 424–32

Spermon JR, Kiemeney LALM, Meuleman EJH, et al. Fertility in men with testicular germ cell tumors. Fertil Steril 2003; 79: 1543–9

Speroff L, Glass RH, Kase NG. Clinical Gynecologic Endocrinology and Infertility, 6th edn. Philadelphia, PA: Lippincott, 1999

Stas SN, Anastasiades AG, Fisch H, et al. Urologic aspects of andropause. Urology 2003; 61: 261–6

Tanji N, et al.Growth factors: roles in andrology. Arch Androl 2001; 47: 1–7. Review

Tesarik J, Balaban B, Isiklar A, et al. In vitro spermatogenesis resumption in men with maturation arrest: relationship with in vivo blocking stage and serum FSH. Hum Reprod 2000; 15: 1350–4

Thonneau PF, Candia P, Mieusset R. Cryptorchidism: incidence, risk factors, and potential role of environment; an update. J Androl 2003; 24: 155–9

Tissot JE, Johnson RH. Pharmacological management of erectile dysfunction. Adv Reprod 2002; 6: 85–7

Tomomasa H, Oshio S, Ashizawa Y, et al. Gonadal function in patients with testicular germ cell tumors. Arch Androl 2002; 48: 405–15

Trent JM, Isaacs WB. Major susceptibility locus for prostate cancer on chromosome 1 suggested by a genome-wide search. Science 1996; 274: 1371–4

Trounson AO, Gardner DK. Handbook of In Vitro Fertilization, 2nd edn. New York: CRC Press, 2000

Tseng CH. Atlas of Ultrastructure, Ultrastructural Features in Pathology. New York, NY: Appleton-Century-Crofts, 1980

Uhler ML, Zinaman, MJ, Brown CC, et al. Relationship between sperm characteristics and hormonal parameters in normal couples. Fertil Steril 2003; 79 (Suppl 3): 535–42

United Nations. HIV/AIDS: Population Impact and Policies, 2001. Washington, DC: United Nations, 2001

Valeri A, Azzouzi I. Early-onset prostate cancer is not associated with specific clinical features. Prostate 2000; 45: 66–73

Vani RG, Rao MR. Cloning of the cDNA encoding rat homologue of the mismatch repair gene MSH2 and its expression during spermatogenesis. Gene 1997; 185: 19–26

Vermeulen A. Androgen replacement therapy in the aging male – a critical evaluation. J Clin Endocrinol Metab 2001; 85: 2380–90

Wakayama T, Perry AC, Zuccotti M, et al. Full-term development of mice from enucleated oocytes injected with cumulus nuclei. Nature Cell 1998; 394: 369–74

Wang HZ, Lee SW, Christ GJ. Comparative studies of the maxi-K (KCa) channel in freshly isolated monocytes of human and rat corpora. Int J Impot Res 2000; 12: 9–18

Wassarman PM. Fertilization in Mammals Sci Am 1988; 259: 18–84

Wespes E, Schulman CC. Male andropause: myth, reality and treatment. Int J Impot Res 2000; 14 (Suppl 1): S93–S98

Westlander G, Ekerhovd E, Bergh C. Low levels of serum inhibin B do not exclude successful sperm recovery in men with nonmosaic Klinefelter syndrome. Fertil Steril 2003; 70: 1680–2

Wilke RJ, Glick HA, McCarron TJ, et al. Quality of life effects of alprostadil therapy for erectile dysfunction. J Urol 1997; 157: 2124–8

Wilmut I, Schnieke AE, McWhir J, et al. Viable offspring derived from fetal and adult mammalian cells. Nature London 1997; 385: 810–13

Wood SA, Allen ND, Rossant J, et al. Non-injection methods for the production of embryonic stem cell embryo chimaeras. Nature London 1993; 365: 87–9

World Health Organization. WHO Laboratory Manual for the Examination of Human Semen and Semen Cervical Mucus Interaction. Cambridge, UK: World Health Organization/Cambridge University Press, 1999

Worrad DM, Schultz RM. Regulation of gene expression in the preimplantation mouse embryo: temporal and spatial patterns of expression of the transcription factor Sp1. Mol Reprod Rev 1997; 46: 268–77

Wroblewski N, Schill WB, Henkel R. Metal chelators change the human sperm motility pattern. Fertil Steril 2003; 79: 1584–9

Xu J. Combined analysis of hereditary prostate cancer linkage to 1q24–25: results from 772 hereditary prostate cancer families from the International Consortium for Prostate Cancer Genetics. Am J Hum Genet 2000; 66: 945

Xu WD, Miao SY, Zhang ML, et al. Expression of the BE-20 epididymal protein gene: in situ hybridization. Arch Androl 1997; 38: 1–6

Yamada Y, Yamamoto H, Yonehara T, et al. Differential activation of the luteinizing hormone beta-subunit promoter by activin and gonadotropin-releasing hormone: a role for the mitogen-activated protein kinase signaling pathway in LbetaT2 gonadotrophs. Biol Reprod 2004; 70: 236–43

Yanagimachi R. Mammalian fertilization. In Knobil E, Neil JD, eds. The Physiology of Reproduction. New York: Raven Press, 1994; 1: 189–317

Zaneveld L. In Hafez ESE, ed. Scanning Electron Microscope Atlas of Mammalian Reproduction. New York: Springer-Verlag, 1975

Zitzmann M, Rolf C, Nordhoff V, et al. Male smokers havea decreased success rate for in vitro fertilization and intracytoplasmic sperm injection. Fertil Steril 2003; 79: 1550–4

Index